# PRIMARY CARE
## OF THE
# CATARACT PATIENT

**Cynthia Ann Murrill, OD, MPH**
Pacific Cataract and Laser Institute
Tacoma, Washington

**David Lee Stanfield, OD**
Pacific Cataract and Laser Institute
Chehalis, Washington

**Michael David VanBrocklin, OD**
Pacific Cataract and Laser Institute
Tacoma, Washington

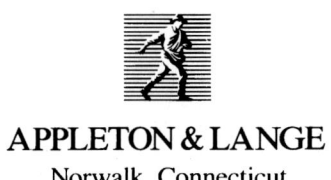

APPLETON & LANGE
Norwalk, Connecticut

Notice: The authors and the publisher of this volume have taken care that the information and recommendations contained herein are accurate and compatible with the standards generally accepted at the time of publication. Nevertheless, it is difficult to ensure that all the information given is entirely accurate for all circumstances. The publisher disclaims any liability, loss, or damage incurred as a consequence, directly or indirectly, of the use and application of any of the contents of this volume.

Copyright © 1994 by Appleton & Lange
Paramount Publishing Business and Professional Group

All rights reserved. This book, or any parts thereof, may not be used or reproduced in any manner without written permission. For information, address Appleton & Lange, 25 Van Zant Street, East Norwalk, Connecticut 06855.

94 95 96 97 98 / 10 9 8 7 6 5 4 3 2 1

Prentice Hall International (UK) Limited, *London*
Prentice Hall of Australia Pty. Limited, *Sydney*
Prentice Hall Canada, Inc., *Toronto*
Prentice Hall Hispanoamericana, S.A., *Mexico*
Prentice Hall of India Private Limited, *New Delhi*
Prentice Hall of Japan, Inc., *Tokyo*
Simon & Schuster Asia Pte. Ltd., *Singapore*
Editora Prentice Hall do Brasil Ltda., *Rio de Janeiro*
Prentice Hall, *Englewood Cliffs, New Jersey*

Library of Congress Cataloging-in-Publication Data
Primary care of the cataract patient / [edited by] Cynthia Ann
  Murrill, David Lee Stanfield, Michael David VanBrocklin.
     p.   cm.
   Includes index.
   ISBN 0-8385-7899-3
   1. Cataract.  2. Cataract—Surgery.  I. Murrill, Cynthia Ann.
II. Stanfield, David Lee.  III. VanBrocklin, Michael David.
   [DNLM: 1. Cataract—therapy.  2. Cataract Extraction.
3. Preoperative Care—methods.  4. Postoperative Care—methods.  WW
260 P952 1994]
RE451.P72  1994
617.7'42—dc20
DNLM/DLC
for Library of Congress                                         93-41307
                                                                    CIP

Acquisitions Editor: Cheryl L. Mehalik
Production Editor: Karen W. Davis
Designer: Penny Kindzierski

PRINTED IN THE UNITED STATES OF AMERICA

*This book is dedicated to our families:*

*Joe, Thomas, and Nicholas Pfeifer,*
*Barb, Zachary, and Matthew Stanfield,*
*and*
*Dana, Bradley, Whitney, and Jennifer VanBrocklin*

# Contributors

**Paul M. Barney, OD**
Pacific Cataract and Laser Institute
Chehalis, Washington
*Corneal Edema*
*Corneal Decompensation*
*Optical Considerations*

**Barbara J. Hetrick, OD**
Pacific Cataract and Laser Institute
La Grande, Oregon
*Ptosis*

**Donald L. Peterson, OD**
Pacific Cataract and Laser Institute
Kennewick, Washington
*Special Instrumentation*
*Nd:YAG Capsulotomy*

**Maynard L. Pohl, OD**
Pacific Cataract and Laser Institute
Bellevue, Washington
*Retinal Break/Detachment*

**Oli I. Traustason, MD**
Pacific Cataract and Laser Institute
Chehalis, Washington
*Patient Preparation*
*Operative Techniques*
*Special Surgical Considerations*
*Intraoperative Complications*

# Contents

*Foreword* ...................................................................................................xi

*Preface* ....................................................................................................xiii

*Color Plates* ..........................................................................................xvii

SECTION I. GENERAL CONSIDERATIONS .......................................1

Chapter 1. Trends in Cataract Care ..................................................3

    Epidemiology of cataracts, cataract surgery, and intraocular lens implants / History of cataract surgical techniques / History of intraocular lens implants / Capsulorhexis / Optometry's role / Studies of comanaged cataract postoperative patients

Chapter 2. Comanagement ................................................................9

    Comanagement defined / Roles of optometrist and ophthalmologist / Medicolegal responsibilities / Patient communication / Doctor communication / Conflict resolution

Chapter 3. Lens Anatomy and Cataractogenesis............................13

Chapter 4. Grading Systems.............................................................17

    Conventional system / Cornea / Cataract / Anterior chamber reaction / Hypopyon / Hyphema / Posterior capsule opacification

SECTION II. PREOPERATIVE CATARACT CARE............................33

Chapter 5. Special Instrumentation ................................................35

    Glare testing / Contrast sensitivity / Interferometer / Super Pinhole / Potential acuity meter / Entoptic phenomena testing / A-scan ultrasonography / B-scan ultrasonography / Endothelial cell counts

Chapter 6. Examination..................................................43

Subjective data / Objective data / Assessment / Plan

Chapter 7. Other Preoperative Evaluations ................................51

Pediatric cataracts / Traumatic cataracts / Subluxated lenses / Secondary intraocular lenses / Intraocular lens repositioning/exchange / Monocular patients / High refractive error / History of iritis / Fuchs' dystrophy / Chronic open-angle glaucoma / Retinal detachment

## SECTION III. OPERATIVE PROCEDURES IN CATARACT SURGERY ............................................59

Chapter 8. History of Intraocular Lenses ................................61

Chapter 9. Patient Preparation..........................................69

Low-stress atmosphere / Preoperative medications / Anesthesia / Pressure on globe / Sterile technique / Instrumentation

Chapter 10. Operative Techniques........................................75

Opening incision / Methods of cataract extraction / Incisional closure / Case conclusion

Chapter 11. Special Surgical Considerations..............................95

Secondary intraocular lens implants / Cataract extraction without intraocular lens / Explantation of intraocular lens / Combined procedures / The traumatic cataract / Congenital lens dislocations

Chapter 12. Intraoperative Complications ................................105

Retrobulbar hemorrhage / Choroidal hemorrhage / Posterior capsular tears/vitreous loss / Zonular rupture / Descemet's detachment

## SECTION IV. POSTOPERATIVE CARE ........................................111

Chapter 13. Uncomplicated Course, Visits, and Procedures..................113

First visit—day 1 / Second visit—3–14 days / Third visit—2–4 weeks / Fourth visit—5–8 weeks

Chapter 14. Early, 1- to 14-day (Emergent) Complications .................125

Ocular hypertension / Wound leak with shallow anterior chamber / Endophthalmitis / Iris prolapse/vitreous to the wound / Intraocular lens dislocations / Retinal break/detachment

Chapter 15. Early, 1- to 14-Day (Less Emergent) Complications.............159

Ptosis / Diplopia / Wound leak with well-formed anterior chamber / Acute corneal edema / Hyphema / Uveitis / Intraocular lens decentration/pupillary capture / Choroidal detachment / Anterior ischemic optic neuropathy

Chapter 16. Intermediate to Late Complications ...........................189

Ptosis / Diplopia / Ocular hypertension/glaucoma / Chronic corneal edema/corneal decompensation / Late hyphema / Chronic iritis /

Posterior capsular opacities/Nd:YAG capsulotomy / Pseudophakic (aphakic) cystoid macular edema / Retinal detachment / Optical considerations

SECTION V.  APPENDICES .................................................................235

    1. Comanagement Patient Communications Aids ...........................237

    2. Standard Abbreviations ...............................................................240

    3. Doctor-to-Doctor Communications Aids ....................................246

    4. Professional Correspondence .....................................................248

    5. Example of Verbal Preoperative Instructions
       to the Patient ..............................................................................251

    6. Informed Consent for Cataract Extraction with
       Posterior Capsule Intraocular Lens ............................................252

    7. Postoperative Instructions to the Patient ...................................255

    8. Nd:YAG Informed Consent and
       Postoperative Instructions ..........................................................256

*Index* ..................................................................................................259

# Foreword

This book is a comprehensive text on the subject of the comanagement of cataract surgery patients between optometrists and ophthalmologists. Due to the increased sharing of these patients in today's ophthalmic community, this textbook is a hallmark in providing the necessary information to clinicians desiring to include this type of eye care in their practices. The authors are clinicians in a busy referral and surgical comanagement cataract practice and their expertise in the subject matter is very evident in each inclusive chapter. The book covers the presurgical considerations and postsurgical complications that optometrists will encounter and describes succinctly the appropriate treatment plans. The authors are to be congratulated for placing into the hands of today's optometrists a text that will help them deliver better care to cataract patients.

**William L. Jones, OD**
Chief of Optometry of
  VA Medical Center
Albuquerque, New Mexico
Adjunct Associate Professor
University of Houston College
  of Optometry
Houston, Texas
and
Southern California College of Optometry
Fullerton, California

# Preface

Doctors of optometry play an important role in caring for the cataract patient. This role often involves having a long-term relationship as the primary eye care provider before a cataract develops and then being the first to detect, diagnose, and manage developing cataracts along with any other eye diseases. The role evolves into that of counselor and advocate for quality surgery and postsurgical care. Finally, if surgical intervention is appropriate, the optometrist today is often intimately involved in providing postoperative and continuing care for cataract patients. This thoughtful initiation and oversight of eye care is important not only to the reassurance of the patient but to the quality of care delivered. In addition, the challenge and satisfaction of the optometrist is an important aspect of contentment in a job well done. The evolution of optometry, with its involvement in all aspects of patient eye care, even when surgery is necessary, reflects the educational and clinical progress of the profession today.

*Primary Care of the Cataract Patient* is designed for optometrists involved in any or all aspects of cataract care. This book provides scientific background on trends in cataract patient care, cataractogenesis, intraocular lenses, surgical intervention, preoperative and postoperative evaluation, assessment, treatment, and management. Equally important, it provides insight into the "art" of caring for a cataract patient based on the editors' and contributors' years of experience with thousands of patients. This book should serve as a text for soon-to-graduate optometry students, as they prepare to provide quality care to their future patients and as a practical reference for busy doctors of optometry with patients "in the chair." Photographs allow clinical teaching and comparison, whether the reader is learning the information for the first time or reviewing for accuracy in a busy clinic. Figures and tables provide quick references for important points. Preoperative care of a cataract patient is common optometric care; therefore, special attention has been paid to postoperative care with its wide range of normal sequelae and complications.

Specific goals of *Primary Care of the Cataract Patient* are to educate students and doctors of optometry about:

- The history and trends of cataract preoperative and postoperative care, surgery, and intraocular lens implants.
- Essential elements of the shared care of the patient by doctors of optometry and ophthalmic surgeons, also called comanagement.
- Clinical evaluation and quantification of common preoperative and postoperative conditions. These common grading systems not only aid ongoing patient care but communication between doctors.
- Practical guidelines for routine preoperative and postoperative patient examination, diagnosis, and treatment.
- State-of-the-art preoperative, intraoperative, and postoperative cataract care procedures, along with practical clinical pearls, based on our experience in a busy comanagement system.
- Presentation, examination, treatment, and management of postoperative dilemmas and complications.

The editors and contributors are optometrists and ophthalmologists who work together in a regional comanagement system dedicated to providing quality cataract care through education and cooperation with a large group of referring doctors of optometry. We strive to provide low-stress state-of-the-art surgery, always considering the needs of referring optometrists and their patients. The system has proven to be successful with the over 40,000 surgeries already provided.

The editors and contributors have relied heavily on this foundation of experience to assimilate information that we would like to share with the optometric community. Therefore, the reader will find frequent reference to "our doctors," "our setting," "our surgeons." We believe the compilation of this practical clinical knowledge will aid optometric students and practitioners in satisfying the needs of their patients as they deliver quality primary care to the cataract patient.

This book is the product of the collective efforts of many doctors and staff within our clinic system. Our appreciation of the talent and assistance of Dorothy Fentress, Kris Lyon, and Angela David as transcriptionists, and Bruce Alves, Gary Swart, Gary Gelder, and Graham Dorland as photographers cannot go unmentioned. All of the staff at our respective offices helped us to complete numerous projects. In addition, family members were sometimes drawn in: specifically Ann Alves for illustrations and Jennifer Jamison for Appendix 2. Doctors Paul Barney, Barbara Hetrick, Donald Peterson, and Maynard Pohl deserve thanks because of their double commitment as both contributors and reviewers. Special heartfelt appreciation goes to Dr Oli Traustason for his considerable involvement in the writing of the intraoperative section and review of all sections. Doctors Robert Ford, Bradley Gardner, Helgi Heidar, Donald James, Ron Sugiyama, Mr. Wayne Carlson, Ms Petrea Dorland, and Ms Sally Riker provided thoughtful comments in review of the book for which we are thankful.

We hesitate to single out one person when so many contributed, but Rose Fischer deserves separate and profound appreciation. Thanks to her knowledge, dedication, enthusiasm, and professionalism we were able to produce illustrations which we hope will serve to better teach the information we have presented. Artist Tom Anderson's talent added a freshness and uniqueness to the illustrations of which we are proud.

The motivation for writing this book provided by the progressive and supportive environment in which we practice as team members at Pacific Cataract and Laser Institute cannot be underestimated. In addition, the Institute provided both direct and indirect financial underwriting in its provision of staff and resources.

We also extend our thank you to Susan Farmer, OD, as an efficient and well-organized research assistant, and Pacific University College of Optometry where she serves as a Fellow.

Finally, our spouses and families gave willing support to our many hours of research, writing, and editing. Without their cooperation and confidence in our ability to contribute a worthwhile effort to our profession, this book would not have been possible.

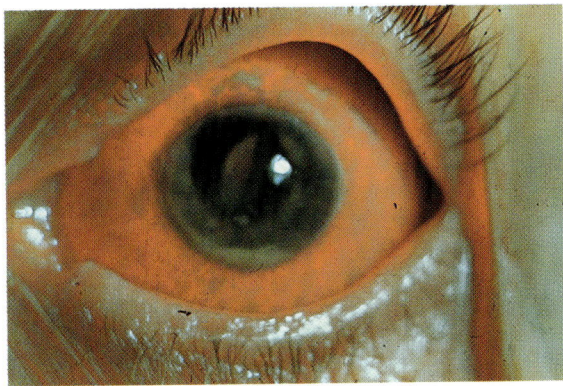

**COLOR PLATE 3–1.** Phacoanaphylactic endophthalmitis. (See page 13.)

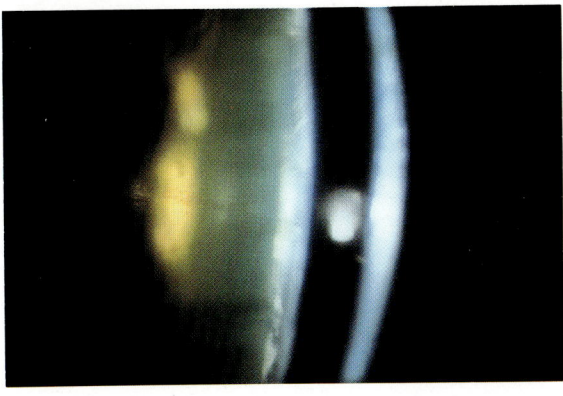

**COLOR PLATE 4–1.** Grade 2+ nuclear sclerosis (NS). (See page 21.)

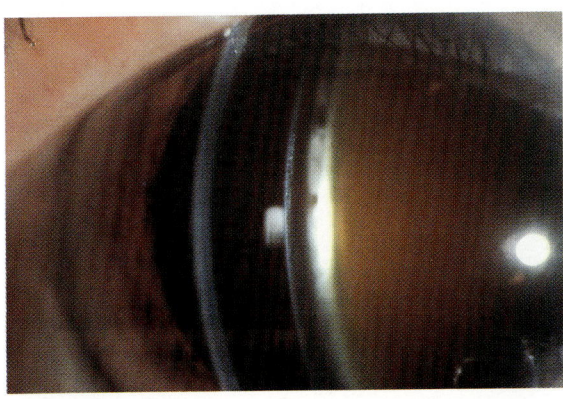

**COLOR PLATE 4–2.** Grade 4+ nuclear sclerosis (NS) with brunescence. (See page 21.)

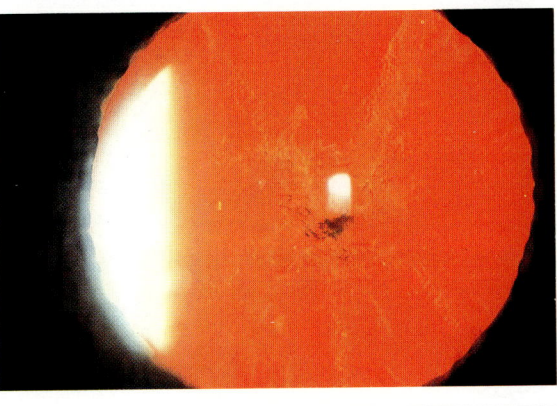

**COLOR PLATE 4–3.** Grade 2+ cortical sclerosis (CS). (See page 21.)

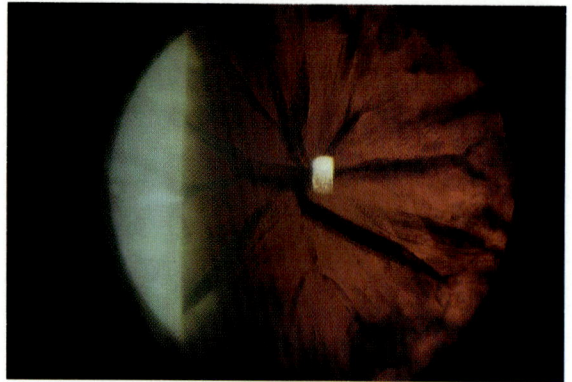

**COLOR PLATE 4–4.** Grade 4+ cortical sclerosis (CS). (See page 21.)

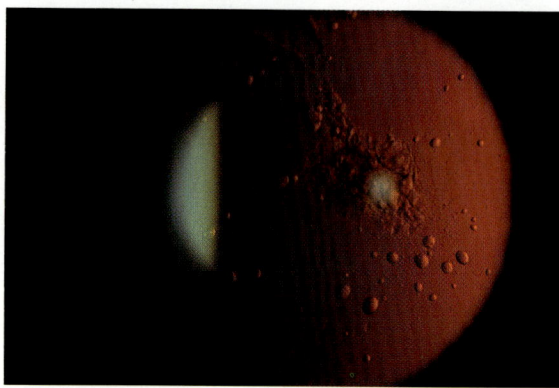

**COLOR PLATE 4–5.** Grade 2+ posterior subcapsular cataract (PSC). (See page 21.)

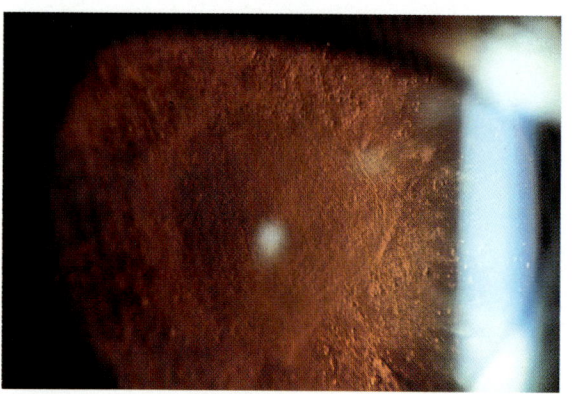

**COLOR PLATE 4–6.** Grade 4+ posterior subcapsular cataract (PSC). (See page 21.)

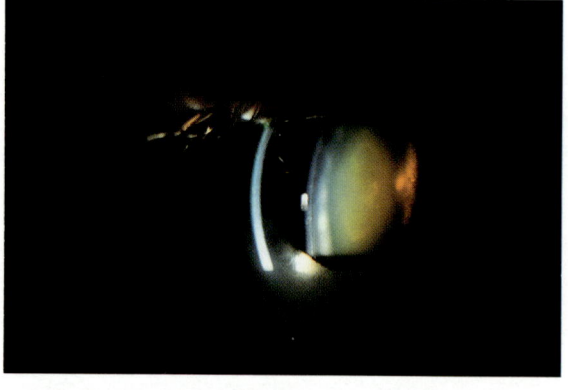

**COLOR PLATE 4–7.** Grade 3+ nuclear sclerotic and 4+ posterior subcapsular cataract in a patient with 20/200 preoperative visual acuity. (See page 24.)

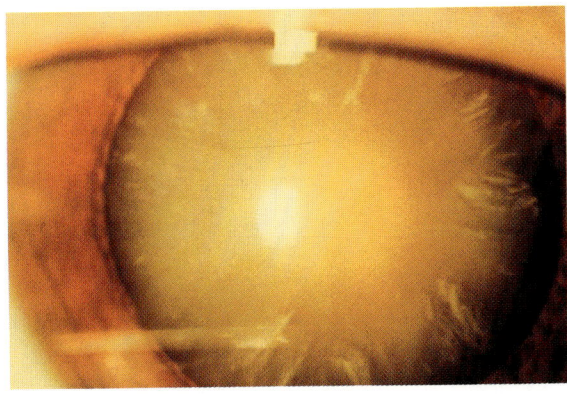

**COLOR PLATE 4–8.** A mature cataract where the entire lens is opacified. (See page 24.)

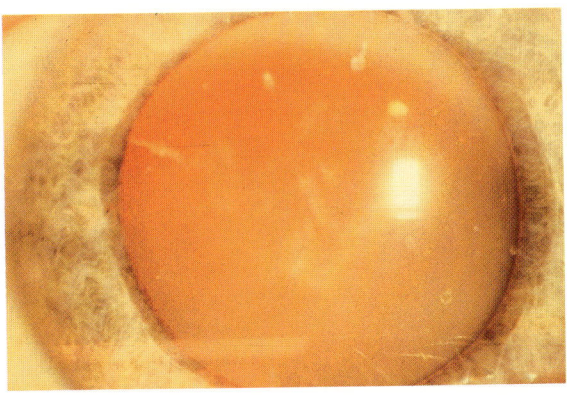

**COLOR PLATE 4–9.** A hypermature or Morgagnian cataract where the cortex has liquified and the nucleus sinks. (See page 24.)

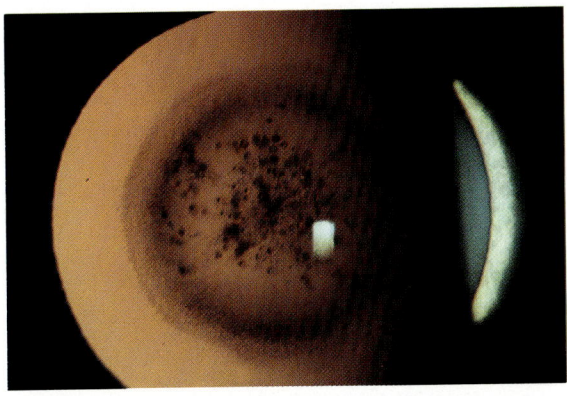

**COLOR PLATE 7–1.** A congenital nuclear cataract with visual acuity of 20/40–3. (See page 51.)

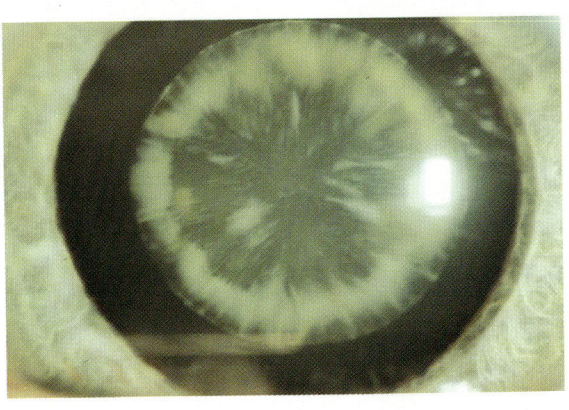

**COLOR PLATE 7–2.** A congenital nuclear cataract in a 45-year-old female with visual acuity of 20/40. (See page 51.)

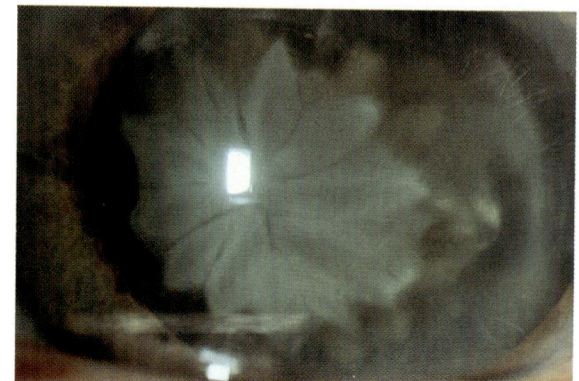

**COLOR PLATE 7–3.** Cortical cataract noted in previously traumatized eye reducing visual acuity to 20/200. (See page 52.)

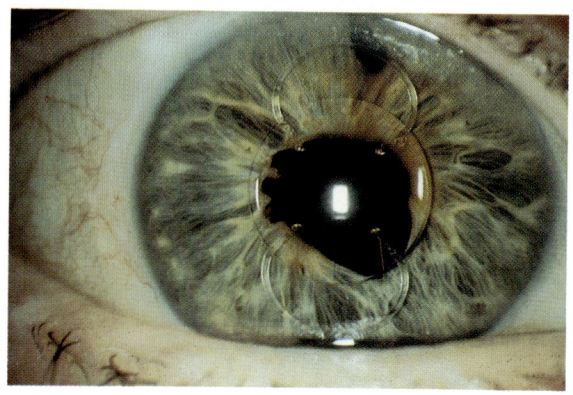

**COLOR PLATE 8–1.** An iris-supported intraocular lens implanted in 1977. After 16 years the lens is well tolerated with visual acuity of 20/20. (See page 63.)

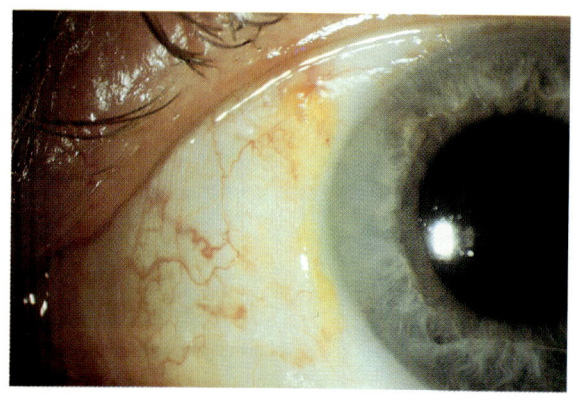

**COLOR PLATE 10–1.** A temporal sutureless limbal incision. This may occasionally be used to try to decrease against-the-rule astigmatism or because the 12 o'clock position is scarred or has a filtering bleb. (See page 75.)

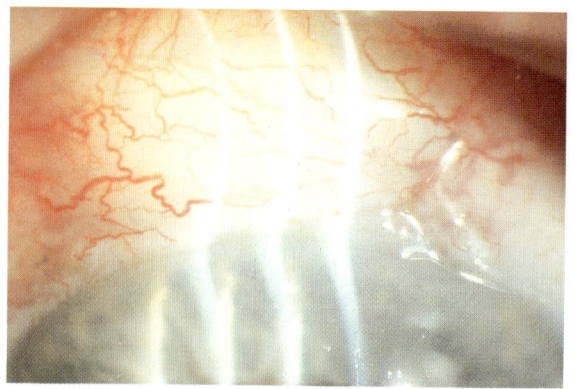

**COLOR PLATE 11–1.** A filtering bleb noted 2 weeks following a combined cataract/trabeculectomy surgery. (See page 100.)

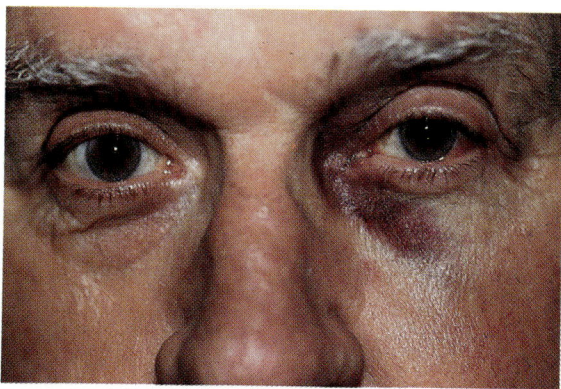

**COLOR PLATE 13–1.** Ecchymosis at 1 day post cataract extraction, secondary to peribulbar anesthesia. (See page 115.)

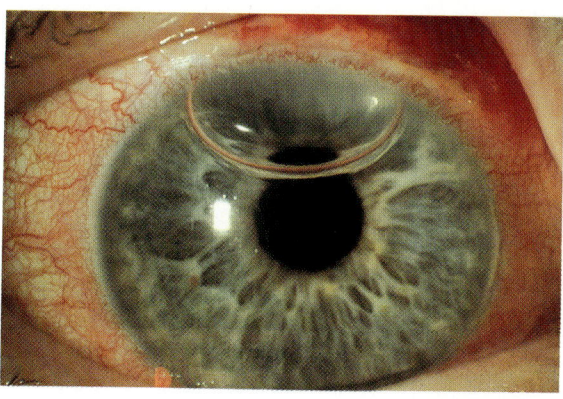

**COLOR PLATE 13–2.** An air bubble noted at the 1-day postoperative examination with normal intraocular pressure and well-sealed incision. This was completely absorbed in 1 week. (See page 116.)

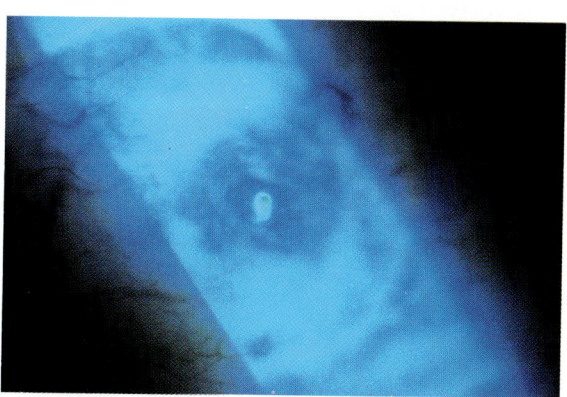

**COLOR PLATE 13–3.** An exposed suture barb following the instillation of sodium fluorescein. Note how the dye pools around the exposed suture end. (See page 124.)

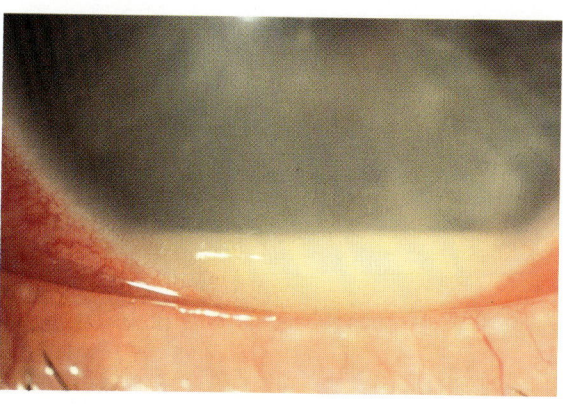

**COLOR PLATE 14–1.** Staphylococcus epidermidis endophthalmitis noted in a patient with an infected glaucoma filtering bleb. (See page 138.)

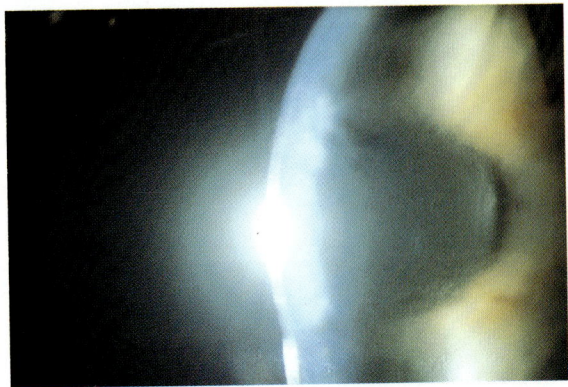

**COLOR PLATE 15–1.** Grade 3–4+ stromal and microcystic edema noted at 1-day postoperative visit in a patient who had a 4+ nuclear sclerotic (NS) cataract. (See page 162.)

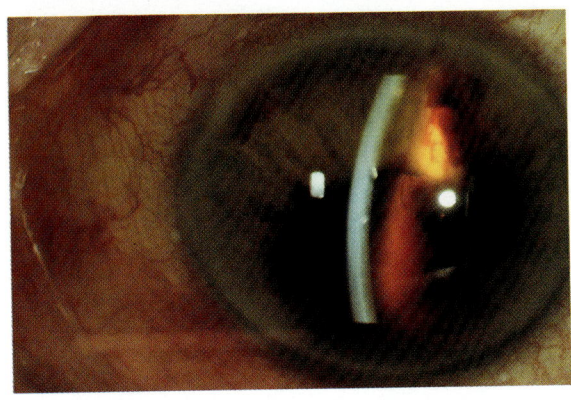

**COLOR PLATE 15–2.** Hyphema following cataract extraction in a 74-year-old man, complicated by vitreous loss. Visual acuity measured Hand Motions. Evacuation of the clot was required since no improvement was noted after 10 days. (See page 165.)

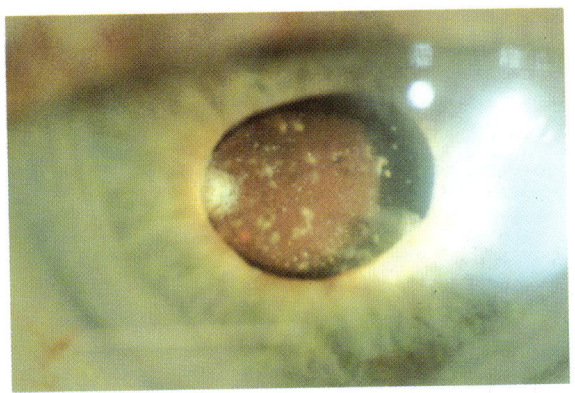

**COLOR PLATE 15–3.** After successful evacuation of the anterior clot in Figure 15–2, the patient's vision remained count fingers due to an endocapsular hematoma. (See page 165.)

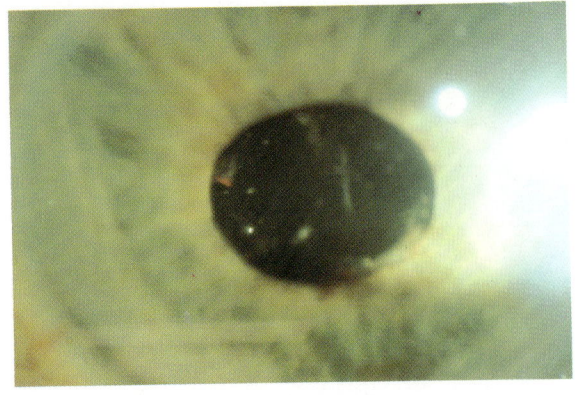

**COLOR PLATE 15–4.** A YAG capsulotomy was performed on the endocapsular hematoma of Figure 15–3, which dispersed the sequestered red blood cells and improved the vision to 20/25. (See page 165.)

COLOR PLATES xxiii

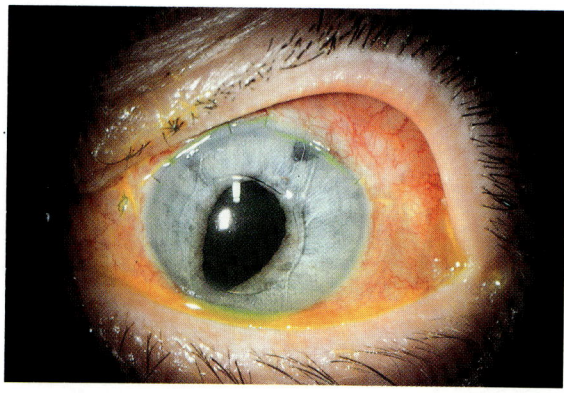

**COLOR PLATE 15-5.** Dislocated superior haptic of an anterior chamber intraocular lens. Patient presented with a history of quiet pseudophakia with an onset of blurred vision, mild photophobia, and ocular discomfort. No iritis was present. (See page 177.)

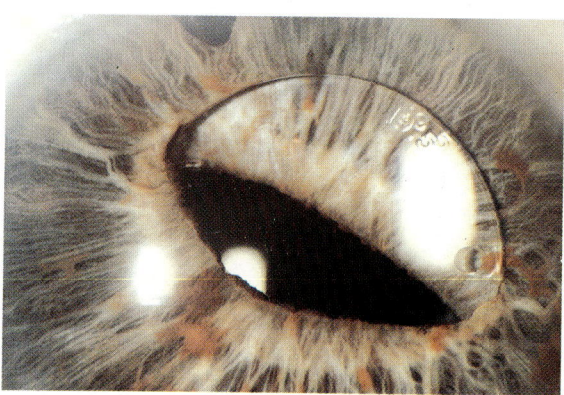

**COLOR PLATE 15-6.** Partial pupillary capture of a posterior chamber intraocular lens. This was surgically repositioned and has since been stable for 4 years. (See page 177.)

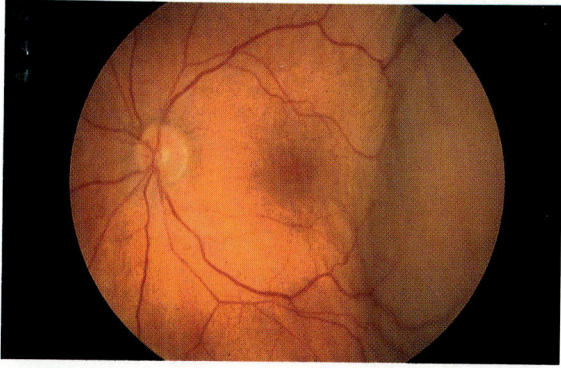

**COLOR PLATE 15-7.** Ciliochoroidal detachment in a 75-year-old female 1 week following cataract extraction, complicated by a torn capsule and vitreous loss requiring an anterior vitrectomy. At the time of presentation, the intraocular pressure was normal with well-sealed incision. The choroidal detachment resolved in 1 month with resulting visual improvement. (See page 179.)

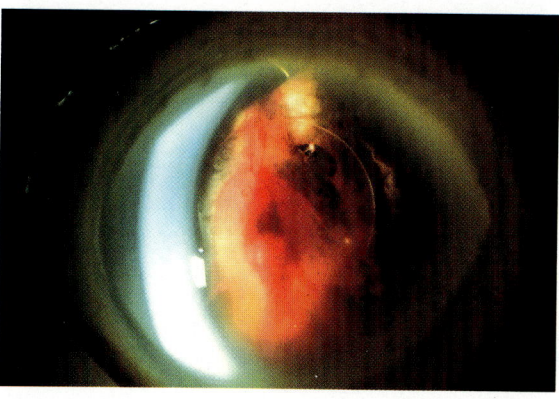

**COLOR PLATE 16-1.** A hyphema noted in a patient with an iris supported intraocular lens implanted 15 years prior. The patient had history of multiple visual white outs over the past few years. The intraocular pressure measured at 35. (See page 205.)

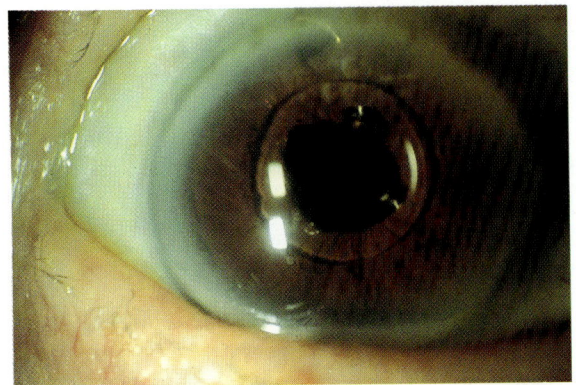

**COLOR PLATE 16-2.** One day later the vision of the patient in Figure 16-1 had returned to 20/30. The patient was scheduled for intraocular lens exchange. (See page 205.)

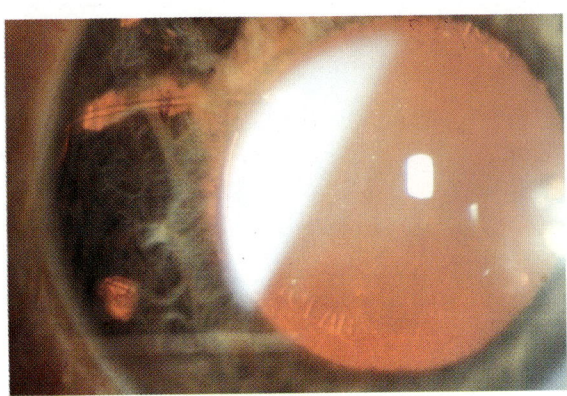

**COLOR PLATE 16-3.** Iris transillumination defects from intraocular lens irritation in a patient with a multiple-piece, sulcus-fixated posterior chamber intraocular lens. This patient experienced multiple microhyphemas and ultimately had the intraocular lens exchanged for a single piece posterior chamber lens. No hyphemas have been noted in over 3 years of follow-up. (See page 205.)

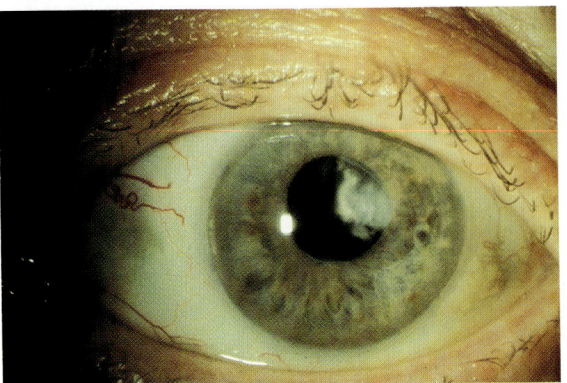

**COLOR PLATE 16-4.** Retained cortex entrapped behind intraocular lens. Note fluffy white texture. (See page 207.)

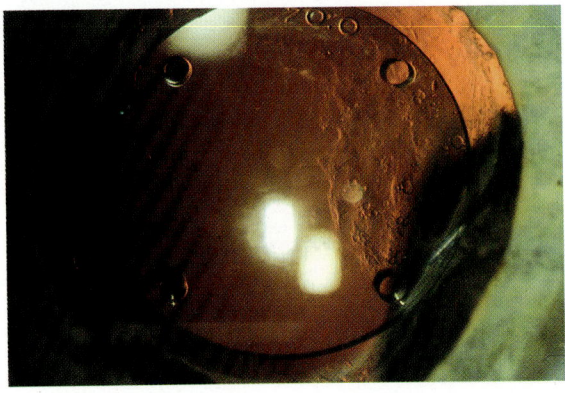

**COLOR PLATE 16-5.** A patient with posterior capsular opacity and ciliary body melanoma. This case illustrates the importance of routine dilation with peripheral fundus examination prior to consideration of referral for YAG capsulotomy. (See page 210.)

# General Considerations

**SECTION I**

# Trends in Cataract Care

## CHAPTER 1

Cataracts are the major cause of blindness in the world and the most prevalent ophthalmic disease. As the median age of the world population increases over the next five decades, the immensity of this eye problem will increase. In the United States, cataracts are the major cause of self-reported visual impairment and are the third leading cause of preventable blindness. Cross-sectional studies show cataract to be present in 10% of all US citizens. The prevalence is 50% in the 65 to 74 age group and 70% in those 75 or older.[1,2] Visual disability from cataract accounts for over 8 million physician office visits per year,[3] and this number does not include optometric visits.

Ultimately, when the disability from cataract begins to affect or alter the patient's functional ability, surgical removal with lens implantation is the most viable alternative to treat these limitations. In the United States, more than 1.2 million cataract procedures are paid for by Medicare yearly, making it the most common surgery for Americans over the age of 65.[1,4-6] In the years between 1987 and 1988, 97% of these cases received intraocular lens implants.[7] The annual cost of cataract surgery and associated care in the United States was approximately 3 billion dollars in 1991.[8] Despite this huge dollar expenditure estimate, the approximate cost per quality-adjusted-life-year (defined as the financial costs of surgery and aftercare balanced against the improved quality of life) for cataract surgery reported in 1988 was $810. This is a better value for the money than other procedures (ie, pacemaker implantation or hospital hemodialysis) assessed in the same way in the United Kingdom.[9]

Remarkable changes have occurred in the care of cataract patients since the first lens implant by Harold Ridley in 1949[10] (Table 1–1). The operating microscope came into routine use during the late 1960s and early 1970s, which allowed development of more intricate microsurgical techniques with lower complication rates. Outpatient surgery in ambulatory surgery centers (ASCs) replaced hospital stays with no apparent adverse effect on surgical outcomes.[11] The use of local anesthesia superseded the use of general anesthesia. Op-

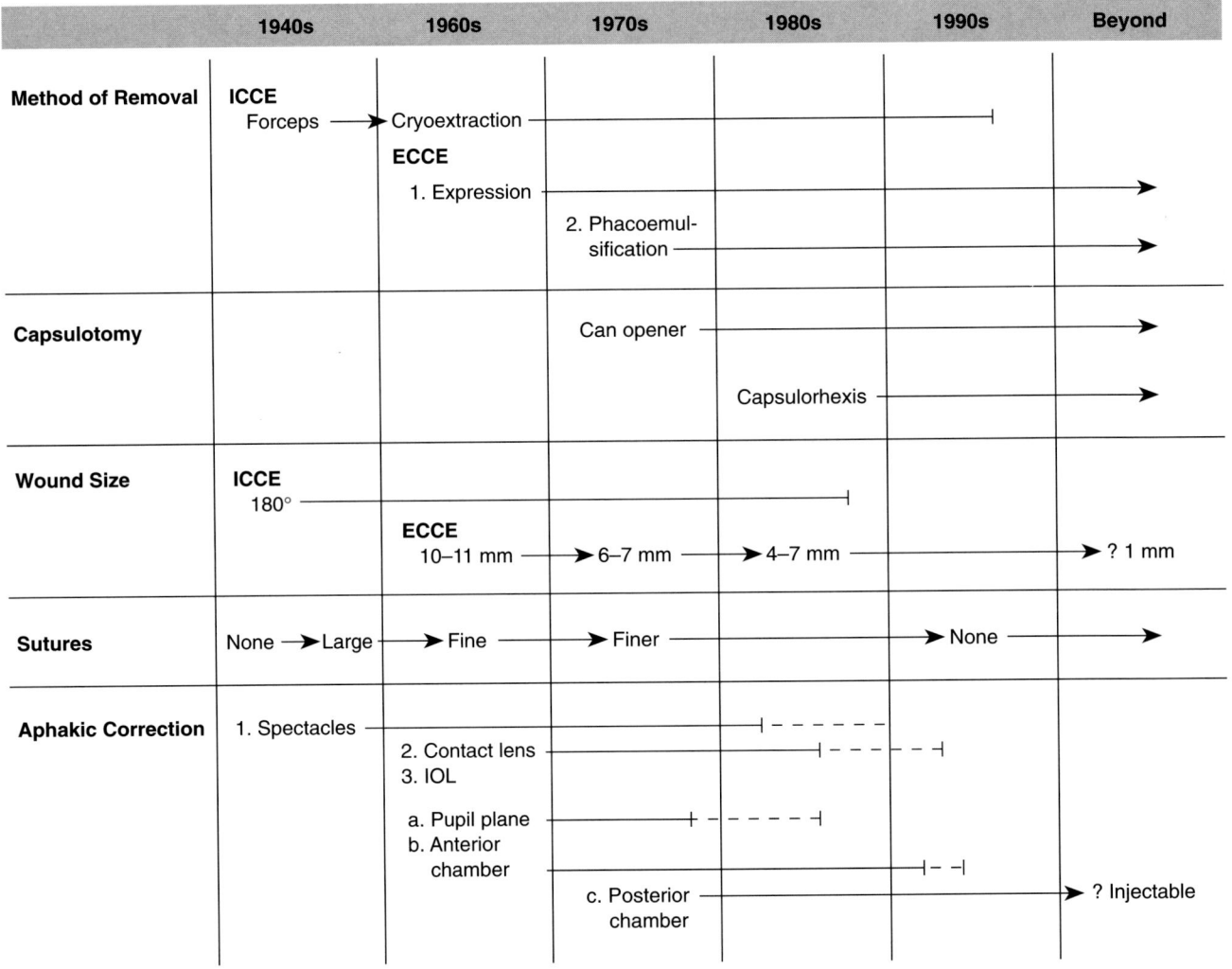

**TABLE 1-1. TRENDS IN ICCE AND ECCE CATARACT SURGERY AND IOL IMPLANTATION**

Courtesy of Oli Traustason, MD.

tometrists came to participate in the preoperative and postoperative care of their patients.

In the 1950s, extracapsular cataract extraction (ECCE) flourished, whereby the anterior lens capsule was grasped and torn centrally with a toothed capsule forceps. The lens nucleus was manually expressed and the anterior and posterior segments were irrigated to remove cortex. The posterior capsule remained intact. The 180-degree (10 mm) wound was then closed with a single silk suture. Extracapsular cataract extraction required a nearly mature cataract because nonopaque portions of the lens were difficult to remove. This meant patients were severely disabled before surgery was performed.

Therefore, intracapsular cataract extraction (ICCE) was met with enthusiasm in the late 1960s to early 1970s, because it allowed removal of the entire lens. Through a large incision, the entire lens, including capsule, was removed by forceps or cryoprobe, sometimes facilitated by the enzyme alpha-chymotrypsin to dissolve the zonules.

Phacoemulsification and a refinement in ECCE were introduced in 1967 by Charles Kelman.[12] With his technique, an ultrasonic vibrating cannula emulsified the lens nucleus and aspirated it through a small incision. The small incision theoretically allowed quicker rehabilitation. Due to difficulty in using the technique, it was performed by only a limited number of surgeons. Nevertheless, due to its anatomically compartmentalized outcome, the theoretical superiority of ECCE has been acknowledged over the years. In addition, the ability to place the intraocular lens into the posterior chamber capsular bag was viewed as potentially reliable and stable. Extracapsular cataract extraction has nearly completely replaced ICCE, with the extracapsular method being used in 95% of all cataract extractions in the United States. About 50% of these are by phacoemulsification.

The idea for modern intraocular lenses came during World War II when fighter plane canopies were shattered by bombs and polymethylmethacrylate fragments occasionally lodged in pilot's eyes without causing great reactivity. This led to experimentation with intraocular lens implants by Harold Ridley. There was a progression from posterior, to anterior chamber, to iris-fixated lenses requiring large incisions for implantation. The trend in the last 10 years has been back to the use of posterior chamber lenses but inserted through a small incision. Today, over 90% of lens implants are posterior chamber lenses.[7]

Another innovation in the 1980s that changed the face of cataract extraction was the introduction of continuous-tear capsulotomy, or capsulorhexis. Previously, the anterior capsule was opened by making small punctures very close to each other that were connected to create the "can-opener" capsulotomy. The resulting jagged edges, however, allowed capsular tears and inhibited the surgeon from visualizing whether or not the intraocular lens (IOL) was in the capsular bag. In capsulorhexis, the anterior capsulotomy has a smooth continuous edge that is extraordinarily strong and easily visible through the operating microscope. This allows visualization of the "bag" and reliable placement of the IOL. Risks of IOL displacement from a torn capsule or inaccurate placement are minimized.[13,14] It is our opinion that cataract extraction through a small incision utilizing capsulorhexis, phacoemulsification, and placing the intraocular lens in the capsular bag provides state of the art cataract surgery with minimal intraoperative, and postoperative complications. There is quick rehabilitation to stable visual acuity.

Finally, the way cataract care is delivered has evolved over the last two decades. Traditionally, optometrists have referred to ophthalmologists for cataract surgery and provided spectacles or contact lenses for these patients after the physician follow-up period of 2 to 3 months. Today, due to expanded scope of practice into the use of diagnostic and therapeutic pharmaceutical agents, as well as Medicare reimbursement for aphakic/pseudophakic care, doctors of optometry play a larger role in diagnosing cataracts and counseling patients as to their options in treatment. Optometrists and ophthalmologists work together to provide a complete preoperative, intraoperative, and postoperative experience that meets the patients' needs. This cooperative care provided by doctors of optometry and ophthalmic surgeons has come to be known as comanagement, which refers to the shared provision of care to patients with eye disease or requiring eye surgery.

As a result of greater optometric involvement in the preoperative and postoperative care of cataract patients, questions have arisen concerning the quality of care delivered to patients undergoing cataract extraction and receiving comanaged follow-up. A report by the Office of Technology Assessment (OTA) expressed concern about this issue.[15] These concerns have been addressed in several other studies that will be explored in the following paragraphs.

Nussenblatt and Murrill described the treatment of cataracts as a process that begins when the patient enters the delivery system, continues through the surgery, and ends when the needed follow-up care is completed at a specific period of time after surgery.[16] The treatment outcome, defined as the patient's postsurgical visual acuity, is dependent on a number of factors that influence this process: the characteristics of the patient, the level of surgical care, and factors affecting the delivery of care to the patient (Figure 1–1). Patient characteristics affecting the surgical outcome include the patient's age and sex, the presence of preexisting ocular conditions, and the visual acuity of the eye prior to surgery. Older patients are more likely to have preexisting ocular conditions and are more likely to be at a higher risk for poorer outcomes than younger patients. Many preexisting ocular conditions, particularly macular degeneration and diabetic retinopathy, affect the patient's preoperative visual acuity and may also impact the patient's postsurgical visual acuity. Both optometrist and ophthalmologist may participate in the care and affect the outcome. Optometrists who refer patients to ophthalmologists frequently may see the patient for postoperative care after the surgery. Patients not referred by optometrists would normally be followed by the surgeon. The doctor who follows the patient could affect the outcome if the patient were not managed properly. The level of surgical care itself also influences the outcome, as the surgeon's skill and the type of surgical procedure performed affect the development of problems. If problems are severe or long lasting, then postsurgical visual acuity will be affected.

In a study of 704 patients who underwent their first eye cataract surgery by ECCE with phacoemulsification, the data from Nussenblatt and Murrill[16] suggest that there is no difference in outcome, judged by postsurgical visual acuity, between patients managed postoperatively by doctors of optometry versus surgeons. The findings were controlled for age, sex, preexisting ocular conditions, presurgical visual acuity, whether the patient was referred by an optometrist or ophthalmologist, and postsurgical conditions; all of which are believed to influence postoperative visual acuity.[16]

Furthermore, a study supported by the American Optometric Association and performed by the Batelle Human Affairs Research Centers, Washington, DC, was designed to describe the practice of comanagement between doctors of optometry and ophthalmic surgeons and to explore any differences in postoperative visual acuity and complications between comanaged cataract surgery patients compared with statistics existing in the medical literature. Records from 2458 consecutive cataract procedures performed between January 1 and July 31, 1988, from five nonrandomized ambulatory surgery centers were reviewed:

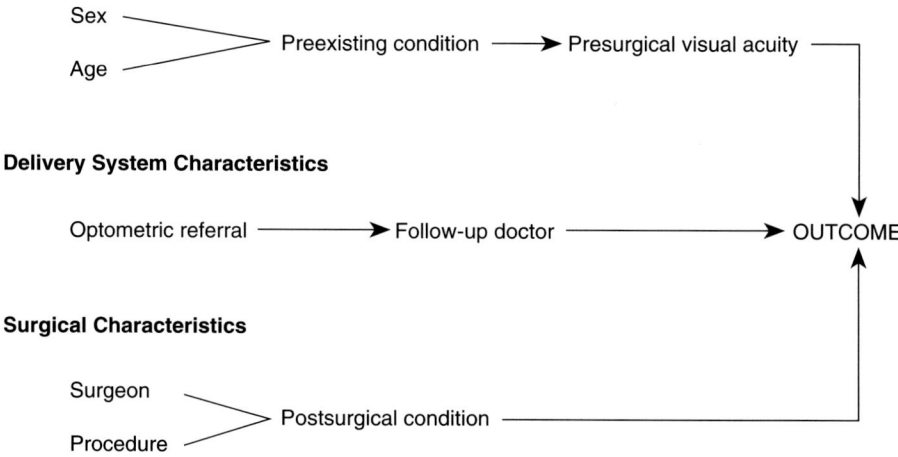

*FIGURE 1–1.* Factors that influence cataract treatment.

"The study findings suggest that patients receiving postoperative care delivered by eye center providers and optometrists located outside of the center have vision outcomes and complication rates that are comparable to those reported in the medical literature" where care is delivered by ophthalmologists.[17] Successful vision outcome, defined as 20/40 or better vision, was experienced by 86% of all comanaged patients regardless of the presence of preexisting conditions. More than 93% of comanaged cases had no postoperative complication; the incidence of postoperative complications fell between 0.04% and 2.0%, depending on the individual complication.

The OTA report on comanaged care implied that optometrists, because of differences in training compared with ophthalmologists, might not deliver acceptable postoperative care following cataract surgery.[15] However, Revicki et al demonstrate that the visual acuity outcomes and complication rates of comanaged patients are not different from the Food and Drug Administration (FDA) CORE study and other published studies.[17] The findings of this study demonstrate that optometrists can and do provide quality patient care following cataract surgery and that patient outcomes are comparable regardless of whether postoperative care is delivered by optometrists and ophthalmic surgeons or by ophthalmic surgeons alone.

## REFERENCES

1. National Advisory Eye Council: *Vision Research: A National Plan.* 1983–1987. Bethesda, MD: US DHHS, PHS Publ (NIH), no. 87–2755; 1987.
2. Leibowitz HM, Krueger DE, Maunder LR, et al: The Framingham eye study monograph: An ophthalmological and epidemiological study of cataract, glaucoma, diabetic retinopathy, macular degeneration and visual acuity in a general population of 2,631 adults, 1973–1975. *Surv Ophthalmol.* 1980;**24**(suppl):335–610.
3. Koch H: *Practice Patterns of the Office-Based Ophthalmologist.* National Ambulatory Medical Care Survey. Advance data from Vital and Health Statistics; no. 162; Hyattsville, MD, National Center for Health Statistics: US DHHS, PHS Publ no. 89–1250; 1985.
4. Based on analysis of Medicare Part-A and Part-B claims files obtained from the US Health Care Financing Administration.
5. Office of the Inspector General: *Medicare Cataract Implant Surgery.* Washington, DC: US DHHS, Publ no. OA1851X046;1986.
6. Obstbaum S: *President of the American Society of Cataract and Refractive Surgery: Testimony before the Physician Payment Review Commission.* Washington, DC; 1987.
7. Jaffe N, Jaffe M, Jaffe G: *Cataract Surgery and Its Complications,* 5th ed. St. Louis, CV Mosby Co; 1990:138.
8. O'Day DM, Adams AJ, Cassem EH, et al: *Cataract in Adults: Management of Functional Impairment.* Clinical Practice Guideline No. 4. US DHHS, PHS, Agency for Health Care Policy & Research; 1993:21.
9. Drummond MF: Economic aspects of cataract. *Ophthalmology.* 1988;**95**:1147–1153.
10. Ridley H: Intraocular acrylic lenses. *Transophthalmol Society, UK.* 1951;**71**:617–621.
11. Holland GN, Earl DT, Wheeler NC, et al: Results of inpatient and outpatient cataract surgery: A historical cohort comparison. *Ophthalmology.* 1992;**99**:845–852.
12. Kelman CD: Phacoemulsification and aspiration: A new technique of cataract removal—A preliminary report. *Am J Ophthalmol.* 1967;**64**:23–35.
13. Assia EI, Apple DJ, Tsai JC, Morgan RC: Mechanism of radial tear formation and extension after anterior capsulotomy. *Ophthalmology.* 1991;**98**:432–437.
14. Wasserman D, Apple DJ, Castenada VE, et al: Anterior capsular tears and loop fixation of posterior chamber intraocular lenses. *Ophthalmology.* 1991;**98**:425–431.

15. Kemp K, Boardman B: *Appropriate Care for Cataract Surgery Patients Before and After Surgery: Issues of Medical Safety and Appropriateness.* Office of Technology Assessment. Washington, DC, US Congress; Oct 1988.
16. Nussenblatt H, Murrill C: *Comanagement of Cataract Patients.* Presented at American Public Health Association annual meeting, New Orleans; 1987.
17. Revicki DA, Brown RE, Adler MA: Patient outcomes with co-managed post-operative care after cataract surgery. *J Clin Epidemiol.* 1993;**46**:5–15.

# *Comanagement*

**CHAPTER 2**

As mentioned in Chapter 1, comanagement is defined as the shared provision of care to patients with eye disease by optometrists and ophthalmologists. In the spectrum of patient management, comanagement fits somewhere between referral (releasing a patient to someone else for care) and consultation (asking another for diagnosis or treatment on a patient in conjunction with care already being provided).[1,2]

In the case of cataract patients, several different providers play important roles in the delivery of care. The optometrist tends to serve as the primary entry point into the eye care system and provides diagnostic and refractive services that allow the patient to reach his or her functional visual expectations. The relationship between the optometrist, clinic staff, and patient tends to be a long-term one, being similar to that between patient and family practice doctor. For that reason, the optometrist also serves as counselor and advocate once a cataract has been diagnosed and consultation or referral for surgery is necessary. As a counselor, the optometrist advises the patient of clinical findings and treatment options, including surgery. The optometrist usually provides information about what a cataract is, how it may be removed, aspects of what quality surgical care is, and makes suggestions about surgeons who provide the level of technical expertise the optometrist prefers for patients. As an advocate, the optometrist not only transfers clinical information to the surgeon but also informs the surgeon and staff of any special needs the patient may have, such as level of anxiety, need for oxygen, hearing impairment, language barriers, or need of a wheelchair. In addition, following any surgical intervention, the optometrist may comanage the patient postoperatively.[3,4]

The ophthalmic surgeon and clinical staff tend to have a shorter but more intense experience with the patient where they provide specific evaluation services, counseling, and surgical care that is unique to their specialty. The surgeon and staff must create an atmosphere of trust for the patient and family that prepares the patient physically and mentally to undergo surgery. Once again, educating the patient and family is very important. Answering all questions, providing information to allow informed consent, and allaying fears are important aspects of care delivered under the surgeon's supervision. Prior to surgery, the surgeon is obligated to advise and receive the consent of the patient concerning who will deliver the postoperative follow-up.[4] Finally, the surgeon and staff provide the surgical care and postoperative follow-up until the patient is stable.

The 1990s were ushered in with an urgency for both the government and professional organizations to develop clinical "guidelines" for delivery of eye care.[5-10] Information and instruction from documents such as these will abound during the next decade, so it is not necessary to reiterate them in this book. As clinicians, however, doctors of optometry should acknowledge their medicolegal responsibilities, which at a minimum are:

1. The responsibility to diagnose coexisting eye disease other than cataract that may result in injury. This necessitates pupil dilation or referral for such care when a patient presents with symptoms of decreased vision in the presence of cataract.
2. The duty to warn the patient of the effect of their decreased vision due to cataracts (as in legal ability to drive a car) or the possible risk of cataract formation secondary to long-term use of certain topical therapeutic agents (ie, topical steroids).
3. The duty to refer exists once a diagnosis of cataract is made. The time at which an optometrist has this duty is both subjective and controversial; however, a prudent criterion for referral might be to refer when the decreased vision from cataract is beginning to hinder the patient's daily activities such that quality of life is affected.

Finally, comanagement may be viewed by the courts as a situation where both the optometrist and ophthalmologist are jointly liable for any negligence, if committed, by either practitioner.[1,11]

In the delivery of comanaged cataract care, there are both advantages and disadvantages. The greatest advantage lies in quality assurance provided by practitioners of different disciplines working together and providing some oversight in the care provided by each type of doctor. The largest disadvantage may lie in practitioner negligence by one doctor or the other and joint liability because both doctors may be providing care concurrently.[1,3,11]

Second only to expert clinical and surgical skills, the most important element of successful primary and comanaged care of a cataract patient is communication. This falls into several categories:

**Patient communication**

- Between optometrist/staff and patient/family
- Between ophthalmologist/staff and patient/family

**Doctor-to-doctor communication**

- Through general education
- Concerning specific patients by phone or by letter

Good patient communication is built on the knowledge of all aspects of preoperative and postoperative cataract care and a sensitivity to the needs and fears of the patient and family. Besides providing information on clinical findings, the optometrist may provide written or video education about what a cataract is and what is involved in quality cataract extraction. Preprinted appointment cards may be used that allow the optometrist's office to clearly convey to the patient any appointments with the surgeon. As a service, the optometric staff may supply the patient with directions to the surgeon's office or surgery center. (See Appendix 1.)

At the surgeon's office, further information, either verbal, written, or videotaped, is necessary. At the least, the patient must read and understand the informed consent for cataract extraction and lens implantation. The patient should be informed as to who will be providing postoperative care.

The communication between doctors is much more involved and occurs at a variety of levels. The first level is through the use of didactic education that establishes a commonality from which the practitioners may discuss patients. As in all other areas of optometric primary care, formal education is the foundation from which clinical expertise builds. Education about cataract care may be obtained through schools and colleges of optometry, institutions such as comanagement or referral centers, or professional organizations at the national, state, and local levels. The educators should be both optometric and medical specialists. In addition, optometrists should speak individually with surgeons to whom their patients may go and learn about the surgeon's preferences and recommendations in preoperative and postoperative care. It is useful to be familiar with the surgeon's delivery of information, examinations, and surgical technique. Better yet, the optometrist should observe a patient or patients receiving care from the surgeon, including surgery, so that he or she is intimately informed as to what patients may experience. This knowledge and familiarity builds respect and trust between the two doctors, which further enhances the exchange of information and quality of patient care.

Written correspondence between the doctors delivering either primary or surgical care is the second level of doctor communication. A knowledge of standard medical abbreviations as well as common ocular abbreviations also expedites most patient reports. (See Appendix 2.) Forms may be used to report quickly on preoperative or routine postoperative visits. In the most organized of comanagement care, the preoperative and postoperative forms from the referring optometrist may be identical to charting forms used by the surgeon's office to aid confirmation of preoperative data gathered and to report postoperative information efficiently. When appropriate, the optometrist uses these forms to convey information to the ophthalmologist postoperatively and vice versa. (See Appendix 3.)

Nonstandardized written correspondence may be most readily organized by utilizing the SOAP (**s**ubjective, **o**bjective, **a**ssessment, **p**lan) format to convey both preoperative and postoperative information exchanged between optometrist and ophthalmologist. (See Appendix 4.)

Telephone conversation is the third level of doctor communication and plays an important role in providing successful cataract care. Preoperatively, the patient may find it convenient for the optometrist to arrange the surgeon appointment(s). In this case, the optometric staff should be educated on the information necessary to make the referral appointment by phone, including patient name, phone number, diagnosis, and any special needs of the patient. On arrival at the surgeon's clinic, the staff or surgeon should feel free to call the optometrist to clarify or confirm any clinical abbreviations in question, as well as to report any discrepancy in observations that may need to be resolved before proceeding with plans for further care. As a courtesy, the surgeon's staff should call to inform the optometrist of the surgery date or other plans made. In the same manner, following surgery, the surgeon's staff should inform the optometrist's staff about how the surgery went. After the surgeon's follow-up, that office should arrange the next follow-up with the optometrist by phone. Following surgery, during the postoperative course, the optometrist should feel free to call the surgeon regarding any unusual clinical findings and expect a phone consultation with the surgeon or staff when necessary.

This intricate system of communication through education, written word, and telephone conversation, is necessary so that both the optometrist and surgeon have a complete set of data while caring for the cataract patient. This allows quality care to be provided no matter what complications arise in the course of care.

Sooner or later, as in all relationships, comanaged care may result in some conflict. The conflicts may relate to discrepancies in patient data gathering, opinions about the best treatment option for the patient, or disagreement in follow-up schedule or location, to name a few. The resolution of conflicts is dependent on the trust and respect between the two practitioners. This trust and respect will lead to honest discussion and decisions made in the best interest of the patient.

## REFERENCES

1. Classé JG: *Legal Aspects of Optometry*. Stoneham, MA: Butterworth; 1989:195–200.
2. Revicki DA, Brown RE, Adler MA: Patient outcomes with co-managed post-operative care after cataract surgery. *J Clin Epidemiol*. 1993;**46**:5–15.
3. *American Medical News. Ethics Answers:* February 23, 1990:23.
4. *Argus:* Revised and Updated Advisory Opinion of the Code of Ethics. March 1992: 6.
5. American Academy of Ophthalmology (Ad Hoc Committee on Ophthalmic Procedures Assessment): *Cataract Surgery in the 1980s*. San Francisco: American Academy of Ophthalmology; 1986.
6. American Academy of Ophthalmology: *Cataract in the Otherwise Healthy Eye (Preferred Practice Pattern)*. San Francisco: American Academy of Ophthalmology; 1989.
7. Foreman J: Federal agency to develop cataract management guidelines by January 1991. *Arch Ophthalmol*. 1990;**108**(Oct):1391.
8. Foreman J: Johns Hopkins outcome study for cataract management. *Arch Ophthalmol*. 1990;**108**(Nov):1533.
9. Foreman J: The clinical appropriateness initiative—Cataract management study. *Arch Ophthalmol*. 1990;**108**(Dec):1678.
10. O'Day DM, Adams AJ, Cassem EH, et al: *Cataract in Adults: Management of Functional Impairment*. Clinical Practice Guideline No. 4. US DHHS, PHS, Agency for Health Care Policy & Research; 1993.
11. Classé JG: *Cataracts and Comanagement: A Clinicolegal View*. Presented at Pacific University College of Optometry Continuing Education "Fun in the Sun"; Maui, HI; January 1990.

# Lens Anatomy and Cataractogenesis

CHAPTER 3

A practicing clinician must have intimate knowledge of the structures examined, diagnosed, and treated for disease. This chapter reviews the anatomy of the lens and some of the established as well as theoretical bases for cataract formation.

## LENS ANATOMY

The natural lens is approximately 14 diopters in power, biconvex, transparent, and suspended by zonules behind the pupil of the eye. The lens increases in weight throughout life but reaches a constant equatorial diameter by age 15. It is 65% water and 35% protein. This protein has antigenic properties such that the body's immune system treats it as "foreign" on exposure and phacoanaphylaxis results.[1] (See Color Plate 3-1.)

Because of its unique embryology, the original basement membrane of the lens proliferates to become an elastic capsule that completely encloses the lens and is the thickest basement membrane of the body. Also, due to the embryology, a single layer of cuboidal surface epithelial cells is completely enclosed behind the anterior surface of the capsule, whereas primary lens fibers from the equatorial and posterior regions form the embryonic nucleus. Secondary lens fibers that form the bulk of the lens arise from the equatorial region and grow anteriorly and posteriorly, meeting other lens fibers to form the Y sutures. The lens fibers that proliferate in utero between the second and eighth months form the fetal nucleus with its fetal Y sutures. The fetal anterior Y suture is erect and the posterior is inverted due to the fact that the lens fibers are approximately one half the lens circumference in length, and those that originate nearest the anterior pole terminate farthest from the posterior pole. These sutures may be viewed with the slit lamp throughout life.

The lens has three zones clinically: capsule, cortex, and nucleus. The cap-

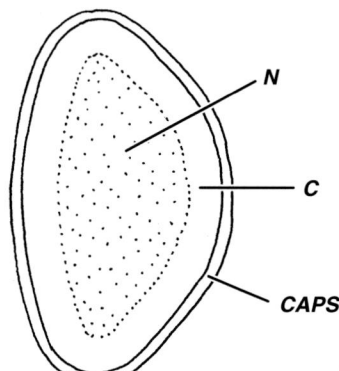

**FIGURE 3–1.** Three clinical zones of the lens. N, nucleus; C, cortex; CAPS, capsule.

sule forms the enclosing "bag" with epithelium attached anteriorly. The nucleus and cortex form the central and more external contents, respectively (see Figure 3–1). There is no sharp distinction between the nucleus and cortex. However, the fetal nucleus may be distinguished by the fetal Y sutures. The nucleus and cortex sometimes may be visualized by "zones of discontinuity" between the various layers. With age, sclerosis, yellowing, or brunescence may allow better distinction between nucleus and cortex.

## CATARACTOGENESIS

A cataract is any opacity of the lens whether it is a small local opacity or complete loss of transparency.[1] Cataracts may occur secondary to hereditary factors, trauma, inflammation, metabolic or nutritional defects, radiation, or the effects of aging. Age-related cataracts are the most common clinically encountered; therefore, we will review their pathogenesis. For in-depth explanation of the other types of cataracts, we refer you to textbooks on the subject.[2,3]

The mechanism of cataract formation is multifactorial, which makes it difficult to study. Oxidation of membrane lipids, structural or enzymatic proteins, or DNA by peroxides or ultraviolet-induced free radicals may be an early initiating event increasing light scattering tendencies in both nucleus and cortex.[2,3] It is known that two specific processes contribute to the loss of transparency following possible initiation by oxidation. In the case of cortical cataracts, an imbalance of electrolytes leads to an overhydration of the lens that leads to liq-

**FIGURE 3–2.** Cortical wedges.

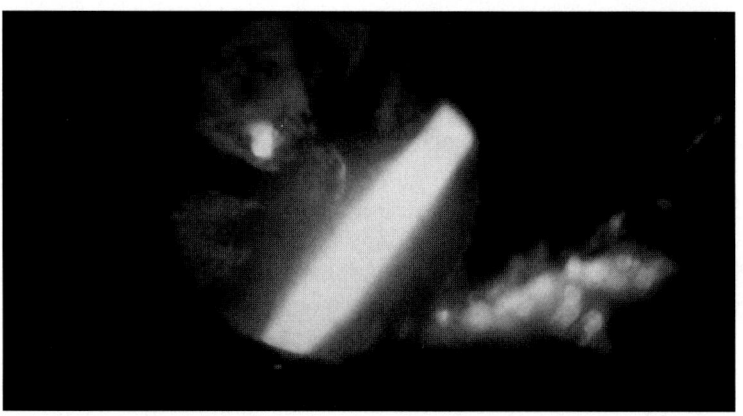

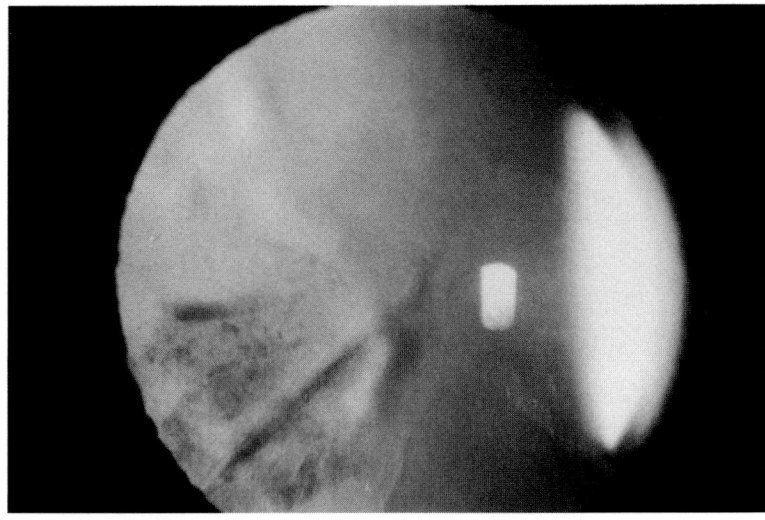

**FIGURE 3–3.** Cortical clefts or spokes.

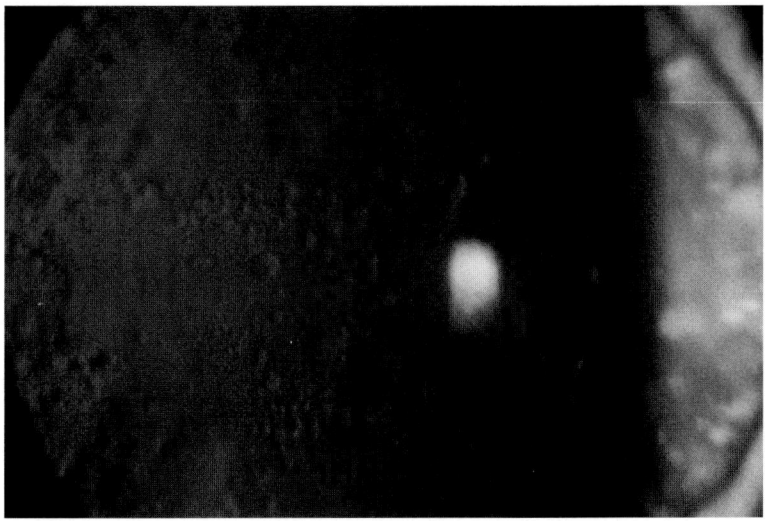

**FIGURE 3–4.** Cortical vacuoles.

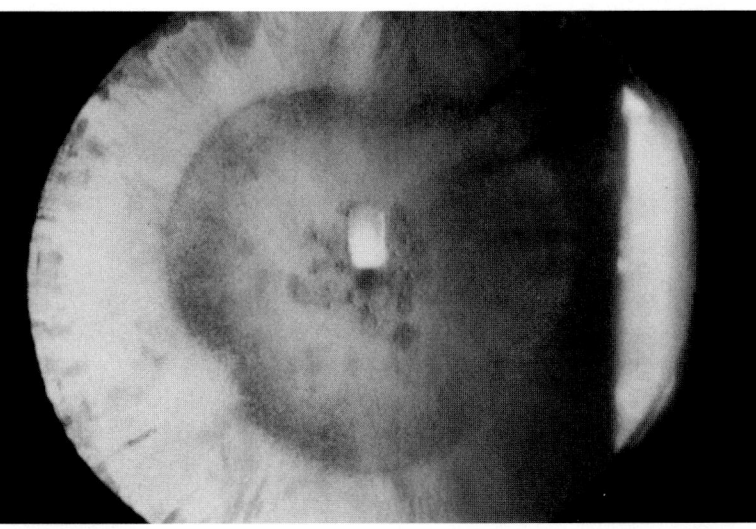

**FIGURE 3–5.** Cortical lamellar separations.

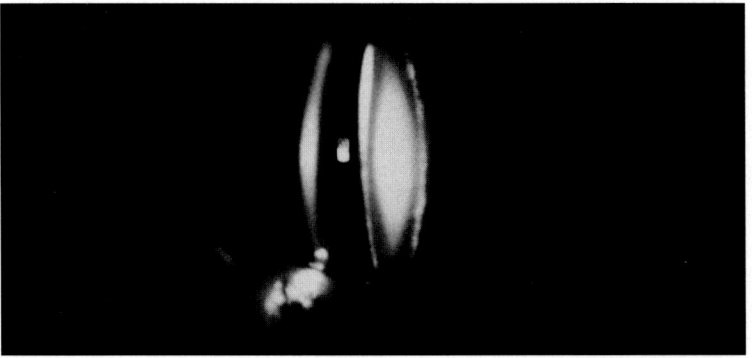

**FIGURE 3–6.** Murky nuclear sclerotic "button."

uefaction of the lens fibers. Clinically, cortical cataract formation occasionally is manifest by refractive error change and by formation of vacuoles, clefts, wedges, or lamellar separations when viewed through the slit lamp (see Figures 3–2 to 3–5).

Nuclear cataracts usually occur secondary to modification of the lens proteins (crystallins) by oxidation, proteolysis, glycation, and deamidation, so that the proteins aggregate into high molecular weight (HMW) particles that scatter light. In addition, colored products are formed from amino acid residues in this process, so that color or pigmentation (urochrome) may occur. The increasing optical density of the nucleus may cause a clinical myopic shift as well as appearing as a murky or yellowish to brunescent central lenticular "button" when viewed by the slit lamp[2,4] (see Figure 3–6).

Age-related posterior subcapsular cataract is created by loss of lens fiber nuclei and replacement by aberrantly migrating epithelial cells toward the posterior pole. These cells cluster, form balloon cells, and interdigitate with adjacent lens fibers and the deep cortical fibers to break them down. The result is the lacy, granular, iridescent appearance of posterior subcapsular cataracts.[5]

## ── REFERENCES

1. Olson L: Anatomy and embryology of the lens. In Tasman E (ed): *Duane's Clinical Ophthalmology*, Vol. 1. Philadelphia: JB Lippincott; 1991:1–8.
2. Datiles MB, Kinoshita JH: Pathogenesis of cataracts. In Tasman E (ed): *Duane's Clinical Ophthalmology*, Vol 1. Philadelphia: JB Lippincott; 1991:1–14.
3. Bunce JE: The role of nutrition in cataract. In Tasman E (ed): *Duane's Clinical Ophthalmology*, Vol 1. Philadelphia: JB Lippincott; 1991:1–9.
4. Luntz MH: Clinical types of cataracts. In Tasman E (ed): *Duane's Clinical Ophthalmology*, Vol 1. Philadelphia: JB Lippincott; 1991:1–20.
5. Eshagian J, Streeten BW: Human posterior subcapsular cataract: An ultrastructural study of the posteriorly migrating cells. *Arch Ophthalmol.* 1980;**98**:134–143.

# Grading Systems

**CHAPTER 4**

Throughout healthcare, a common method of communicating the range of disease is necessary. In this book, we want to describe preoperative and postoperative conditions in a uniform manner. Therefore, though subjective, we have chosen to define the standard grading systems that may apply to clinical findings described in this text and in the care of cataract patients.

## CONVENTIONAL SYSTEM

The conventional system of grading usually uses a series of pluses (+) to describe severity with a grade one plus (1+) condition being most mild and grade four plus (4+) being most severe (see Table 4–1). Additionally, one may also indicate even milder conditions by using the terms *rare, occasional,* or *trace*. One may also classify a finding outside of the plus system with use of the less than symbol (<), as in < grade 1+ corneal striae.

Preoperatively, there are corneal, anterior chamber, and lenticular findings that commonly affect the clinician's decision making, counseling, and prognosis for a cataract patient. Postoperatively, corneal, anterior chamber, posterior capsule, vitreous, and macular findings may be directly related to the surgery.

**TABLE 4–1. CONVENTIONAL GRADING SYSTEM**

| | |
|---|---|
| Mild | + or grade 1+ |
| Moderate | ++ or grade 2+ |
| Marked | +++ or grade 3+ |
| Severe | ++++ or grade 4+ |

Quantifying these findings is important for monitoring progress and communicating with the surgeon. In the following sections, observations and grading of these entities are described.

## CORNEA

Cornea guttata, or Fuchs' dystrophy, is an important preoperative finding that must be detected and graded or ruled out in every cataract case. When present, depending on the severity, corneal edema or corneal decompensation (where the cornea loses its ability to remain deturgesced), may occur postoperatively. Corneal guttae are excrescences of Descemet's membrane that appear as tiny water droplets or as ground glass when observed at the slit lamp by retroillumination. Marked or severe (grade 3+ to grade 4+) preoperative corneal guttae may require an endothelial cell count by specular microscopy and special counseling regarding the risk of postoperative corneal decompensation (see Chapter 5). Special intraoperative precautions to protect the cornea may be taken by the surgeon, such as use of a viscoelastic material.

Corneal edema is manifested in numerous ways. Central corneal clouding was a common finding secondary to the use of polymethylmethacrylate (PMMA) hard contact lenses but may also be seen in postoperative cataract patients. It may be described as circumscribed anterior stromal edema that is best observed at the slit lamp by the use of sclerotic scatter. Diffuse epithelial edema appears as microcysts that, in the most severe form, may coalesce to become corneal bullae. Stromal edema may be observed as striae or folds in the deep stroma and Descemet's membrane and causes an actual thickening of the cornea observable at the slit lamp or measurable by pachymetry.

For the purposes of preoperative and postoperative cataract patients, we have blended these findings to describe the cornea (Table 4–2; Figures 4–1 to 4–6).

## CATARACT

Each anatomic type of cataract appears to be initiated by different factors and has unique biochemical properties (see Chapter 3). Therefore, the three common cataract types—nuclear, cortical, and posterior subcapsular—should be examined through a dilated pupil and graded separately. We recommend evaluating all three major areas of the lens with a variety of lighting and viewing angles, but for final grading, we use a 45-degree slit angle for nuclear assessment and a 0-degree angle (retroillumination) for cortical and subcapsular as-

**TABLE 4–2. GRADING SYSTEM FOR CLINICAL CORNEAL FINDINGS**

| Grade | Clinical Description |
|---|---|
| 0 | Clear cornea |
| 1 | Occasional guttae or fold in Descemet's membrane without stromal thickening |
| 2 | Mild guttae or folds in Descemet's membrane, mild thickening of the stroma, mild epithelial edema |
| 3 | Frequent guttae or folds in Descemet's membrane, moderate thickening of the stroma, moderate epithelial edema |
| 4 | Thick guttae, many folds in Descemet's membrane, markedly thickened stroma, epithelial microcysts and bullae |

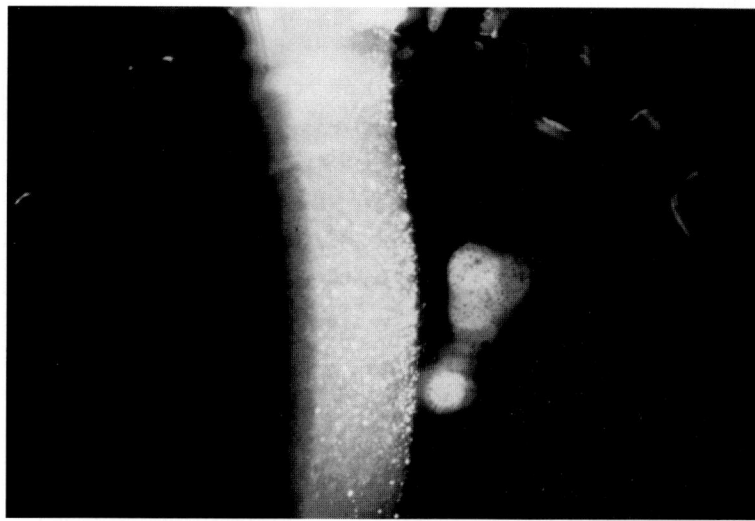

**FIGURE 4–1.** Corneal microcystic edema.

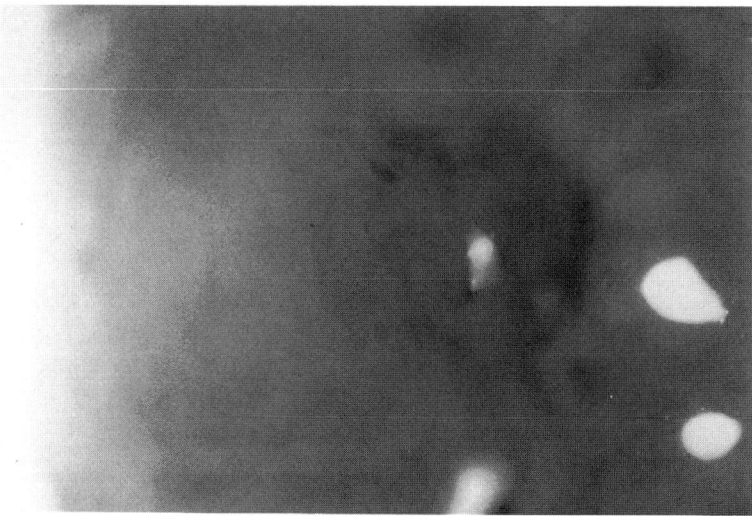

**FIGURE 4–2.** Corneal bullae.

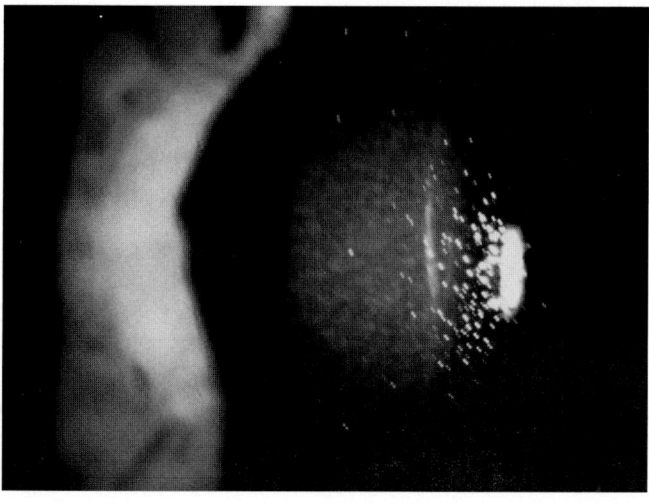

**FIGURE 4–3.** Grade 1+ corneal striae.

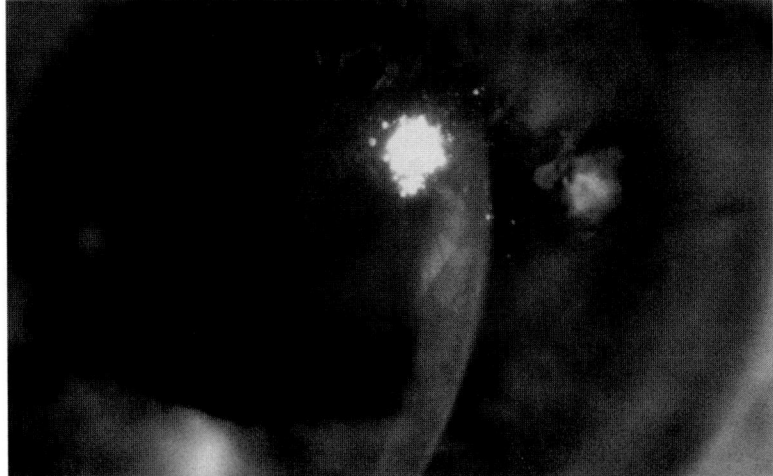

**FIGURE 4–4.** Grade 3+ corneal edema with stromal thickening and folds.

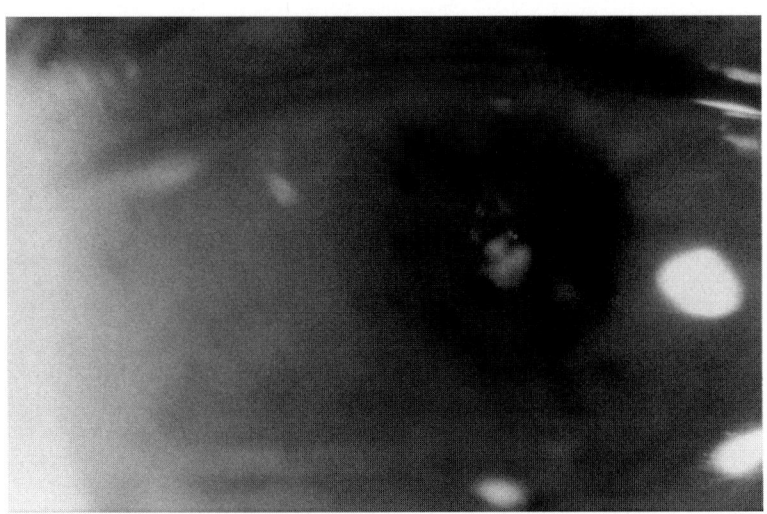

**FIGURE 4–5.** Grade 4+ corneal edema with stromal thickening, folds, and epithelial bullae.

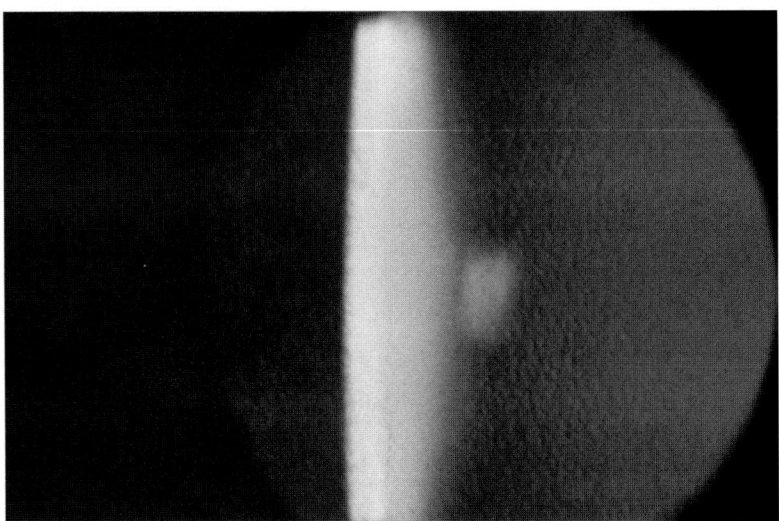

**FIGURE 4–6.** Grade 3+ corneal guttae.

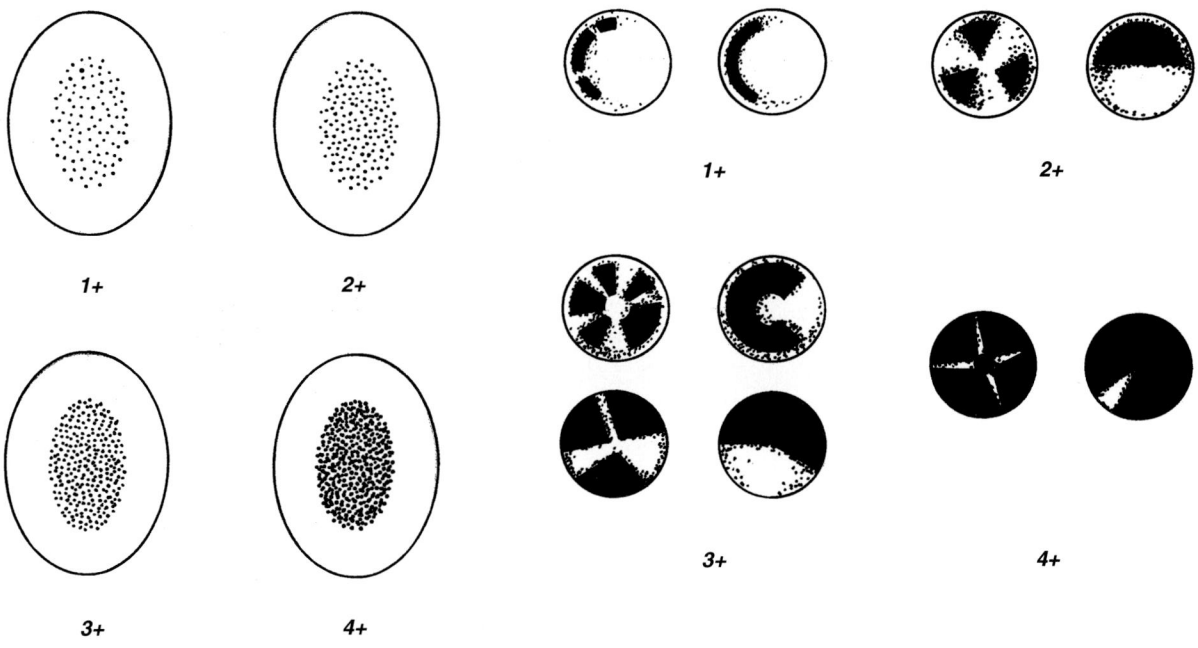

**NUCLEAR SCLEROSIS**

**CORTICAL SCLEROSIS**

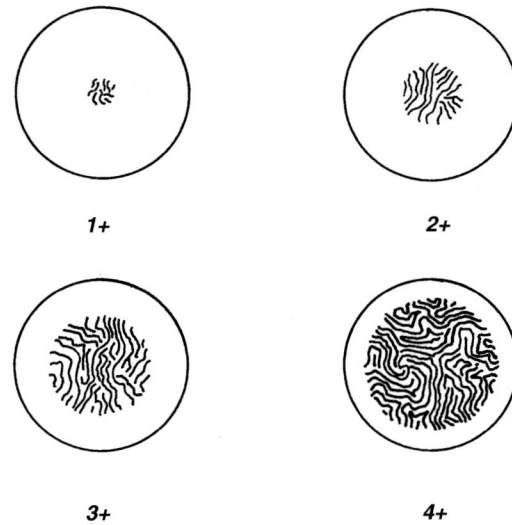

**POSTERIOR SUBCAPSULAR CATARACT**

*FIGURE 4–7.* Grading the three common types of cataracts: **Top left.** Nuclear sclerosis. **Top right.** Cortical sclerosis. **Bottom.** Posterior subcapsular cataract.

sessment. For clinical use, we employ a modification of the Lens Opacities Classification System II (LOCS II).[1-3]

First, a clear lens is one where the nucleus, cortex, and subcapsular area are free of opacities. The subcapsular and cortical zones are free of dots, flecks, vacuoles, and waterclefts. The nucleus is transparent and the embryonal nucleus may be visible. Opacities in all three major zones are graded 1+ to 4+ (Figures 4–7 to 4–13; Color Plates 4–1 to 4–6). To put quantification of the opacities into perspective, nuclear sclerosis (NS) is graded by evaluating the average color and opalescence of the nucleus as a continuum from grade 1+ (mild or early nuclear sclerosis) to grade 4+ (severe or advanced nuclear sclerosis with milky brunes-

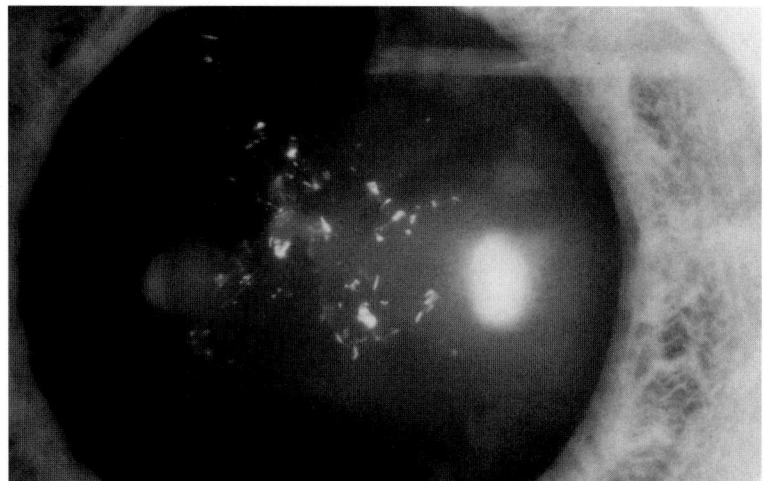

**FIGURE 4–8.** Cortical (Christmas tree) cataract under diffuse illumination.

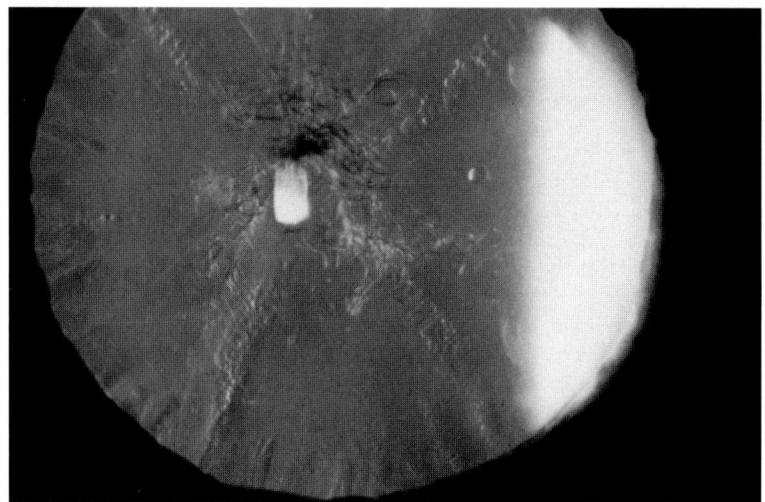

**FIGURE 4–9.** Cortical (Christmas tree) cataract under retroillumination.

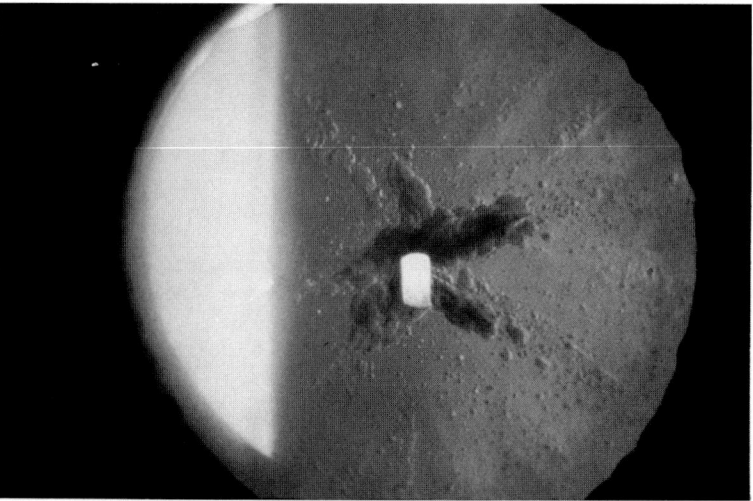

**FIGURE 4–10.** Grade 3+ sutural cataract.

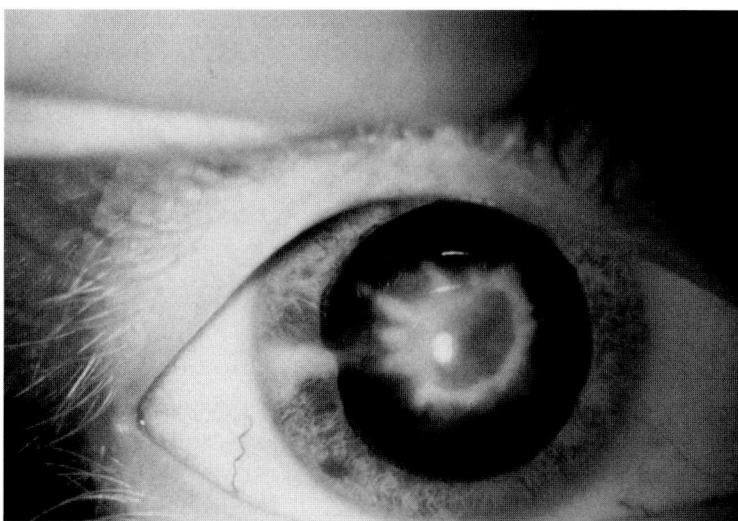

**FIGURE 4–11.** Grade 3–4+ traumatic cataract.

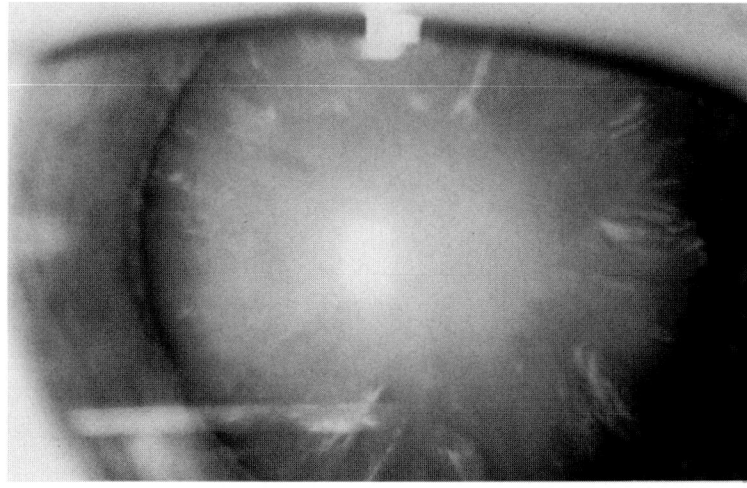

**FIGURE 4–12.** Grade 4+ nuclear, cortical, and posterior-subcapsular cataract (also called "mature" cataract).

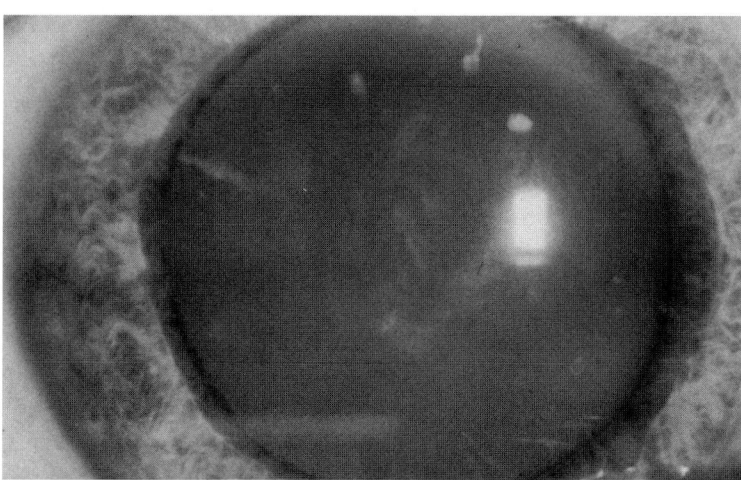

**FIGURE 4–13.** Completely opaque cataract with liquified cortex and sunken nucleus (also called hypermature or morgagnian cataract).

cence). Cortical and posterior subcapsular opacities should be visualized as "aggregate" and quantified. In the case of grade 2+ cortical sclerosis (CS), the cortical changes may obscure parts of two full quadrants of the lens. Grades 3+ and 4+ cortical sclerosis obscure an aggregate of more than approximately 50% and 90% of the intrapupillary zone, respectively. Cortical changes in the visual axis are more debilitating and therefore should be specifically described or the grade should be weighted to reflect the clinical relevance (eg, grade 1 + CS with spokes in the visual axis). Posterior subcapsular cataract (PSC) grade 1+ fills approximately 3% of the posterior zone, grade 2+ approximately 30%, and grade 3+ approximately 50%. Again, posterior subcapsular cataract in the visual axis is much more debilitating and the description or grading should reflect this (example: grade 2+ PSC in visual axis). (See Color Plates 4–7 through 4–9.)

## ANTERIOR CHAMBER REACTION

During both the preoperative and postoperative evaluation, the anterior chamber should be examined for inflammatory cells and flare. Cells and flare become visible when inflammation of the iris or ciliary body is significant enough to spill over into the aqueous. Cells are primarily lymphocytes with some neutrophils. They should be differentiated from pigmentary and red blood cells. Flare is increased protein in the aqueous due to alteration of the blood aqueous barrier.

The examination technique for counting cells involves creating a high-intensity, high-magnification field with a 1 mm by 1 mm slit beam at a 30- to 60-degree angle in a darkened room. Table 4–3 describes one grading system's recommendations for quantities of cells for each grade of severity[4] (Figures 4–14 to 4–16).

A slit beam that is visible when aimed obliquely across the anterior chamber demonstrates proteinaceous flare. The greater the visibility of the beam, the greater the concentration of protein in the aqueous. Flare may be quantified by aiming the slit beam obliquely across the anterior chamber[4] (Table 4–4; Figures 4–17 to 4–19).

## HYPOPYON

Hypopyon, although rare, may occur postoperatively. It is a collection of white blood cells that settle in the lower anterior chamber angle. It should be considered the hallmark of endophthalmitis until proven otherwise. Hypopyon is quantified by describing the percentage of the anterior chamber that is occupied (ie, 10%, 30%) (Figures 4–20 and 4–21).

**TABLE 4–3. GRADING SYSTEM FOR ANTERIOR CHAMBER CELLS**

| | |
|---|---|
| Grade 0 | No cells in field[a] |
| Trace | 2–4 cells in field |
| Grade 1 | 5–15 cells in field |
| Grade 2 | 16–25 cells in field |
| Grade 3 | 26–60 cells in field |
| Grade 4 | Over 60 cells in field |

[a] Field: 1 mm × 1 mm slit beam at 30- to 60-degree angle.
From Nussenblatt RB, Palestine AG: *Uveitis Fundamentals and Clinical Practice.* Chicago: Year Book Medical; 1989:65–66; with permission.

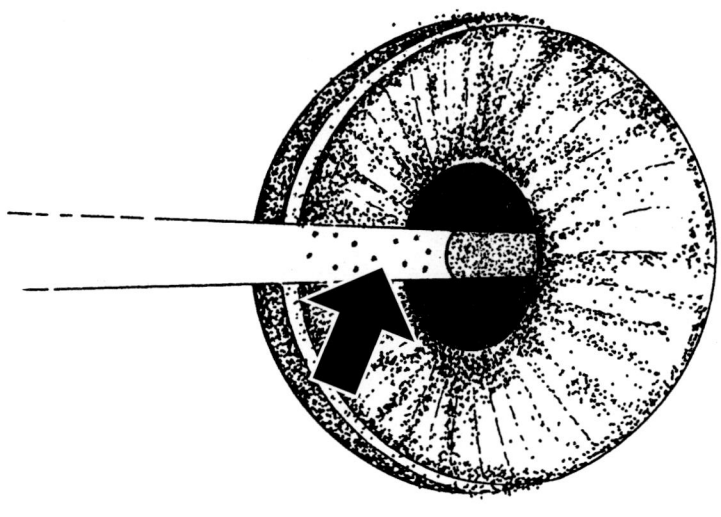

**FIGURE 4–14.** Grade 1+ cells in anterior chamber.

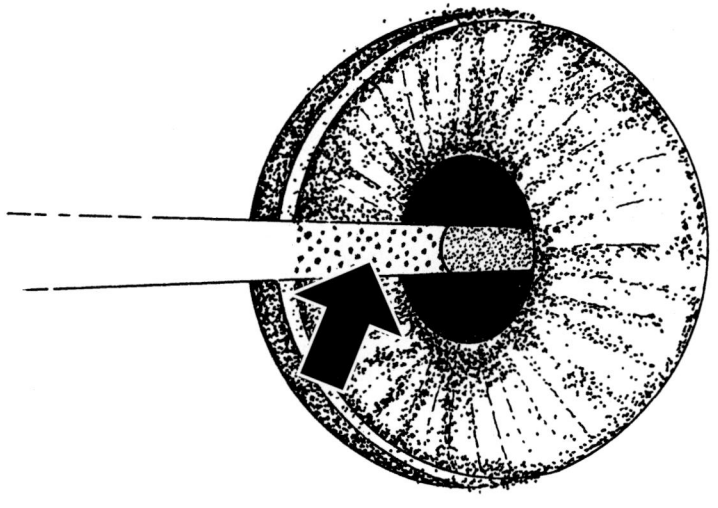

**FIGURE 4–15.** Grade 3+ cells in anterior chamber.

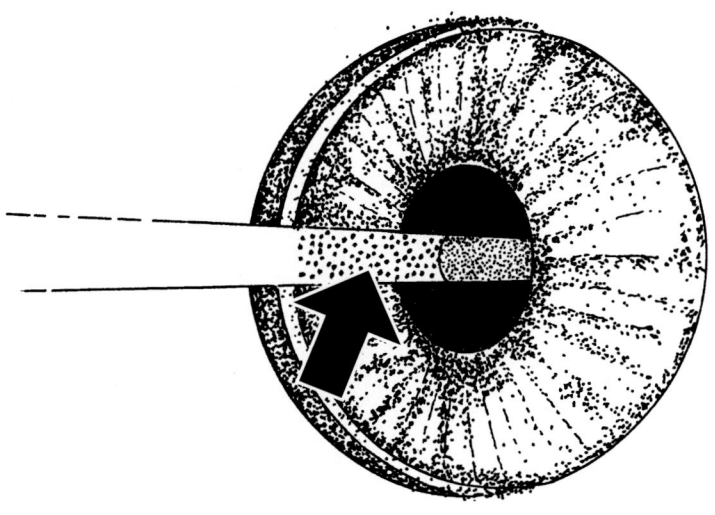

**FIGURE 4–16.** Grade 4+ cells in anterior chamber.

### TABLE 4-4. GRADING SYSTEM FOR ANTERIOR CHAMBER FLARE

| | |
|---|---|
| Grade 0 | Complete absence |
| Grade 1 | Mild—barely detectable |
| Grade 2 | Moderate—iris and lens details clear |
| Grade 3 | Marked—iris and lens details hazy |
| Grade 4 | Intense—fixed, coagulated aqueous |

From Nussenblatt RB, Palestine AG: *Uveitis Fundamentals and Clinical Practice*. Chicago: Year Book Medical; 1989:65–66; with permission.

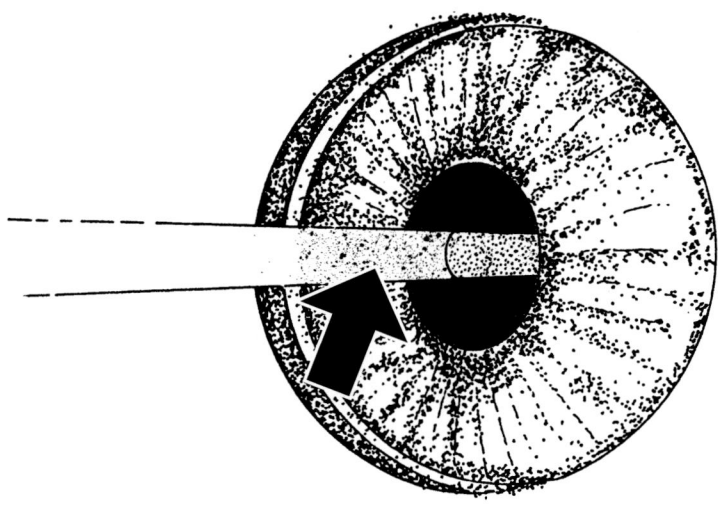

**FIGURE 4–17.** Grade 1+ flare.

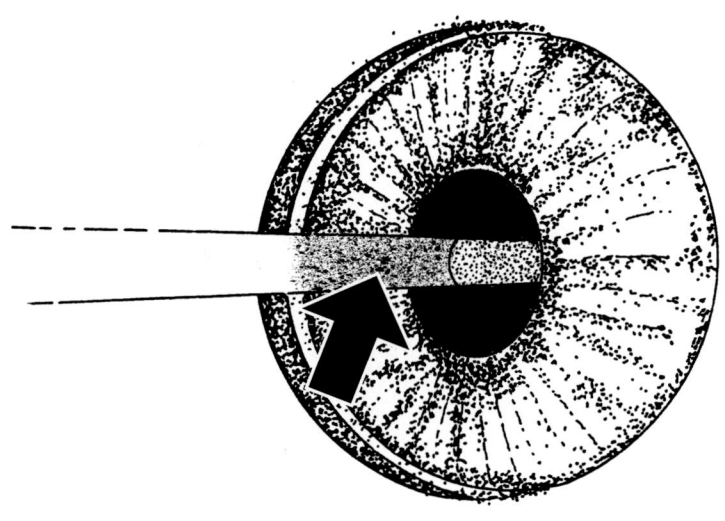

**FIGURE 4–18.** Grade 2+ flare.

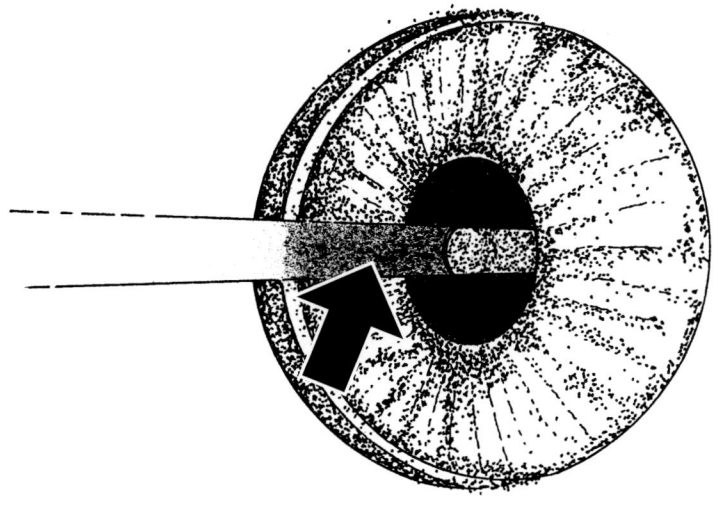

**FIGURE 4–19.** Grade 4+ flare.

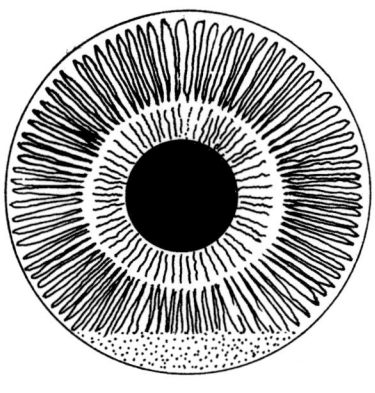

A

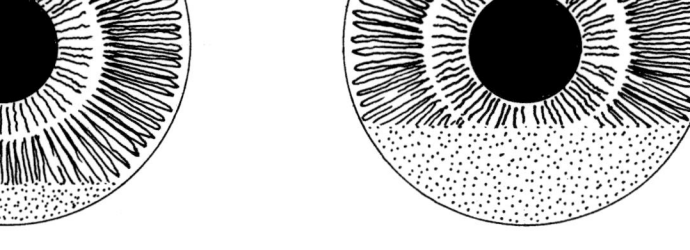

B

**FIGURE 4–20. A.** 10% hypopyon. **B.** 30% hypopyon.

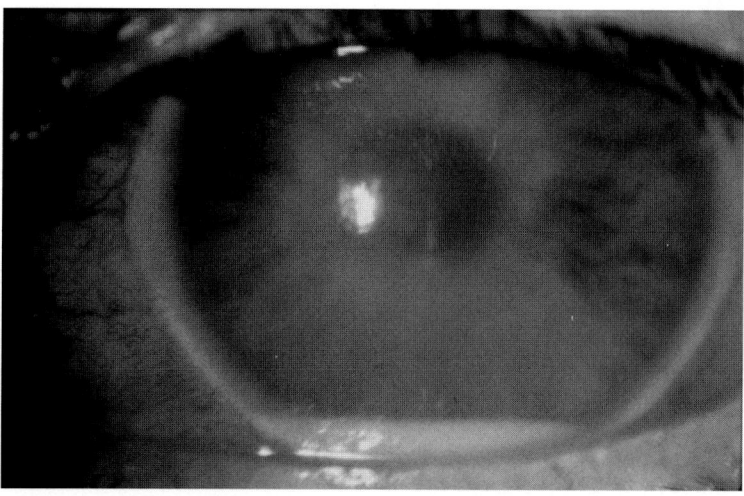

**FIGURE 4–21.** 10% hypopyon.

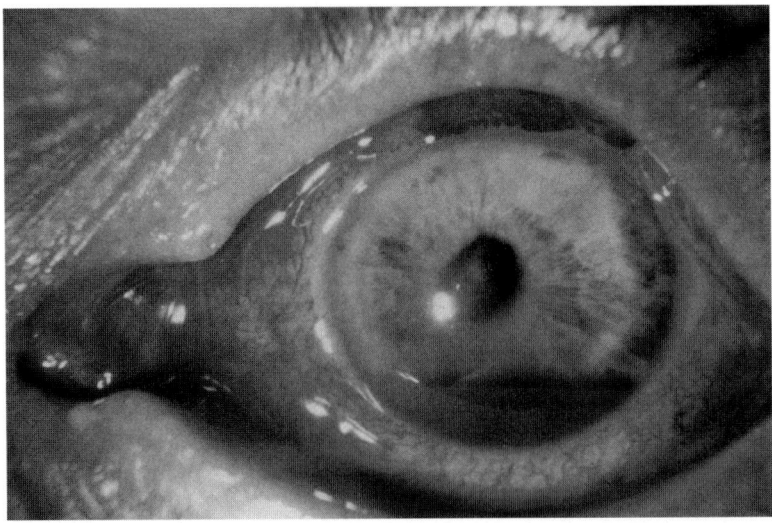

**FIGURE 4–22.** 20% layered hyphema.

## HYPHEMA

Hyphema may be observed in the immediate postoperative period. Grading the extent of hyphema is necessary in order to monitor its resorption. Three types of hyphema are commonly observed: diffuse hyphema (microhyphema) due to circulating erythrocytes, layered hyphema in the inferior anterior chamber, and vertically oriented coagulated blood from the wound site. In general, the diffuse type may be graded in the same way as anterior chamber cells (see Table 4–3), the layered type quantified in the same manner as hypopyon (Figure 4–22), and the vertical coagulums are described by location and dimensions (eg, grade 2+ diffuse hyphema, 20% layered hyphema, and nasal vertical 1 mm by 6 mm coagulum from internal wound site). The term *eightball hyphema* is used to describe an anterior chamber filled with a fibrin clot of blood (see Figure 4–23).

**FIGURE 4–23.** Eightball hyphema.

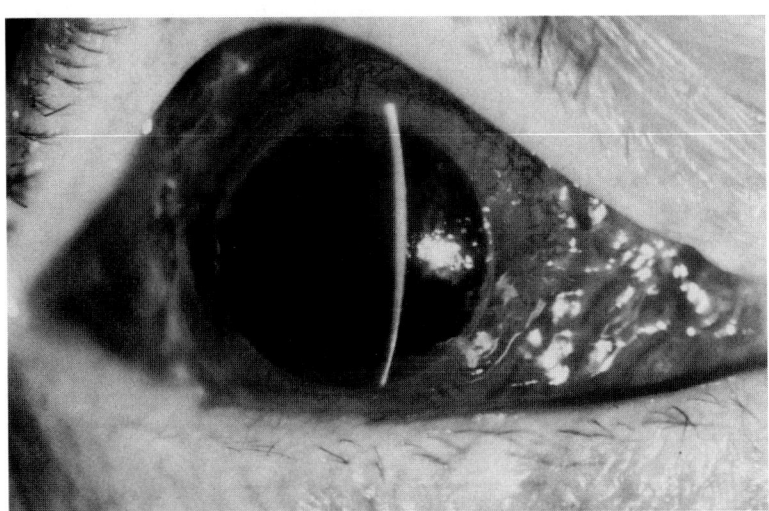

## TABLE 4-5. GRADING SYSTEM FOR POSTERIOR CAPSULE OPACIFICATION (PCO)

| | |
|---|---|
| Grade 1+ | Mildly observable clouding, fibrosis, or thickening that fills approximately 3% to 10% of the posterior capsule. The patient is usually unaware of visual difficulties at this level. |
| Grade 2+ | Moderate clouding, fibrosis, or thickening of the capsule that fills approximately 10% to 30% of the posterior capsule. The patient complains of minimal to moderate visual difficulties. |
| Grade 3+ | Marked clouding, fibrosis, or thickening that fills 30% to 50% of the capsular area. The patient reports moderate to significant reduction in vision and/or glare symptoms. |
| Grade 4+ | Severe clouding, fibrosis, or thickening of the capsule that fills more than 50% of the posterior capsule. The patient reports significant vision and/or glare problems. |

## POSTERIOR CAPSULE OPACIFICATION

The postoperative finding of posterior capsule opacification (PCO) may be present in up to 50% of patients and is usually noted by observing wrinkling, thickening, or the formation of Elschnig's pearls on the posterior capsule. One should examine the posterior capsule with direct and retroillumination and quantify the amount of opacity in the same fashion as in posterior subcapsular cataract. The presence of the opacity in the visual axis is, of course, more important clinically, so it should be specifically noted or the grade should be weighted to reflect this (Table 4–5; Figures 4–24 to 4–27).

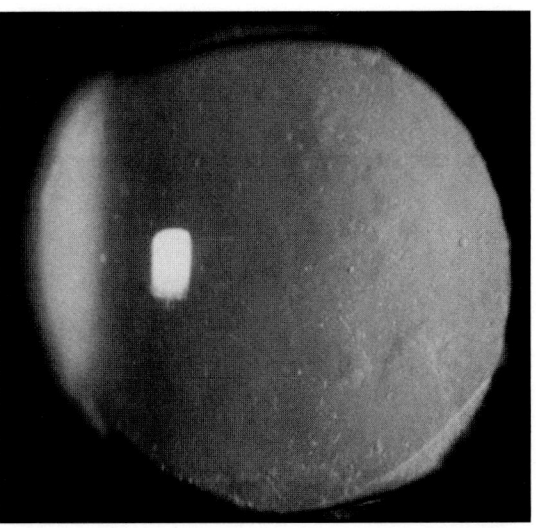

*FIGURE 4–24.* Grade 1+ posterior capsular opacification (PCO).

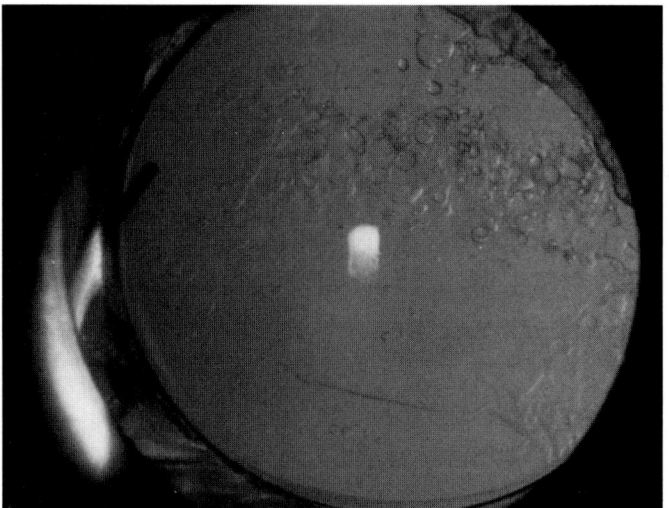

**FIGURE 4–25.** Grade 2+ posterior capsular opacification (PCO).

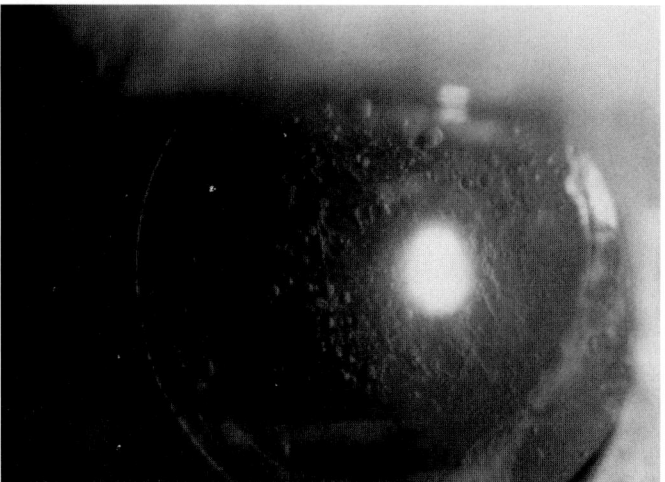

**FIGURE 4–26.** Grade 3+ posterior capsular opacification (PCO).

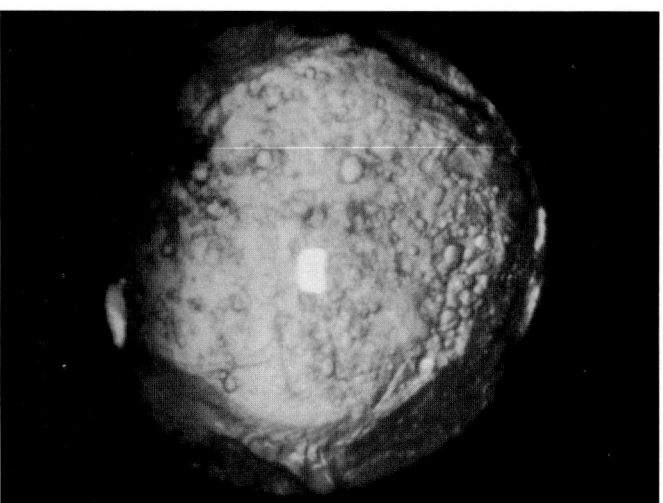

**FIGURE 4–27.** Grade 4+ posterior capsular opacification (PCO); note thickness of the opacifications.

## REFERENCES

1. Chylach LT: *Instructions for Applying the Lens Opacity Classification Systems (LOCS) in Grading Human Cataractous Changes at the Slit Lamp.* Center for Clinical Cataract Research. Boston: 1987:1–7.
2. Chylach LT, Leske CM, Sperduto R, et al: Lens opacities classification system. *Arch Ophthalmol.* 1988;**106**:330–334.
3. Chylach LT, Leske CM, McCarthy D, et al: Lens opacities classification system II (LOCS II). *Arch Ophthalmol.* 1989;**107**:991–997.
4. Nussenblatt RB, Palestine AG: *Uveitis Fundamentals and Clinical Practice.* Chicago: Year Book Medical; 1989:65–66.

# Preoperative Cataract Care

## Section II

# Special Instrumentation

## CHAPTER 5

In the course of examination of cataract patients, special instrumentation may be necessary to determine the extent of visual dysfunction, to quantify acuity or structural limitations, and to calculate the intraocular lens power. These instruments and their applications and limitations will be described.

## VISUAL FUNCTION TESTS

### Glare Testing

Glare testing is a method for isolating vision loss due to intraocular light scatter. Increased glare sensitivity is known to occur in the presence of anterior segment disorders and specifically cataracts.[1] Clinically, this means a patient with mild Snellen visual acuity reduction from cataracts may perform much worse when a bright light source (glare) causes a "veiling luminance" that further degrades the retinal image.[2] By adding glare testing to the clinical history and other objective findings in a cataract patient, it is possible to better correlate the patient's symptoms with the amount of cataract present and to determine if cataract extraction would benefit the patient.

Glare testing may be performed simply by aiming a penlight into the pupil from below the line of sight while the patient is reading an acuity chart. A slightly more elaborate test involves attaching a movie or camcorder light above an acuity chart and measuring the acuity. This has the advantage of providing more uniform patient testing conditions.

A commercially available instrument called the Brightness Acuity Tester (BAT) (Mentor, Inc, Norwell, MA) is a small, illuminated, hemispherical shell through which the patient looks at an acuity chart (Figure 5–1). This allows measurement of the disability glare by Snellen equivalent. It has the advantage of portability and a selectable range of brightness.

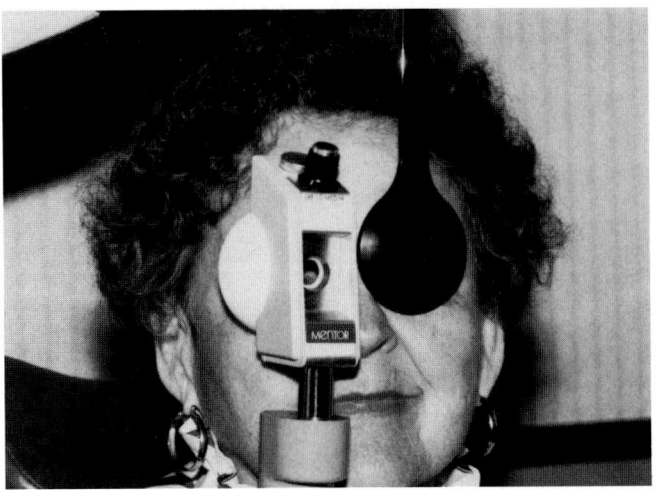

**FIGURE 5–1.** Brightness acuity tester (BAT).

Other testing instruments may incorporate glare testing into their normal operation. Some interferometers and autorefractors, for example, have glare-testing capabilities.

## Contrast Sensitivity

Contrast sensitivity is a measure of the degree of contrast required to detect or recognize a target.[1] It is relatively nonspecific but may help differentiate acuity loss due to refractive error versus reduced acuity caused by a cataract in the absence of other ocular or neurologic diseases.

Bar grids are commonly used to estimate contrast sensitivity. Contrast is defined as the difference in illumination between the light and dark areas of a grid. The frequency of a bar grid in cycles per degree (cpd) is determined by the width of the bars and the space between them. Fine, closely spaced bars are referred to as high frequency and coarse, widely spaced bars are referred to as low frequency. The contrast threshold for a given frequency is the lowest level of contrast for which a patient can detect the presence of the dark bars against the light background. A contrast sensitivity function is usually a bell-shaped curve for a given individual, with the highest sensitivity occurring in the middle of the range (usually between 3 and 10 cpd) and dropping off at both ends in the highest and lowest frequencies. Low-frequency visual data define the shape and position of large objects. High-frequency data define fine details.

Acuity charts and most other measures of visual acuity reflect sensitivity to high frequencies only. Contrast sensitivity testing is able to differentiate high- and low-frequency visual responses. In general, optical blur reduces high-frequency information, and diffraction from a cataract reduces both high- and low-frequency information. The degree of low-frequency loss may be a reasonably good measure of the visual impairment caused by a cataract in the absence of other ocular and neurologic diseases.

Contrast sensitivity, measured before and after adding a glare source, is probably the most specific and sensitive means of documenting disability from mild cataracts.[1]

## VISUAL POTENTIAL DEVICES

### Interferometer

Interferometry may provide predictive information concerning acuity following cataract surgery. Interferometers produce a Moiré interference pattern on the retina with two fine beams of coherent light (white or laser light) directed through a dilated pupil. The spacing of the fringe pattern is controlled by varying the separation between the two light beams and gets coarser as the beams are moved closer together. The ability of an interferometer to produce observable fringes on the retina is affected more by light amplitude than flux density. This means that fringes can be produced through fairly dense cataracts, which allows an examiner to obtain a relatively accurate potential acuity measurement through significant opacities. In general, although this instrument may overestimate visual potential, especially in the presence of macular disease,[3] it may provide a better estimate of potential acuity in the presence of dense cataracts than some other methods.

### Super Pinhole

The Super Pinhole (Micro-Surgical Technology, Inc, Kirkland, WA) potential acuity test has been found to be effective in estimating postsurgical visual outcome in a fairly wide range of cataract densities. The Super Pinhole is a black box with intensely back-lighted white letters, which are observed through a multiple pinhole occluder (Figure 5–2). The contrast between the bright letters and the dark background is approximately 1000 times greater than a normal projected chart. Clinically, we have found that there is good agreement between predicted acuity and the actual postsurgical outcome with this instrument, and it has the advantage of being relatively inexpensive and easy to use compared with other potential acuity devices. In our experience, the disadvantage of the instrument is that it tends to overestimate acuity in the

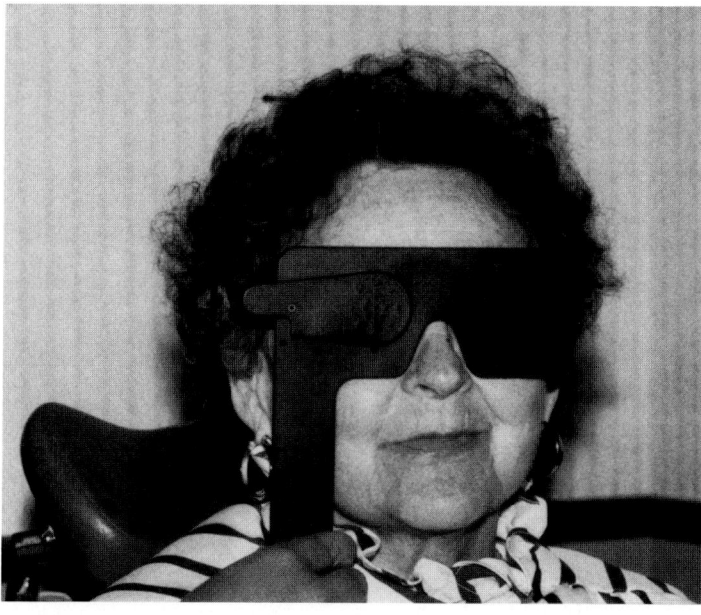

**FIGURE 5–2.** Performing Super Pinhole on a patient.

presence of early macular disease and to underestimate acuity in the presence of dense cataracts.

## Potential Acuity Meter

The potential acuity meter (PAM) is useful in measuring potential acuity in patients with mild to moderate cataracts. The PAM is a slit lamp–mounted instrument that projects an acuity chart onto the retina in a Maxwellian view (see Figure 5–3). In a Maxwellian view, light is focused at the entrance pupil of an observing eye so that illumination is relatively independent of pupil size. The advantage of the PAM (Mentor, Inc, Norwell, MA) is that the beam is only 0.1 mm in diameter and can be projected through small, clear areas in a cataractous lens to measure potential acuity. The disadvantage of the PAM is that results are dependent on illumination intensity, which limits its effectiveness in dense cataracts.

## Entoptic Phenomena Testing

Entoptic phenomena may be used to obtain a gross assessment of potential acuity in cases of very dense cataracts. The results are variable and should be interpreted with caution; however, this may be the only measure of potential acuity obtainable in the presence of severe cataracts. There are two entoptic phenomena that are useful in obtaining potential acuity data: the Purkinje tree and the blue field flying corpuscle test.

The Purkinje tree phenomenon is elicited by shining a transilluminator through the sclera toward the macula, which allows a person with a functioning macula to see the shadows of his or her own blood vessels. If a patient with an opaque cataract is able to appreciate the Purkinje tree, this implies some level of macular function.

The blue field entoptic phenomenon, also known as Scheerer's phenomenon or the flying corpuscle test, allows a patient with good macular function to see the movement of white blood cells in the retinal circulation. This test is

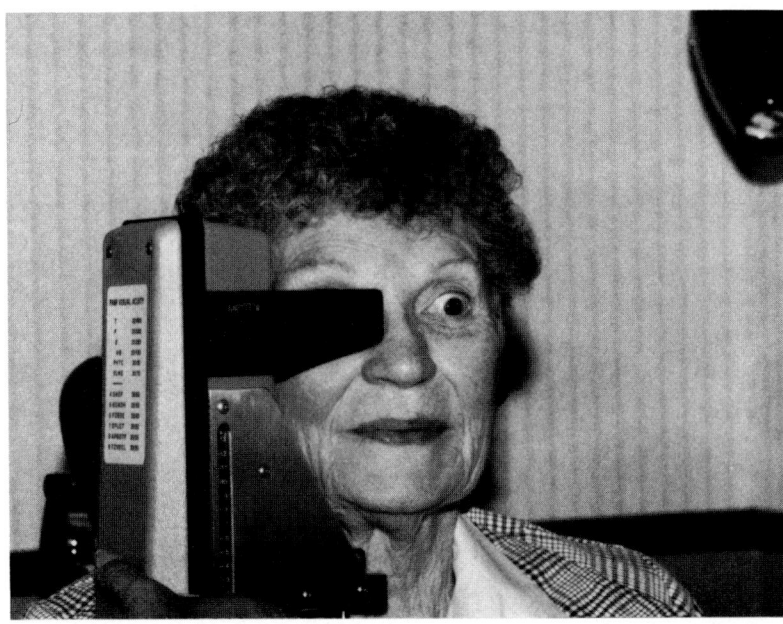

**FIGURE 5–3.** Potential acuity meter (PAM).

performed by shining a diffuse, bright light at the patient through an interference filter with a transmittance of 430 nm.

## LENS IMPLANT POWER CALCULATION

### A-Scan Ultrasonography

A-scan ultrasonography and keratometric data are essential measurements for determining the power of the implant to be inserted during cataract surgery. A-scan utilizes an ultrasound transducer, emitting a linear beam of sound waves, to measure relative distances between surfaces of ocular elements in the eye (Figure 5–4). The A-scan may be used to measure texture, thickness, distances between surfaces, and vascularity.

A variety of formulas are used to derive intraocular lens powers from A-scan and keratometric readings. Theoretical formulas calculate the power based on optics and specific measurements. The original Binkhorst formulas are theoretical. Regression formulas use a "fudge factor" based on statistical constructs, as well as optical laws and empirical data. The SRK formula (developed by Drs D. R. Sanders, J. Retzlaff, and M. C. Kraff) is a regression formula that assigns a statistical constant to each type of implant to correct for differences between results obtained in actual patients and results predicted by theoretical models. The Holladay formula (developed by Dr Jack T. Holladay) assigns a statistical constant to each surgeon based on past surgical results. All of these formulas require A-scan ultrasonography as the key measurement in determining intraocular lens power.

## AUXILIARY TESTS

### B-Scan Ultrasonography

B-scan ultrasonography is useful for detecting retinal detachments, hemorrhages, and neoplastic growths in patients whose cataracts are too dense to allow ophthalmoscopic observation. The B-scan ultrasonograph works by projecting a broad beam of sound waves to create a sonar picture of ocular structures. The B-scan is useful in assessing shapes, locations of lesions, and

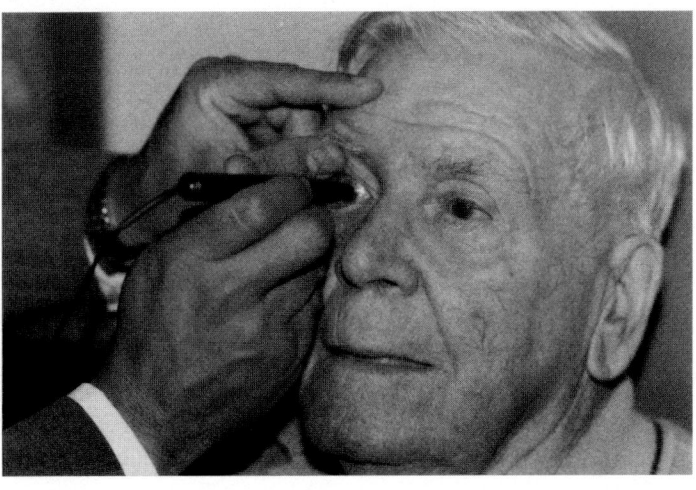

*FIGURE 5–4.* Performing A-scan ultrasonography on a patient.

lateral size of lesions (not thickness). It is not useful in assessing most types of macular disease, nor does it help predict functional visual outcome.

## Endothelial Cell Counts

A compromised endothelium, either preoperatively or postoperatively, may lead to postsurgical corneal edema, bullous keratopathy, and corneal decompensation. Endothelial cell counts and observation of cell morphology have value in predicting these problems. Preoperatively, a compromised endothelium should be suspected in the presence of Fuchs' endothelial dystrophy (cornea guttata), history of trauma, or any other preexisting endothelial disease. The endothelium may be damaged intraoperatively by prolonged phacoemulsification time or other surgical trauma (cell losses of 8% to 33.8% are possible); contact with an intact, prolapsed vitreous face; a flat anterior chamber; any contact between an intraocular lens and the endothelium (cell losses of 24% to 62% are possible); epithelial downgrowth; secondary glaucoma; endophthalmitis; and mechanical trauma from surgical instruments.

Although endothelial cells may be viewed through a special high-magnification slit lamp ocular lens, the most accurate endothelial cell counts require an anterior segment camera capable of obtaining highly magnified specular photographs of the corneal endothelium. The eye is topically anesthetized and then applanated with a lens attached to the camera. The endothelial cells are viewed through the view finder and photographed (Figure 5–5). The cells are then counted on the photograph utilizing a superimposed measuring scale. The normal range of cell counts for adults is 1400–2500 cells per mm$^2$. A minimal cell count is in the range of 400–700 cells per mm$^2$. Additionally, examination of the cell morphology is important because a uniform endothelial mosaic will generally have a lower incidence of postoperative corneal edema than one with marked polymegathism regardless of the cell count.[4]

It is important that the endothelial layer be intact. If the endothelial cell count is low enough that spaces appear between the endothelial cells, postoperative corneal decompensation is very likely.

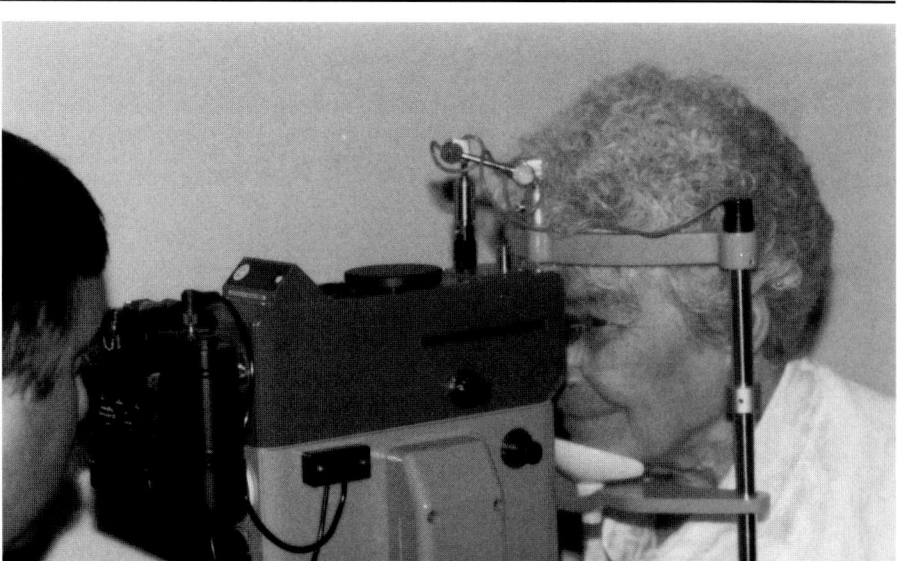

**FIGURE 5–5.** Performing an endothelial cell count on a patient.

## REFERENCES

1. American Academy of Ophthalmology: Contrast sensitivity and glare testing in the evaluation of anterior segment disease. *Ophthalmology.* 1990;**97**:1233–1237.
2. Lasa MSM, Datiles MB, Podgor MJ, Magno, BV: Contrast and glare sensitivity: Association with the type and severity of the cataract. *Ophthalmology.* 1992;**99**:1045–1049.
3. Severin TD, Severin SL: A clinical evaluation of the potential acuity meter in 210 cases. *Ann Ophthalmol.* 1988;**20**:373–375.
4. Rao GN, Aquavella JV, Goldberg SH, Berk SL: Pseudophakic bullous keratopathy: Relationship to preoperative corneal endothelial status. *Ophthalmology.* 1984;**91**:1135–1140.

# Examination

## CHAPTER 6

Preoperative care of a cataract patient begins when the patient complains of reduced vision. The clinician's goal is to identify all possible sources of the patient's complaints and ascertain which, and to what extent, they are contributing to the disability. If the disability is secondary to cataract, the clinician must determine if it is such that the patient cannot perform the daily activities he or she desire or are required. The clinician should take the time to understand the patient's ocular complaints and personal needs and desires, as this understanding will be combined with the objective clinical findings to plan the course of treatment most appropriate for the patient.

We favor approaching all patient examinations, including evaluation of the cataract patient, with the SOAP format—that is, obtain the patient's **s**ubjective complaints and history; gather **o**bjective data; combine these to make an **a**ssessment of the patient's case, which allows development of a **p**lan for action in the treatment and management of the patient. Utilizing the SOAP format provides a framework within which every patient is systematically evaluated (Table 6–1).

## SUBJECTIVE DATA

Because the clinician must decide whether or not the disability of which the patient complains is due to cataract or not, a careful history is one of the most important aspects of the examination. The history for a cataract patient is not unlike that of any other optometric patient. Three main areas should be explored: the chief complaint, ocular health history, and general medical history.

One should listen to the patient's chief complaint after a nonleading question such as, What brought you in today? or What problems are you having with your eyes? Then more specific questions may be asked such as, Did the problem come on gradually or suddenly?; Is the problem worse at near or far?;

**TABLE 6-1. NORMAL PREOPERATIVE EXAMINATION**

| | Elements of a SOAP Examination | | |
|---|---|---|---|
| **Subject** | **Objective** | **Assessment** | **Plan** |
| Chief complaint<br>Ocular history<br>Medical history | Vision<br>Pupils<br>Refraction<br>Intraocular pressure<br>Slit lamp evaluation (SLE)<br>Dilated fundus examination (DFE)<br>Other neurologic and binocular testing | Assessment of all significant diagnoses and evaluation of their contribution to complaints and/or vision loss | Plan of treatment for each diagnosis: may include further study of coexisting conditions before deciding on cataract surgery |

Are there specific tasks where the problem is worse?; Is there a difference during the day or nighttime?; and Do you specifically have problems with glare or halos? A cataract patient may describe a general blur at distance and/or near of gradual onset. Specifically, they frequently have reading or driving complaints, with worsening symptoms when driving at night or on sunny days. They often describe variable vision with special problems under glare conditions. The ultimate question that may be asked later in the examination, in assessing the extent of disability from cataract, is Does the problem affect your everyday activities or lifestyle?

The ocular history is critical in determining the patient's need for cataract surgery and prognosis. Coexisting disease may alter the timing for cataract surgery, contraindicate cataract surgery, or affect the necessary preoperative testing and counseling (see Chapter 7). Specifically ask:

- Have you had any serious injuries to your eyes?
- Do you have a lazy eye or history of crossed eyes?
- Is there history of eye disease in yourself or family?
- Have you had any eye surgeries?
- Do you use any medications for your eyes?

Special note should be made of any abnormalities such as inflammation, glaucoma, or optic nerve or retinal disease, because the ensuing examination, assessment, and plan for care may be modified based on the patient's reported history.

The medical history should explore the presence of significant health problems such as:

- Do you have high blood pressure, diabetes, or heart disease?
- Do you have breathing problems or predisposition to coughing?
- Do you have history of major surgeries?
- Do you take any medication?
- Do you have any medication allergies?

At some point it may be necessary to determine if the patient's mental state allows him or her to participate in the decision whether or not to have surgery.

## OBJECTIVE DATA

The objective portion of a cataract evaluation is similar in scope to most optometric examinations with special attention to documenting the extent of disability from cataract and identifying any other pathologic conditions that may be contributing to visual loss.

Visual acuity should be tested by Snellen at distance and near, as cataract may affect performance more at one distance than the other. In addition, vision in dim compared with bright illumination may be tested, glare vision created by penlight, contralight (placing a light near the chart or placing a chart on a brightly lit window), or other special instrumentation may be helpful. Contrast testing with a loss at all frequencies supports a diagnosis of cataract or other disease process. Poor contrast acuity at only high frequencies usually indicates refractive error but has also been documented with early glaucomatous optic atrophy (see Chapter 5).

The findings from retinoscopy and refraction play a large role in making the decision to remove a cataract. Retinoscopy not only gives a starting point for the refraction but close observation of the retinoscopic reflex helps determine if symptoms mostly originate from the lens. Occasionally, a patient may have significant symptoms such as blur or monocular diplopia under certain conditions and the eye examination including biomicroscopy of the lens appears normal. The diagnostic use of the retinoscope in this situation may uncover the lenticular refractive or diffractive abnormalities in an otherwise clear lens that explain the symptoms. Significant nuclear sclerosis may also be noted. It appears as a murky central "button." This is seen by sweeping the dilated pupil with the retinoscope and observing the altered red reflex. The refraction itself may initially require large steps (eg, 3 diopters) initially to determine the direction of testing to obtain best vision in the case of severe (grade 4+) cataracts. The results of refraction should be used for ancillary visual acuity tests (glare, contrast, potential) if it is significantly different from the habitual refraction (see Chapter 5). Binocularity and motility should be reviewed. Occasionally, a significant cataract may disrupt binocularity enough to cause a tropia in a patient without history of strabismus. This in itself may justify surgical intervention. However, if cataract is not clearly the etiology of the tropia, a systemic evaluation to rule out other sources of idiopathic strabismus should be considered.

At the very least, visual fields may be evaluated by confrontation. In severe or grade 4+ cataract with visual acuity of light perception or light projection, the method of testing called light projection may be useful in establishing gross retinal function. (Method: Hold a bright transilluminator in the eight major meridians, randomly selected, and have the patient point to the light while maintaining straight gaze. The test may be made more sensitive by holding a red filter over the eye being tested.) If more formal visual fields are used, moderate to advanced cataracts may cause general depression or an arcuate scotoma that mimics glaucomatous changes.

Pupillary testing should be performed to evaluate for anisocoria and direct and consensual reflexes. One may identify a relative afferent pupillary defect, but cataracts never cause afferent pupillary defect.[1] Pupil size is significant because a pupil that dilates poorly may make surgery more difficult.

The anterior segment examination with slit lamp should include a systematic scanning of all structures. Particular attention should be paid to the lids, cornea, anterior chamber, and lens (see Chapter 4). Observe the presence of any lid disease. This should be treated and controlled preoperatively. The cornea should be examined for scars and pterygia. The highest magnification should be used to examine the stroma for striae and thickening and the endothelial mosaic for guttae and polymegathism (Figure 6–1). Grades 3–4 guttae with stromal thickening may require endothelial cell count or pachymetry preoperatively (see Chapter 5). In the least, the patient counseling should address this finding. The anterior chamber depth should be evaluated for risk of

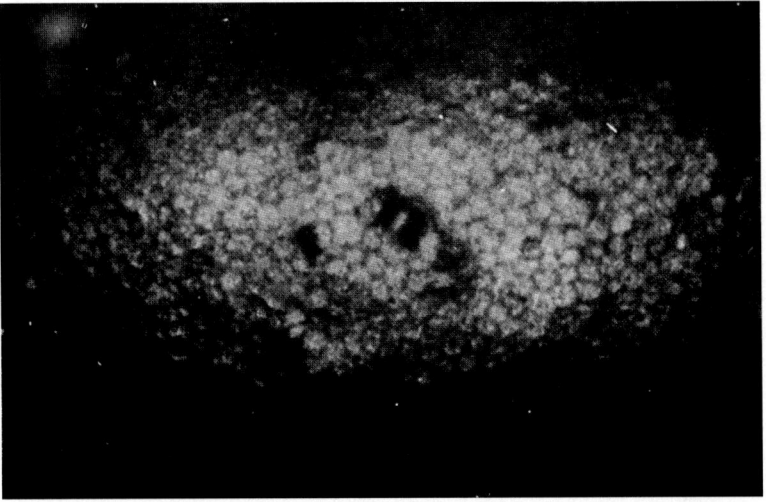

FIGURE 6–1. Corneal guttae.

pupillary block (noted by observation of a convex iris, narrow angle by Von Herrick's technique and gonioscopy) and signs of old or present inflammation (look for old keratic precipitates on the cornea, iris synechiae, or atrophy) (Figures 6–2 to 6–5). Acute anterior uveitis should be controlled for several months before surgery[2] and chronic uveitis should be worked up for systemic etiology.

Lenticular evaluation should include examining nucleus, cortex, and anterior and posterior subcapsular areas by diffuse illumination, optic section, and retroillumination. Observe both color and opalescence. Quantify the amount of cataract in each region and consider if the amount of cataract justifies the visual complaints (see Chapter 4). Also, examine the anterior lens capsule for signs of previous inflammation (synechiae), narrow-angle glaucoma attacks (glaukomflecken), and pseudoexfoliation (Figure 6–6). Pseudoexfoliation is significant because not only is the patient at risk for glaucoma but may have weak zonules that may affect the outcome of extracapsular cataract extraction with intraocular lens placed in the capsular bag[3] (see Chapter 12). In the case of grade 4+ nuclear with grade 4+ cortical sclerotic cataract (also called mature) where the entire lens is opacified and/or has a hard nucleus, the surgery may be more difficult if phacoemulsification is utilized. Planned extracapsular cataract extraction by expression may be used as an alternative (see Chapter 10).

Intraocular pressure (IOP) should be evaluated and controlled at the time of surgery. In most cases, we recommend lowering pressures over 30 mm Hg by medication, even in an eye without glaucomatous changes. Intraocular pres-

FIGURE 6–2. Convex iris; note shallow anterior chamber between the illuminated cornea and illuminated iris.

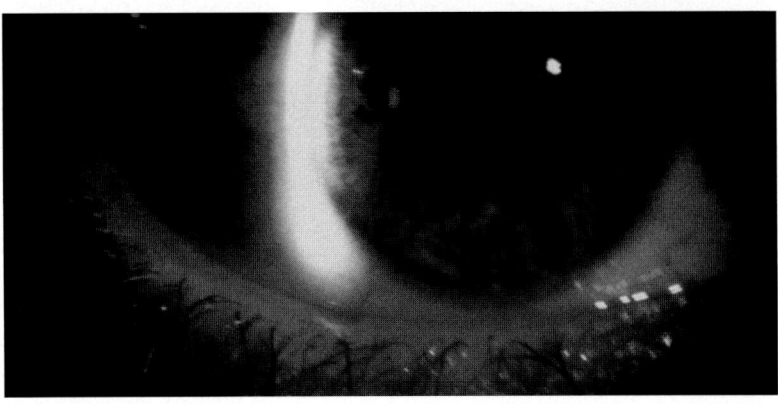

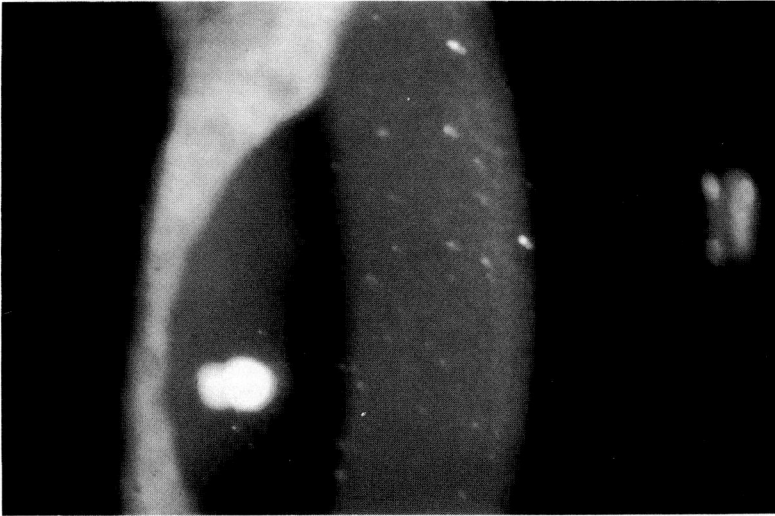

FIGURE 6–3. Old keratic precipitates.

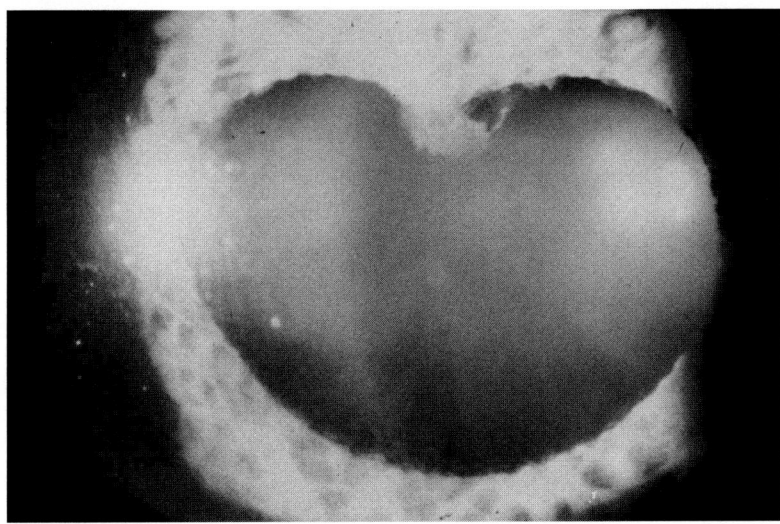

FIGURE 6–4. Posterior iris synechia at 12 o'clock position.

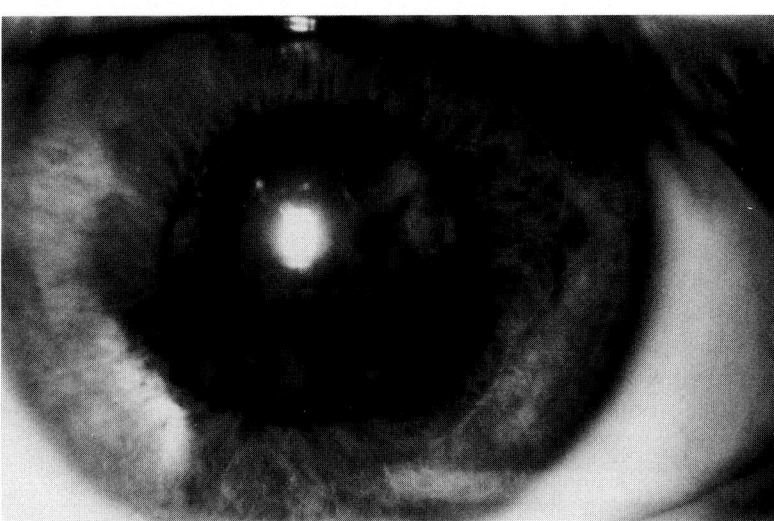

FIGURE 6–5. Iris atrophy at 8 o'clock position, secondary to trauma.

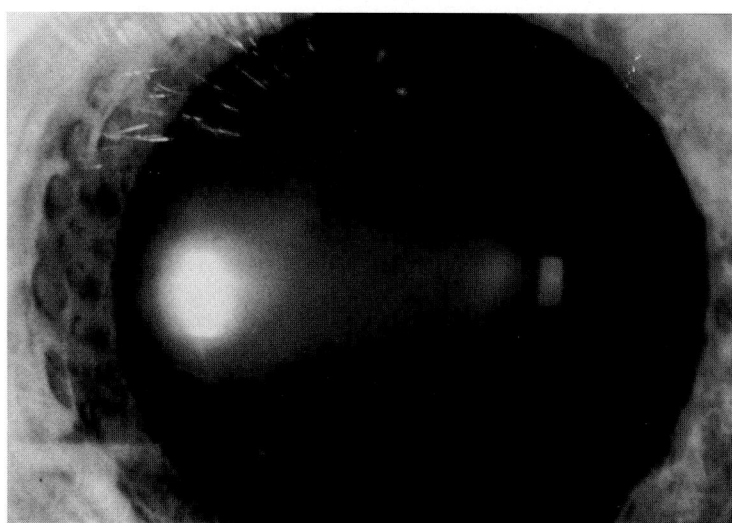

**FIGURE 6–6.** Pseudoexfoliation on the anterior lens surface.

sure control is even more important in patients with glaucoma. More aggressive medical treatment may be instituted and evaluated preoperatively and perioperatively or a combined procedure of cataract extraction, intraocular lens implantation, and trabeculectomy may be considered (see Chapter 11).

Macular function or potential acuity may be evaluated by PAM (Mentor, Inc, Norwell, MA), laser interferometry, Super Pinhole (Micro-Surgical Technology, Inc, Kirkland, WA), Amsler grid, or photostress test. Ophthalmologists commonly include one or more of these tests in their preoperative evaluations. However, recent guidelines have recommended these evaluations in limited cases only where prediction of macular function is ambiguous from physical examination or visual acuity measurements.[4]

Posterior segment/retinal examination should include viewing the vitreous at the slit lamp with and without a fundus lens such as a Hruby, 60-, 78-, or 90-diopter lens. The posterior pole should be examined stereoscopically with the same lens(es) to observe any other etiology for decreased vision, such as optic nerve disease or macular disease. Complete this evaluation with the binocular indirect ophthalmoscope and again scanning the posterior pole as well as closely examining the peripheral retina, observing for holes, tears, and degenerations that may place the patient at greater risk for preoperative or postoperative retinal complications. In the case of dense and/or mature cataracts, a definitive evaluation of the retina may not be possible. In this situation, additional simple ancillary tests for retinal function may be attempted: light projection (the patient locates the light from a transilluminator with eyes in straight-ahead position), two-point discrimination (the patient reports when two lights are first noted, as the doctor separates them), Maddox rod, or entoptic phenomenon (the patient describes what he or she sees when the transilluminator is applied to lids).[5] The more sophisticated A- and B-scans may be used to rule out tumor, retinal detachment, vitreous opacities or severe macular elevation as in severe disciform scarring (see Chapter 5). In the case of high myopia with peripheral changes such as significant retinal holes, tears, or degenerations, scleral depression is indicated. Significant macular degeneration or chronic inflammation with cystoid macular edema (CME) in the presence of a cataract makes the decision as to the source of vision loss more difficult. Fluorescein angiography in the surgeon's office or by retinal consultation may be ordered to help clarify the appropriateness of cataract extraction.

Table 6–2 reviews the additional preoperative tests that may be indicated for a patient with coexisting disease who is considering cataract surgery.

**TABLE 6-2. ADDITIONAL PREOPERATIVE TESTS THAT MAY BE INDICATED IN THE PRESENCE OF COEXISTING EYE DISEASE**

| Preoperative Test(s) for Coexisting Eye Disease | |
|---|---|
| **Corneal Disease** | **Optic Nerve Disease and Glaucoma** |
| • Endothelial cell count | • Contact lens examination |
| • Pachymetry | • Gonioscopy |
| | • Visual fields[a] |
| **Macular Disease** | • Stereophotographs |
| • Contact lens examination | • Nerve fiber layer photographs |
| • Fluorescein angiography | • Fluorescein angiography |
| • Amsler grid | |

[a] However, some cataracts may cause arcuate visual field loss.

When a cataract is the proven source of the visual complaints and coexisting diseases have been controlled or treated, keratometry, A-scan, and intraocular lens calculations are performed. Our experience is that the most accurate calculations occur when data are taken by experienced examiners.

A preoperative physical assessment should be performed. As directed by the surgeon, the extent of this may range from an immediate preoperative survey of blood pressure, pulse, respiration, and electrocardiogram to routine complete physical examination with appropriate laboratory testing performed by the family physician, general practitioner, or internist[6] (see Chapter 9).

## ASSESSMENT

The assessment of a cataract patient involves reviewing all information from the subjective and objective portions of the examination and identifying significant findings. These findings form a list of either historically important problems or current findings/problems. This list then must be evaluated for its impact on the patient's symptoms, needs, and desires. If a cataract is present, with or without other diseases, ask, Will vision be improved significantly by removal and will this help remedy the patient's problems and complaints? In addition, an assessment of the patient's mental capacity and physical needs is necessary in deciding whether or not the patient should undergo cataract extraction.

## PLAN

When all the subjective and objective data have been evaluated and an assessment of these findings has been made, a treatment plan must be formulated by discussion with the patient and his or her family. We recommend asking the patient if he or she would like family member(s) to be present for counseling or ask if there is anyone whom we should contact concerning the discussion.

Counseling the patient is another critical aspect of cataract care. Patients should be advised of the findings succinctly and in language they understand. They should be given their options. In the case of cataracts with no coexisting disease, one of their options is to do nothing (with the exception of the most advanced intumescent cataract or hypermature cataract). They should understand that the cataract extraction is an elective surgery, and the decision whether or not to do it is ultimately theirs. They should understand that there are risks involved, even in the hands of the most experienced surgeon. In addition, in the presence of coexisting disease, other limitations to their potential vision exist, and patients must be counseled concerning these limitations. They should receive several recommendations on the best surgeon to see, based on technical quality of care delivered, quality of emotional care delivered, and your personal trust and respect of the surgeon. If you favor one surgeon because of quality of overall outcome, you should advise the patient, or consider advising the patient, of the surgeon to whom you would send your family. You should advise the patient of the expected preoperative, operative, and postoperative visits with the surgeon and yourself. Consideration and discussion of the desired postoperative refractive error outcome is important. In general, in the presence of low refractive error and/or bilateral cataracts, we aim for emmetropia to low myopia postoperatively. Occasionally, in patients with previous monovision contact lens experience or in patients with myopias accustomed to reading without glasses, we explain and aim for a monovision type of outcome. A monocular cataract in a patient with high refractive error and/or special visual needs requires careful counseling and decision making as to postoperative refractive error (see Chapter 7). It is essential to emphasize that spectacles are usually necessary postoperatively. It may also be necessary, depending on the surgeon's preference, to discuss possible preoperative discontinuance of certain medications such as pilocarpine or anticoagulants. The surgeon, ultimately, will determine the need for this counseling. It is our policy to discontinue pilocarpine 1–3 days prior to surgery and to continue use of anticoagulants and aspirin unless the patient's general physician advises discontinuance.

Many of these topics will be repeated by the surgeon or his or her staff, but their introduction allows the patient time to consider all aspects of the process and discuss them with the family. Finally, details such as location of the surgeon's office, where the surgery will be performed, what to eat, how to dress, transportation or housing arrangements if necessary, restrictions before or after surgery, other special testing, and cost considerations may be mentioned, although the surgeon's staff should provide that information as they provide care to the patient (see Appendix 5).

In addition to verbal counseling, written information is useful. Consider providing a packet to cataract patients including: (1) Explanation of what a cataract is. (2) Explanation of modern cataract surgery. (3) Brochure from selected surgeon, map to the office. (4) Card to list medications. (5) Preoperative information.

Video information is also valuable and may be available generically from professional optometric or ophthalmologic organizations, commercial marketing/practice management firms, or the surgeon's office.

## REFERENCES

1. Lam BL, Thompson HS: A unilateral cataract produces a relative afferent pupillary defect in the contralateral eye. *Ophthalmology*. 1990;**97**:334–338.
2. Hooper PL, Rao NA, Smith RE: Cataract extraction in uveitis patients. *Surv Ophthalmol*. 1990;**35**:142.
3. Tarkanen A: Exfoliation syndrome (pseudoexfoliation of lens capsule). In Percival P (ed): *Color Atlas of Lens Implantation*. St Louis: Mosby-Year Book; 1991:215–216.
4. O'Day DM, Adams AJ, Cassem EH, et al: *Cataract in Adults: Management of Functional Impairment*. Clinical Practice Guideline No. 4. US DHHS, PHS, Agency for Health Care Policy & Research; 1993:21.
5. Weinstein GW. Cataract surgery. In Tasman W (ed): *Duane's Clinical Ophthalmology*. Philadelphia: JB Lippincott; 1991:6–7.
6. Bartley GB, Narr BJ: Preoperative medical examinations for patients undergoing ophthalmic surgery. *Am J Ophthalmol*. 1991;**112**:725–727.

# Other Preoperative Evaluations

## CHAPTER 7

There are some patients who require special consideration in their preoperative evaluation and counseling.

## — PEDIATRIC CATARACTS[1]

Cataracts in children are generally due to congenital malformation, trauma, or some other insult to the eye. The challenge associated with congenital and infantile cataracts is not only early detection but removal of the cataract at a time when visual rehabilitation may be optimal. Consultation with a pediatric ophthalmologist is recommended for evaluation of the surgical, refractive, and antiamblyopic options. Axial length of preteens is equal to that of adults; therefore, in selected cases, preteens with cataracts may undergo standard cataract extraction with intraocular lens (IOL) placement. However, long-term follow-up on any series of patients receiving modern cataract extraction with lens implant is unavailable. (See Color Plates 7–1 and 7–2.)

## — TRAUMATIC CATARACTS

Traumatic cataracts may arise secondary to blunt or perforating injury. In the case of blunt trauma, the cataract may develop quickly and be noted soon after the injury or may gradually develop over weeks or months following the trauma. The opacities are usually stationary, localized, and often not associated with visual loss (Figure 7–1). In a series of 212 eyes with contusions,[2] blunt trauma was associated with an incidence of angle recession in 80%, iris abnormalities in 37%, and lens subluxation or cataracts in 25%. Therefore, if vision is affected by a contusion cataract, detailed examination of the anterior chamber angle and zonules must be performed gonioscopically. Findings of

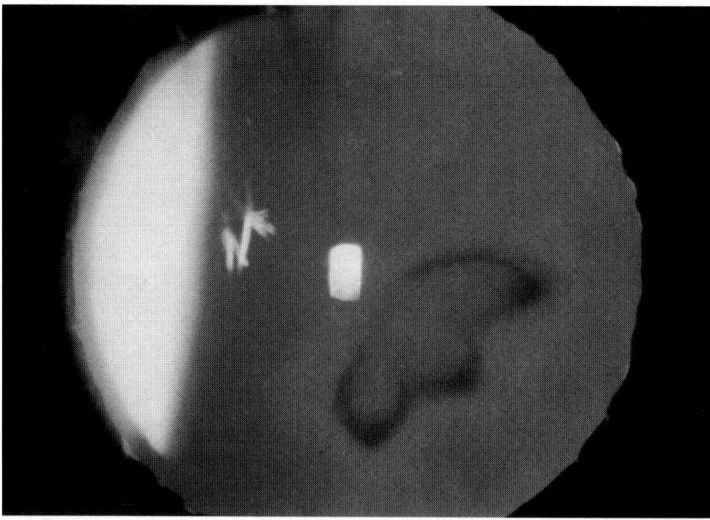

FIGURE 7-1. Traumatic cataract secondary to blunt trauma.

zonular rupture and capsule injury may necessitate intracapsular cataract extraction (ICCE) with sutured, sulcus-placed, or anterior chamber intraocular lens if appropriate.

Perforating trauma, on the other hand, is an ocular emergency. If the lens is penetrated, the lens fibers imbibe aqueous and opacification occurs quickly. A penetrated or perforated eye should be stabilized and protected with a shield and immediately referred.

The history of significant but old blunt or perforating trauma requires careful examination, including gonioscopy and retinal function tests, knowledge of past surgical procedures if possible, and then case-by-case determination of the appropriate intervention based on patient needs and status of the eye's potential for vision (Figure 7–2). (See Color Plate 7–3.)

## SUBLUXATED LENSES

If a patient has nonemergent subluxated lens(es) secondary to trauma or systemic or ocular disorders,[3] then the decision as to whether or not to remove

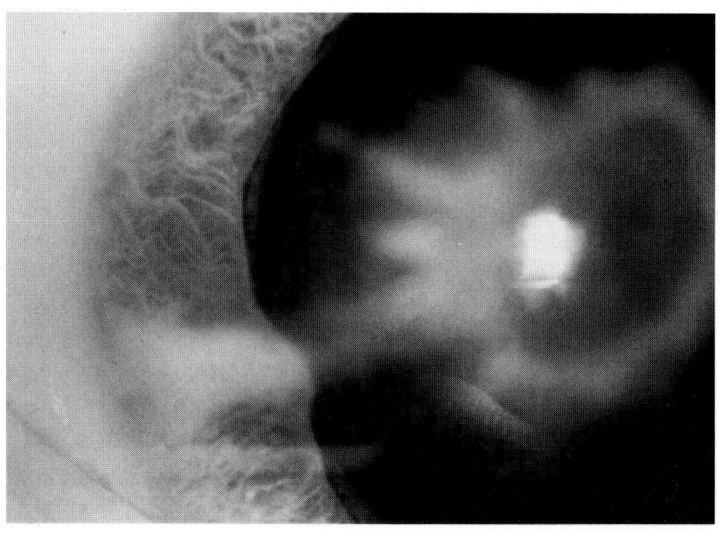

FIGURE 7-2. Traumatic cataract secondary to perforating trauma; note: corneal and iris scarring at 8 o'clock position.

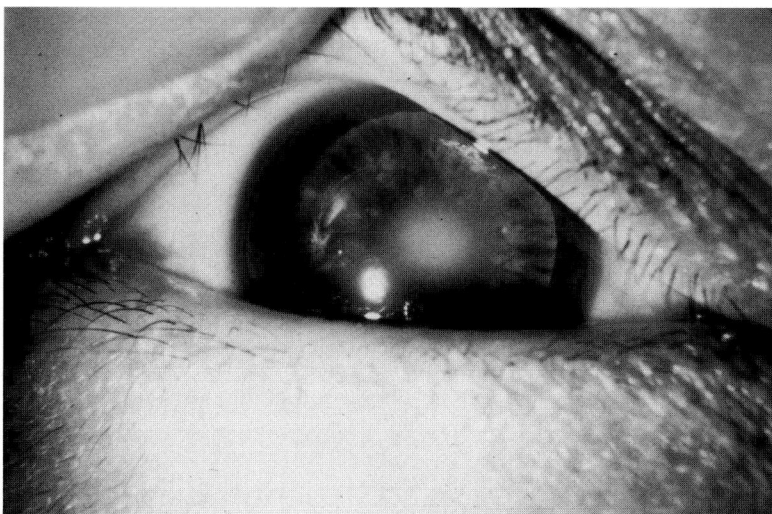

**FIGURE 7–3.** Luxated lens in anterior chamber in 11-year-old girl with Marfan's syndrome. The lens dislocated following a blow to the eye during a soccer game.

the lens(es) is based on the patient's needs (Figure 7–3). Some patients do well with spectacles or contact lenses. Others require lens extraction to function well. By definition, these are zonular abnormalities, so intracapsular cataract extraction is usually required and sutured, sulcus-placed, or anterior chamber intraocular lenses may be used.

## — SECONDARY INTRAOCULAR LENSES —

Secondary intraocular lenses (IOLs) may be indicated in patients with aphakia who are failing with their present spectacles or contacts or who are at risk for strabismus or amblyopia (Table 7–1).[4] Preoperative subjective evaluation should carefully explore the patient's difficulty with aphakia and history of potential contraindications to surgery such as chronic uveitis or proliferative diabetic retinopathy. The objective evaluation requires special attention at the slit lamp to corneal endothelial integrity because the eye has already undergone one surgery. Examine the anterior segment for traumatic scars, inflammation, and persistent corneal edema. Specifically, note the presence or absence of the posterior capsule. Vitreous prolapse or evidence of vitreous attached to the initial wound is also important because it may necessitate vitrectomy. If the posterior capsule is intact, this is a good prognostic factor for the patient because a pos-

### TABLE 7–1. PREOPERATIVE CONSIDERATIONS FOR SECONDARY INTRAOCULAR LENS IMPLANTATION

| Favorable | Unfavorable |
| --- | --- |
| Uncomplicated, well-tolerated first surgery | Well-tolerated contact lens wear |
| History of contact lens complication/handling problems | History of chronic anterior uveitis |
| | Persistent corneal edema |
| At risk for amblyopia or strabismus | Low endothelial cell count |
| Normal endothelial cell count | Proliferative diabetic retinopathy |
| Normal angle structure | Absence of posterior capsule |
| | Vitreous in anterior chamber or wound |
| | Large sector iridectomy |
| | Angle synechia, fibrosis, and/or neovascularization |

terior chamber IOL may be placed. In most cases, however, the posterior capsule is not intact. Therefore, an anterior chamber or sutured posterior chamber IOL will be necessary.[5] The presence of a large-sector iridectomy should therefore be noted. The anterior chamber angle should be examined for damage, peripheral anterior synechia (PAS), or neovascularization. Examine the fundus for signs of previous cystoid macular edema (CME). Examine the optic nerve for signs of atrophy secondary to ischemia. Any visual limitations must be determined and assessed. The treatment plan should include education of the patient on the option of secondary IOL implant, as well as other findings and sources of visual limitations. If secondary IOL implantation (probably anterior chamber IOL) is preferred, advise the patient of the risks, especially those of CME, retinal detachment, persistent postoperative iritis, increased IOP/glaucoma, and uveitis, glaucoma, and hyphema (UGH) syndrome (see Chapters 14–16).

## INTRAOCULAR LENS REPOSITIONING/EXCHANGE

An IOL is *decentered* if its optical center is partially or totally off the visual axis but maintains most of its tissue support. A *dislocated* lens may be subluxated, luxated, expelled, or extruded. It is subluxated when it is partially moved from its proper position but remains attached to some tissue. It is luxated when it lies free of any tissue support. If the lens suddenly moves to a new position, it is expelled. If it moves slowly, it is extruded[4] (see Chapters 14 and 15). Finally, pupillary capture occurs when the pupillary margin becomes located partially or completely anterior to an anterior chamber lens or posterior to a posterior chamber lens.

If a patient presents to your office with any of these IOL conditions, a careful history should be taken to decide if this is an acute or chronic problem and to determine the amount of related discomfort and/or visual symptoms. If the lens implant is iris-fixated, pupil dilation is contraindicated because of the risk of dislocation secondary to dilation (see Chapter 8). Otherwise, slit lamp and dilated fundus examinations should be performed to observe the extent of the problem and to observe closely for signs of active or chronic inflammation in the anterior segment, lens movement in the case of a small anterior chamber lens, or CME. Refraction may determine if an optical problem exists. All these factors must be assessed to determine if the lens decentration or dislocation warrants intervention.

In the optometric office, when an IOL decentration or dislocation is identified, the patient should be advised and counseled that one of three treatment options exists:

1. No treatment
2. Repositioning
3. Exchange

If the condition is long standing, the eye is quiet, refraction is stable, and the patient has few, if any, complaints, the patient should be advised of the findings but no action should be taken. In the case of one-piece or closed-loop anterior chamber IOLs and flexible anterior chamber lenses sized too small, chronic inflammation, pseudophakic bullous keratopathy, glaucoma, or hyphema may result, and lens exchange must be considered.[4,6] If the anterior chamber lens is too large, chronic inflammation, tenderness, or frank extrusion may result, and lens exchange is appropriate. If a posterior chamber lens is decentered or dislocated so that chronic inflammation, glare, symptomatic anisometropia, or astigmatism results, repositioning or exchange of the lens may be considered. Finally, if the lens is of a power such that intolerable anisometropia results, exchange may be considered. In our practice, we have attempted to identify this error as early as possible and perform the exchange if appropriate.

The decision to do nothing may be made in the optometric office. The surgeon who performed the surgery should be advised if the lens has decentered or dislocated in the early to intermediate postoperative period. If the condition is more long standing, the original surgeon or a surgeon experienced in reparative work may be consulted by phone or patient visit. The ultimate decision to reposition or exchange lies in the hands of the surgeon and should only be undertaken after careful counseling and consent of the patient.

## COEXISTING CONDITIONS

There are certain coexisting conditions in which cataract extraction with intraocular lens implantation are contraindicated[7,8]:

- Active proliferative diabetic retinopathy
- Rubeous iridis and/or neovascular glaucoma
- Active chronic iritis, except heterochromic cyclitis
- Ectopia lentis
- Microphthalmos
- Buphthalmos

There are other conditions that may require more extended evaluation and counseling before proceeding with cataract extraction and lens implantation[7,8]:

- Monocular patients
- High refractive error, especially myopia
- Past history of iritis
- Traumatic cataract
- Fuchs' dystrophy (cornea guttata)
- Glaucoma
- History of retinal detachment or lattice degeneration

### Monocular Patients

Cataract extraction with a posterior chamber IOL placed in the capsular bag in a one-eyed patient is believed to be a reasonable and beneficial option today.[8] Preoperative counseling, especially the risks of ocular surgery, should be carefully reviewed and understood by the patient (see Chapter 6).

### High Refractive Error

Postoperative refractive error may be calculated to remain similar to the preoperative value or may be altered to meet the needs and desires of the patient. The patient should be advised of the options and participate in deciding the postoperative refractive goal. In the case of bilateral cataracts, the patient should be counseled concerning the potential for change in refractive error toward emmetropia. Experience has taught us that individuals with hyperopia are happy with a myopic shift but those with myopia may choose to remain slightly myopic. We carefully question the patient concerning their visual needs and may leave a person with moderate to high myopia slightly myopic owing to their visual habits. In the case of monocular cataract and high refractive error, we recommend advising the patient that the refractive error may be slightly decreased toward emmetropia but will still "match" the other eye. We calculate a

**TABLE 7-2. SPECIAL PREOPERATIVE CONSIDERATIONS: HIGH REFRACTIVE ERROR**

Patient's lifelong refractive error
Patient's habits, avocations, and lifestyle
Patient's needs and desires
Determine proposed postsurgial refractive error based on above considerations and the presence of monocular versus binocular cataract
Patient should participate in deciding proposed best postsurgical refractive error and amount of anisometropia

postoperative refractive error that is within 2.00–2.50 diopters of the other (unoperated) eye in the vertical meridian[9,10] (Table 7–2).

In the case of high myopia, not only should the refractive error results be discussed with the patient but counseling about the possibility of retinal detachment should occur. If there is any question as to the integrity of the retina, consider a preoperative retinal consultation.

## History of Iritis

With the exception of heterochromic cyclitis, which reportedly is unaffected by cataract extraction with intraocular lens implant, cataract patients with a history of iritis deserve special consideration.[11] The history of an iritis patient should establish the patterns of recurrence and chronicity. Examine the patient for signs of chronic iritis and its complications: old keratic precipitates (KPs) on the endothelium, active anterior chamber inflammation, posterior synechia, PAS, active or old chronic CME, secondary steroid-induced glaucoma. In the assessment, one must sort out if vision loss is secondary to cataract or the complications of chronic iritis: chronic CME and secondary glaucoma. The plan for this type of patient may include considering ordering an internal medicine work-up for the iritis if there are signs of chronicity or bilaterality without knowledge of underlying systemic diseases.

Theoretically, if inflammation can be controlled preoperatively, it should also be controllable postoperatively. Therefore, in order to recommend cataract extraction, the rule of thumb that we use is that the eye should be free from inflammation 2–3 months prior to cataract removal. In conjunction with the surgeon, the patient may be pretreated with anti-inflammatories and given additional dosages intraoperatively and postoperatively. The patient should be advised that the postoperative course of treatment and extent of inflammation is somewhat unpredictable. Anterior chamber IOLs are contradicted in patients with iritis (Table 7–3).

**TABLE 7-3. SPECIAL PREOPERATIVE CONSIDERATIONS: CHRONIC UVEITIS**

Establish chronicity by history and examination
Examine for complications: PAS, posterior synechia, CME, steroid-induced glaucoma
Is vision loss secondary to cataract?
Pretreat uveitis and maintain quiet eye for 2–3 months prior to surgery
Work up systemic causes of uveitis
Counsel patient concerning the unpredictability of postoperative inflammation

**TABLE 7-4. SPECIAL PREOPERATIVE CONSIDERATIONS: FUCHS' DYSTROPHY**

Observe and treat epithelial edema
Quantify the corneal thickening (endothelial cell count, pachymetry)
Counsel patient carefully concerning additional risks, possiblity of postoperative corneal edema and potential need for PK

## Traumatic Cataracts

(See pages 51–52.)

## Fuchs' Dystrophy

Patients with Fuchs' dystrophy, or cornea guttata, may or may not know of its presence. History should determine specific symptoms, such as variable vision, which may not be attributable to the cataract. The amount of guttae, corneal thickening, and epithelial microcystic edema (if present) should be observed and treated. Quantification of the extent of the condition may be done by endothelial cell counts (specular photomicroscopy) and pachymetry. In general, we favor cataract extraction with implantation of an IOL after careful counseling of the patient as to the additional risks, possibility of postoperative edema, and potential future need for penetrating keratoplasty (PK). Our experience shows us that recovery from cataract extraction with IOL and separate penetrating keratoplasty, if necessary, is more rapid (Table 7–4).

## Chronic Open-Angle Glaucoma

If both glaucoma and cataract are present, the patient should be evaluated, counseled, and treated for each of these conditions. Preoperatively, intraocular pressure should be controlled, if possible, and current visual field loss and optic nerve information should be available and supplied to the surgeon. We advise the patient that in our experience, the cataract extraction may favorably affect the intraocular pressure at least initially. However, in the case of poorly controlled glaucoma, consideration of combined procedure of cataract extraction with IOL implantation and trabeculectomy should be made in concert with the surgeon. Preoperatively, miotics in use may be discontinued and preoperative and postoperative treatment with additional antiglaucoma drops or oral medications may be prescribed. The patient should be advised preoperatively that even in the case of a combined procedure, antiglaucoma medications may be necessary postoperatively (Table 7–5).

**TABLE 7-5. SPECIAL PREOPERATIVE CONSIDERATIONS: CHRONIC OPEN ANGLE GLAUCOMA**

Supply surgeon with current visual fields
Evaluate anterior chamber angle
Cataract extraction may affect glaucoma favorably
Counsel about need to do combined procedure versus cataract extraction only
Counsel patient that glaucoma medications may still be necessary postoperatively

## Retinal Detachment

A history of retinal detachment in the fellow eye and the existence of lattice degeneration statistically place an eye at greater risk for retinal detachment following cataract extraction. However, recent studies have reported retinal detachment rates and results of repair to be uninfluenced by intraocular lens implantation, although repair may be more difficult.[8]

## REFERENCES

1. Morgan KS: Congenital and infantile cataracts. *Curr Opin Ophthalmol.* 1990;**1**:20–24.
2. Kwitko ML, Kwitko GM: Management of the traumatic cataract. *Curr Opin Ophthalmol.* 1990;**1**:25–27.
3. Gressel MG: Lens induced glaucoma. In Tasman WT (ed): *Duane's Clinical Ophthalmology,* Vol 3. Philadelphia: JB Lippincott; 1991:54A:6.
4. Alpar J, Choyce P: Complications of anterior chamber lenses and management. In Percival P (ed): *Color Atlas of Lens Implantation.* St Louis: Mosby-Year Book; 1991:235–244.
5. Stark WJ, Gottsch JD, Goodman DF, et al: Posterior chamber intraocular lens implantation in the absence of capsular support. *Arch Ophthalmol.* 1989;**107**:1078–1083.
6. Jaffe NS, Jaffe GS, Jaffe MF: *Cataract Surgery and Its Complications,* 5th ed. St Louis: CV Mosby; 1990:186.
7. Noble B, Hayward M: Contraindications to intraocular lens implantation. In Percival P (ed): *Color Atlas of Lens Implantation.* St. Louis: Mosby-Year Book; 1991:147.
8. Bernitsky DA, Stark WJ, McCartney DL, et al: Changing indications for intraocular lenses: Guidelines (legal and ethical) for cataract surgery. In Caldwell DR (ed): *Cataracts: Transactions of the New Orleans Academy of Ophthalmology.* New York: Raven Press; 1988:1–8.
9. Holladay JT, Rubin ML: Avoiding refractive problems in cataract surgery. *Surv Ophthalmol.* 1988;**32**:357–360.
10. Ford RO: Memorandum to the authors concerning postoperative refractive error, March 1989.
11. Hooper PL, Rao NA, Smith RE: Cataract extraction in uveitis patients. *Surv Ophthalmol.* 1990;**35**:120–144.

# Operative Procedures in Cataract Surgery

## SECTION III

# History of Intraocular Lenses

## CHAPTER 8

The idea of using an intraocular lens (IOL) following cataract extraction was conceptualized in England during World War II. In air battle, the polymethylmethacrylate (PMMA) canopy of English fighter planes occasionally was shattered by enemy fire and created small projectile fragments that entered the eyes of the pilots. When this happened, the foreign body was found to be remarkably well tolerated and often surgical removal was avoided. With this in mind, Harold Ridley, an English ophthalmologist, became the first person to implant an IOL in 1949.[1-3] Following this monumental procedure, surgeons have continued to develop IOLs which are consistently safer and more effective. Most will agree that the desired level of performance was not attained until the late 1970s when modern posterior chamber IOLs were introduced.

Although most modern surgeons use posterior chamber IOLs almost exclusively for uncomplicated primary cataract procedures, many patients are still "wearing" the earlier designed IOLs. For this reason, it is essential that the practicing optometrist be able to recognize the various lens designs, be knowledgeable of their drawbacks, and be observant of potential complications (Figure 8–1).

## — EARLY POSTERIOR CHAMBER IOLS

The original IOL implanted by Ridley was a posterior chamber intraocular lens IOL. Ridley had the foresight to realize that in order to minimize complications, the lens should be implanted in a position where there was minimal contact to adjacent vascularized tissues. Therefore, his original intent was to place the lens in the capsular bag.[1] Ridley also believed that the ideal intraocular lens should duplicate the dimensions of the physiologic lens.[4] This proved to be the downfall of early posterior chamber IOLs, since this resulted in a large and bulky lens without a fixation device that was prone to dislocation. An additional fac-

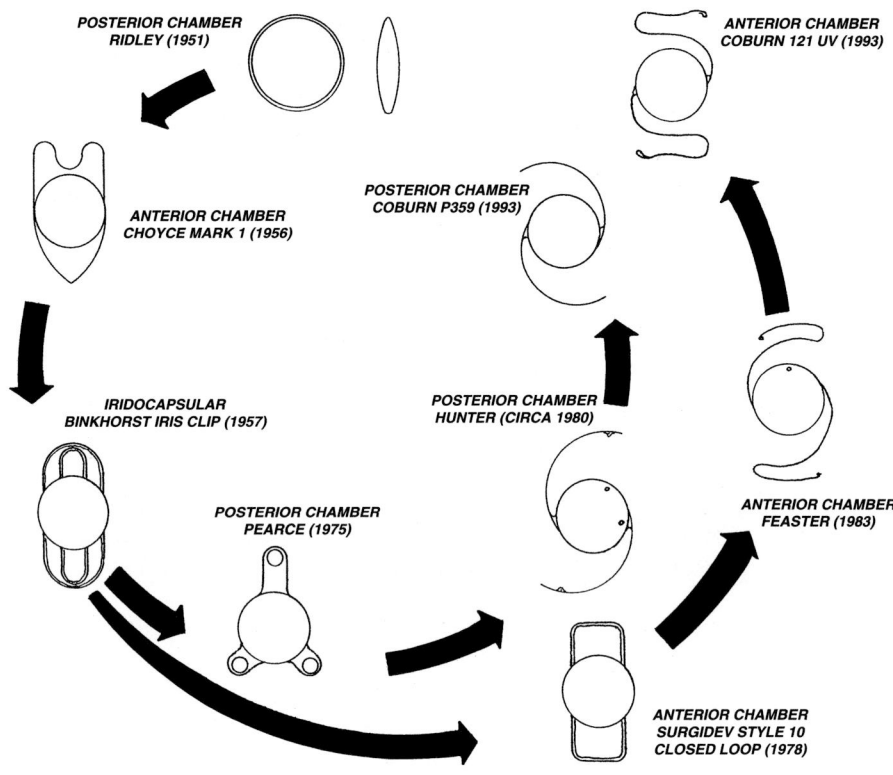

**FIGURE 8–1.** Evolution in the design of IOL implants.

tor that led to the discontinuation of the use of this type of lens was that with the standard surgical technique of the time, a large anterior capsulotomy was made that exacerbated the problem of lens dislocations.[1]

## — EARLY ANTERIOR CHAMBER IOLS —

Since lens dislocations were the major drawback of the early posterior chamber IOLs, surgeons directed their efforts toward developing lenses that were less likely to dislocate (Figure 8–2). The anterior chamber was a logical site for fixation, as the iris was a barrier to posterior dislocation. André Baron im-

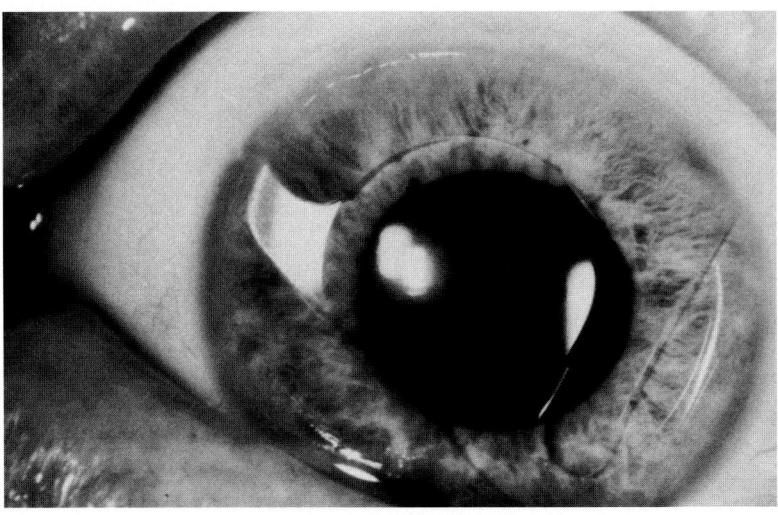

**FIGURE 8–2.** Pregnant 7 anterior chamber IOL.

planted the first anterior chamber lens in 1952. Shortly afterward, B. Strampelli and Peter Choyce developed anterior chamber intraocular lenses (IOLs) and began implanting them following cataract extraction.[1] Numerous problems were encountered with these early anterior chamber IOLs, primarily due to their primitive design.[1,2,5] These early lenses were rigid, had poorly finished edges that often irritated the tissue of the angle, and were improperly vaulted causing iris and/or corneal contact. Since the early anterior chamber IOLs were rigid, it was difficult to size the implant correctly, as there was little margin for error.

An IOL sized too small could "propeller" in the angle damaging the tissues and increasing the risk of uveitis, glaucoma, and hyphema (UGH syndrome).[5] An undersized lens was also likely to shift anteriorly resulting in endothelial contact and corneal edema. An oversized lens was apt to become embedded in the angle structures causing discomfort, tenderness to touch, uveitis, glaucoma, hyphema, or even total erosion through the angle.[5] Many early anterior chamber lenses had poorly finished edges that exacerbated the problem of incorrect lens sizing. The vault of the lens also was critical. If the lens vaulted forward excessively, endothelial touch occurred resulting in corneal edema and if there was insufficient vaulting, the iris was irritated.[1,6]

Another one of the many flaws of the early anterior chamber IOLs could be found in the design of the fixating loops, or haptics. Many of the earlier designs had closed loops and broad areas of contact with the uveal tissues. This increased the incidence of glaucoma and uveitis, and quite commonly PAS would form around the haptics causing them to be firmly adhered to the angle.[6] When these lenses required explantation due to complications, it was often a difficult procedure due to the closed-loop design.[1,6] Synechiae would cocoon around the haptics creating the need to cut the haptics in order to remove the lens. Since most early anterior chamber lenses caused excessive anterior segment damage based on their rigid design, unfinished edges and poor vaulting characteristics, surgeons then directed their attention to capsular and iris-fixated lens designs.

## IRIS-SUPPORTED INTRAOCULAR LENSES

At the time, this concept seemed appealing to surgeons, since theoretically two major problems could be alleviated: The lens would be less likely to dislocate, and the lens would be farther away from the cornea and the trabecular meshwork (Figure 8–3). (See Color Plate 8–1.)

Epstein implanted the collar stud lens in 1953, which was the first iris-fixated IOL.[1] Following this, numerous visually fascinating designs were manufactured such as the Worst Medallion, Binkhorst, and Copeland IOLs. In general, the lenses were designed with either the optic and/or one haptic anterior to the iris and a second haptic posterior, using the iris as the sole means for support.[1,7] Some of these lenses were designed with small holes so that a suture could aid in fixation. Although there were some advantages to iris-fixation, these lenses were inadequate for a variety of reasons[1]:

1. Stability was dependent on iris fixation; therefore, pupillary dilation could dislocate these lenses.
2. Constant uveal contact resulted in uveal chafing and inflammation. Complications included UGH syndrome.
3. Intermittent corneal touch increased the risk of pseudophakic bullous keratopathy (PBK).
4. Some iris-fixated IOLs utilized metals such as platinum for a fixation element. This further increased the incidence and severity of iritis and glaucoma.

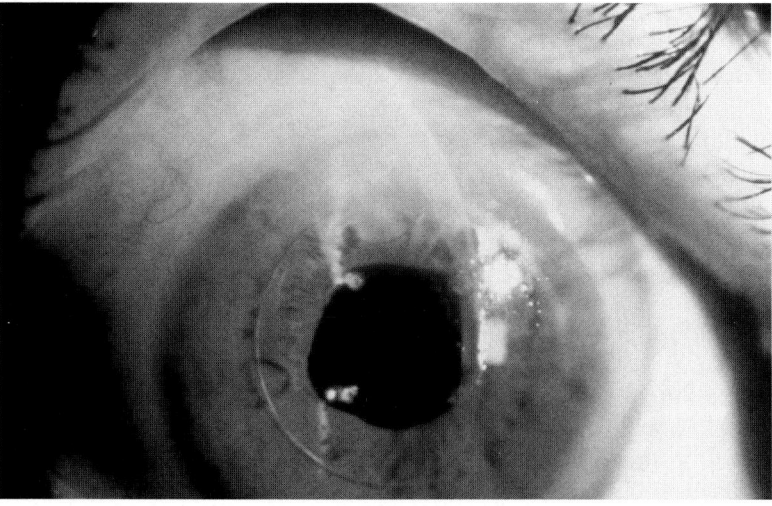

FIGURE 8–3. Iris-fixated IOL.

## IRIDOCAPSULAR INTRAOCULAR LENSES

C. D. Binkhorst is credited as a pioneer in modern cataract surgery. He began performing extracapsular cataract surgery and modified his original four-loop iris-fixated design into a two-loop IOL (Figure 8–4). He placed the two haptics within the capsular bag, which left only the optic anterior to the iris.[8] This iridocapsular IOL is considered by most to be the forerunner of modern posterior chamber IOLs.

## MODERN ANTERIOR CHAMBER LENSES

Following the many failures observed with the iris-fixated lenses, IOL designers began to address the many flaws inherent with the early anterior chamber IOL designs. Modern anterior chamber IOLs are the culmination of these efforts (Figures 8–5 and 8–6).

The major flaws of the early anterior chamber IOLs included their rigidity, which made lens sizing difficult, poorly finished edges, faulty vaulting charac-

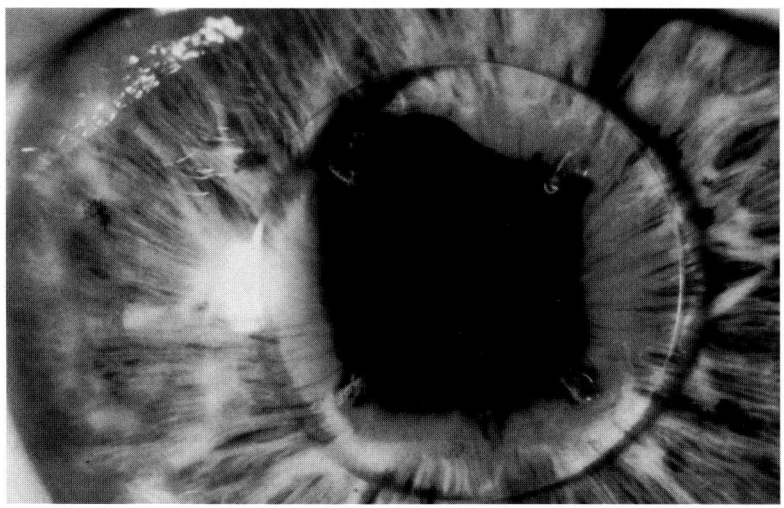

FIGURE 8–4. Binkhorst iridocapsular supported IOL.

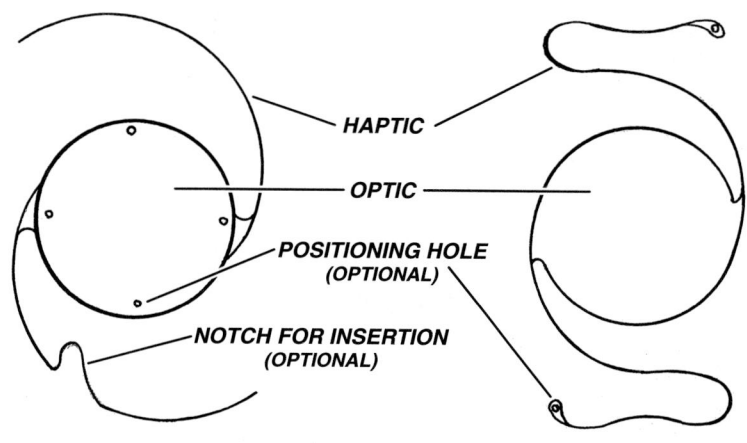

**FIGURE 8–5.** Anatomy of modern anterior and posterior chamber IOLs.

teristics, and faulty loop designs.[1-3,5,6,9] All of the above have been addressed and the modern anterior chamber lens is much improved. The following are good characteristics found in most modern anterior chamber IOLs:

1. Lens haptic flexibility. This makes sizing less critical and reduces the number of complications associated with improperly fitted IOLs.
2. Finely polished edges. This reduces ocular damage at the point of contact with the lens.
3. Point fixation. In most modern anterior chamber IOLs, the loop is designed such that contact with the structure of the angle is minimized to several small points.
4. Open-loop design. With this design, if the lens requires explantation, the haptics may be left intact in most cases.

The modern anterior chamber lenses represent a significant improvement over earlier designs (Figure 8–6). Most surgeons today utilize these lenses for secondary implants and when implantation of a posterior chamber IOL is not advisable due to the lack of capsular support.[9]

Even with the marked improvements that have been made with the ante-

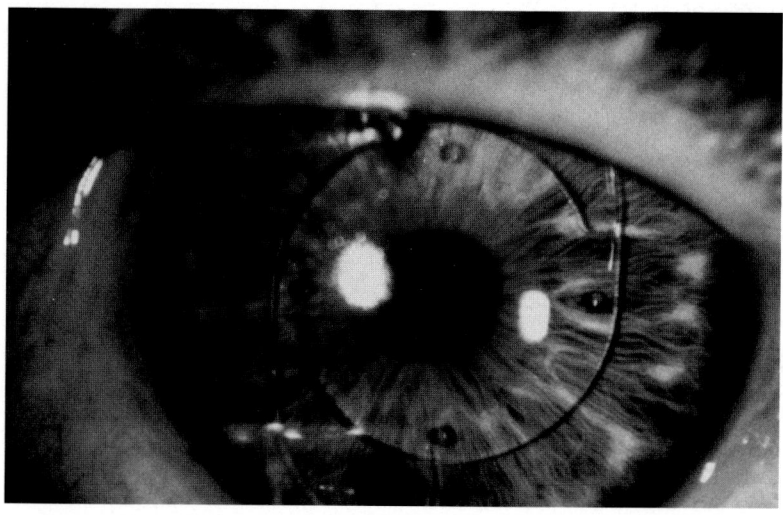

**FIGURE 8–6.** Open-loop duo-lens in anterior chamber (may be placed in the posterior chamber).

### TABLE 8-1. INTRAOCULAR LENS CHARACTERISTICS

| Type | Favorable | Unfavorable |
| --- | --- | --- |
| **Anterior Chamber** | Flexible | Rigid |
| | Polished edge | Rough-finished edge |
| | Point fixation | Broad-based fixation |
| | Open loop | Closed loop |
| **Posterior Chamber** | Capsular bag fixation | Ciliary sulcus fixation |
| | Flexible haptics | Rigid haptics |
| | One-piece manufacture | Multipiece manufacture |
| | Angulated haptics | Nonangulated haptics |

rior chamber IOLs, they are not the lens of choice for uncomplicated primary cataract extraction, since there is a greater incidence of complications compared with posterior chamber IOLs (Table 8–1).

## MODERN POSTERIOR CHAMBER IOLS

It seems logical to infer that the most natural place to implant a lens would be the same position as the physiologic lens. Ridley noted the advantages of lens fixation at this site; however, his original lens was too large and heavy for reliable fixation. Unlike Ridley's lens, modern flexible posterior chamber lenses seldom dislocate and if proper capsular fixation is achieved, seldom decenter. Other complications found with the iridocapsular, iris-fixated and anterior chamber lenses such as iritis, corneal edema, iris chafing, hyphema, and glaucoma also are reduced in frequency.

The two possible locations for the haptics when implanting posterior chamber IOLs are the ciliary sulcus and the capsular bag. In the 1970s and 1980s, many surgeons advocated sulcus fixation; however, recently most state of the art surgeons recognize the importance of capsular fixation. The disadvantage of sulcus fixation is that ciliary tissue may be irritated by the haptics and the IOL is in closer proximity to the iris increasing the risk of pupillary capture, iris chafing, and pupillary block.[1,2]

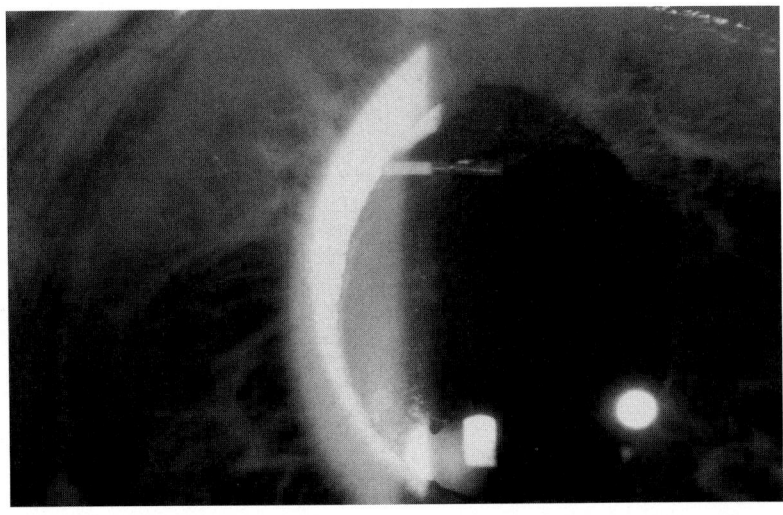

*FIGURE 8–7.* Three-piece posterior chamber IOL. Note haptic attachment to optic at 12:00.

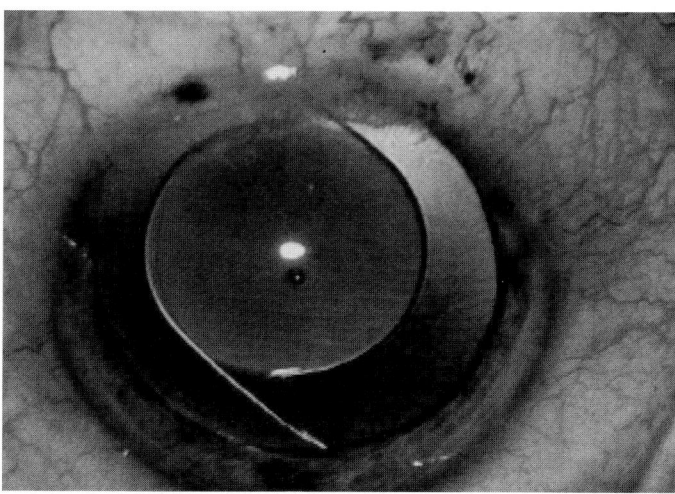

*FIGURE 8–8. One-piece PMMA posterior chamber (taken at time of surgery).*

Modern posterior chamber lenses have flexible **J** or **C** loop haptics. The lens is manufactured in one or multiple pieces (see Figure 8–7). One-piece IOLs are made of PMMA (Figure 8–8) or silicone. The optic section of a multiple piece lens may be PMMA or silicone with monoabsorbable surgical suture material (Prolene) or PMMA haptics (Figure 8–9). The posterior surface of the IOL is usually convex, which inhibits lens epithelial cell migration across the posterior capsule and thus reduces capsular opacification.[1,2]

A variable number of positioning holes that aid the surgeon in centering the lens may be found at the perimeter of the optic. In order to position the implant away from the iris, the haptics are angled approximately 10 degrees, which reduces the risk of iris irritation and pupillary block. Although lens finishing is less critical with the posterior chamber IOL, since the lens does not contact iris tissue, its edges should be smoothly polished.[1,2]

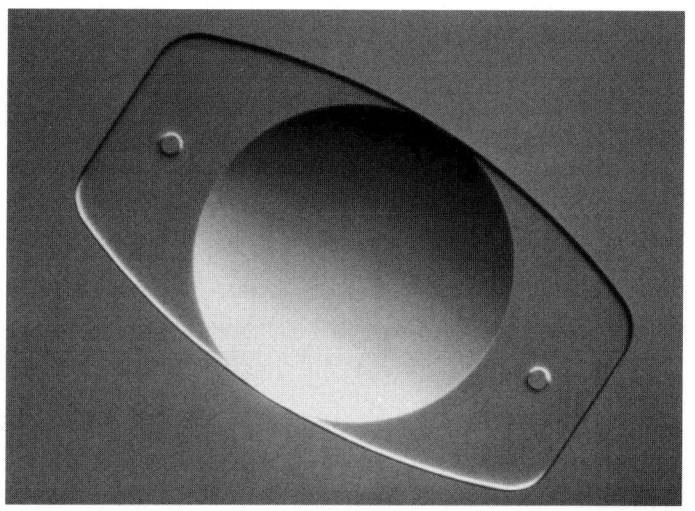

*FIGURE 8–9. Silicone (foldable) IOL.*

## REFERENCES

1. Apple DJ: Evolution and classification of intraocular lenses. In *Intraocular Lenses*. Baltimore: Williams & Wilkins; 1989:11–44.
2. Alpar JJ, Fechner PY: History of modern lens implantation. In *Intraocular Lenses*. New York: Thieme; 1986:6–34.
3. Apple DJ, Mamalis N, Loftfield K, et al: Complications of intraocular lenses. A historical and histopathologic review. *Surv Ophthalmol*. 1984;**29**:1–54.
4. Ridley H: Intraocular acrylic lenses. *Trans Ophthalmol Soc UK*. 1951;**71**:617–621.
5. Moses L: Complications of rigid anterior chamber implants. *Ophthalmology*. 1984;**91**:819–825.
6. Kornmehl EW, Steinert RF, Odrich MG, Stevens JB: Penetrating keratoplasty for pseudophakic bullous keratopathy associated with closed-loop anterior chamber intraocular lenses. *Ophthalmology*. 1990;**97**:407–414.
7. Binkhorst CD: Iris supported artificial pseudophakia. A new development in intraocular artificial lens surgery (iris clip lens). *Trans Ophthalmol Soc UK*. 1959;**79**:569–584.
8. Binkhorst CD: The iridocapsular (two-loop) lens and the iris-clip (four-loop) lens in pseudophakia. *Trans Am Acad Ophthalmol Otol*. 1973;**77**:589–617.
9. Lim ES, Apple DJ, Tsai JC, et al: An analysis of flexible anterior chamber lenses with special reference to the normalized route of lens explantation. *Ophthalmology*. 1991;**98**:243–246.

# Patient Preparation

CHAPTER 9

In-depth explanations of patient preparation immediately before cataract extraction are available in other texts.[1,2] Therefore, this chapter reviews our "philosophy" of providing that care in our surgery center.

## LOW-STRESS ATMOSPHERE

We believe patient preparation for cataract surgery begins when the patient hears about a surgery facility or surgeon from another patient or a referring doctor. This encounter sets the tone for how the patient views the experience to follow. The active part of patient preparation begins when the patient calls for an appointment. From this first encounter until completion of follow-up, the patient's experience and management need to be as low stress as possible. Teamwork is necessary to create this. The philosophy that the patient comes first also is very important (Figure 9–1).

Our surgery center is divided into the preoperative/postoperative area and the actual surgical suites (Figure 9–2). We have found that separating the two areas creates a quiet, comfortable environment. The preoperative/postoperative area has a somewhat private section for anesthesia. Otherwise, patients waiting for their preoperative anesthesia, those who have had their anesthesia, and postoperative patients are seated and cared for near each other. Staff members constantly pay attention to all the patients and see to their needs. Family members are allowed in the preoperative/postoperative area in order to maintain familiar ties for the patient. Surroundings are made pleasant and well lit to increase the patient's level of emotional comfort. Soothing music may be played to reduce anxiety.

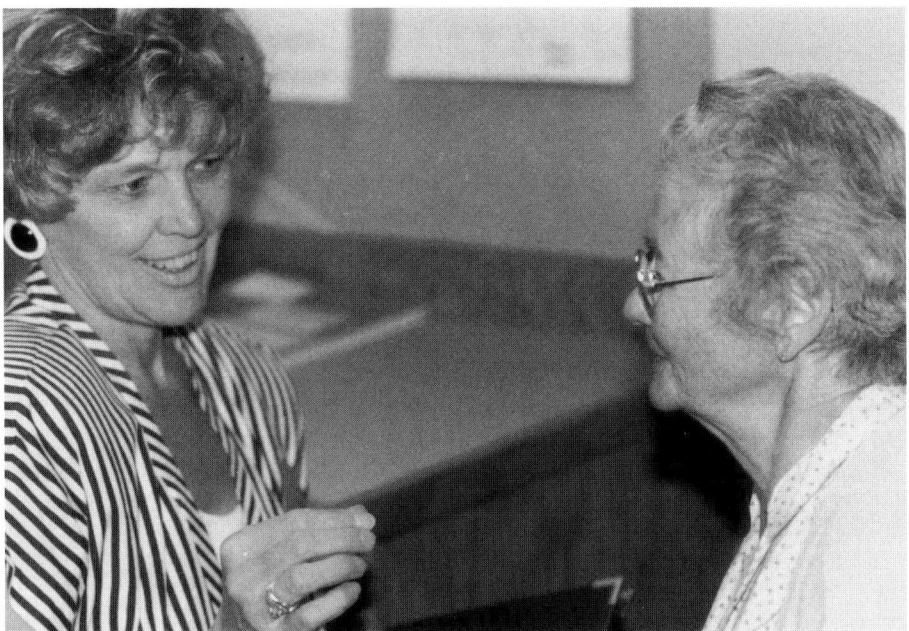

FIGURE 9–1. Patient counselor with patient and family.

## HISTORY AND MEDICATIONS

On entering the preoperative/postoperative area, the patient's head, clothing, and feet are covered. Their medical and ocular history is reviewed, with special attention to medication allergies, the presence of systemic disease, and medications in use.

The main classes of medications used immediately preoperatively are anesthetics, mydriatics/cycloplegics, intraocular pressure–lowering agents, anti-inflammatories, sedatives, and antibiotics. Some or all of these may be used at any one time. As an example, if there are no contraindications, we routinely administer topical xylocaine HCl 4%, cyclopentolate HCl 1%, phenylephrine

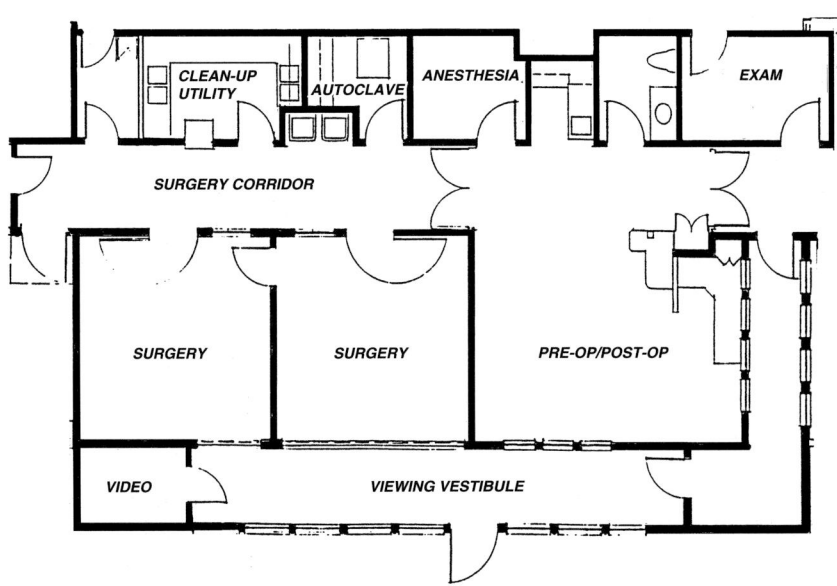

FIGURE 9–2. Floor plan of preoperative/postoperative area and operating suites.

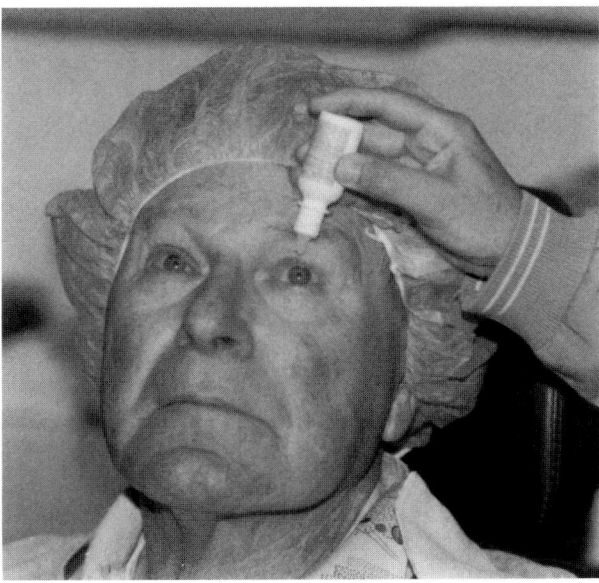

FIGURE 9–3. Instilling topical medications.

HCl 2.5% or 10%, tropicamide 1%, and suprofen 1% (Figure 9–3). Orally, we give 250 mg each of acetazolamide and cephalexin.

Preoperative sedation is rarely used in our setting. If it is given, it is usually in the form of an oral sedative such as diazepam (Valium). Rarely is an intravenous agent given.

## ANESTHESIA

Local anesthesia is most commonly used in an ambulatory surgery center (ASC) (Figure 9–4). This consists of 4–8 mL of 50:50 mix of xylocaine HCl 4% and marcaine HCl 0.75%, which is pH neutralized for comfort. Hyaluronidase is added for enhancement of anesthetic penetration and epinephrine (adrenaline) is added for blood vessel constriction. The conjunctiva is anesthetized with a topical anesthetic a couple of minutes prior to the injection. The injection is given in a modified peribulbar fashion, transconjunctivally, from the inferior

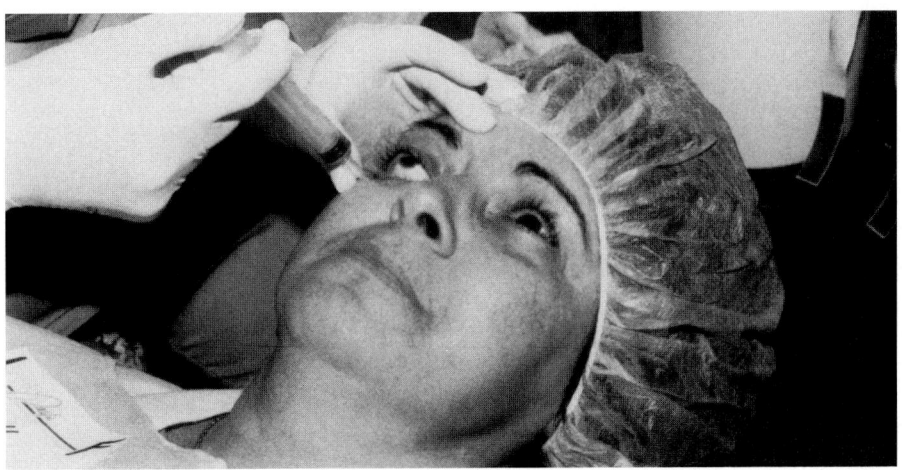

FIGURE 9–4. Peribulbar block.

temporal area. A small percentage of patients will require a second injection for complete immobility of the eye. Generally there is less sensation with the second injection. Akinesia (paralysis of the extraocular muscles) is the desired endpoint.

Retrobulbar as well as facial blocks are rarely used in our ambulatory surgery center because of the safety and effectiveness of the peribulbar blocks.[3] Complications from peribulbar anesthesia are rare. Occasional hemorrhages tend to be limited to the peribulbar area and do not interfere with surgery or delay surgery. Persistent diplopia beyond a day or so is extremely uncommon. Ocular perforations also are rare. Subconjunctival hemorrhages, chemosis, and lid ecchymoses are seen from time to time.

## PRESSURE ON THE GLOBE

Following the anesthetic injection, pressure is generally applied to the globe in order to soften the eye prior to surgery (Figure 9–5). The benefits of softening the eye have to do with egress of fluid from the vitreous and the orbit, as well as retarding any bleeding that might have occurred following anesthetic injection.

Traditionally, pressure was applied by the anesthetist's fingers (digital pressure) with intermittent release of pressure to allow for recirculation of the retina through the central retinal artery. With the advent of "mechanical" compressors, such as the Honan balloon and the Loyd Superpinkie (a rubber ball) (Tom Loyd, Newport Richey, FL), constant pressure could be applied. Initially this resulted in concern over the possibility of ischemia to the globe, but the Honan balloon has a built in pressure gauge to preclude that possibility. The Superpinkie has no built in safeguards, so the person that applies it must ensure that excess pressure on the globe is avoided. Periodic checks on the Superpinkie throughout the immediate preoperative period may be performed to avoid significant problems. Unfortunately, the possibility of ocular ischemia does exist and its effects would not be seen until the postoperative period. This, however, has not been seen in our practice.

Pressure is kept on the eye from the time of the anesthesia until the pa-

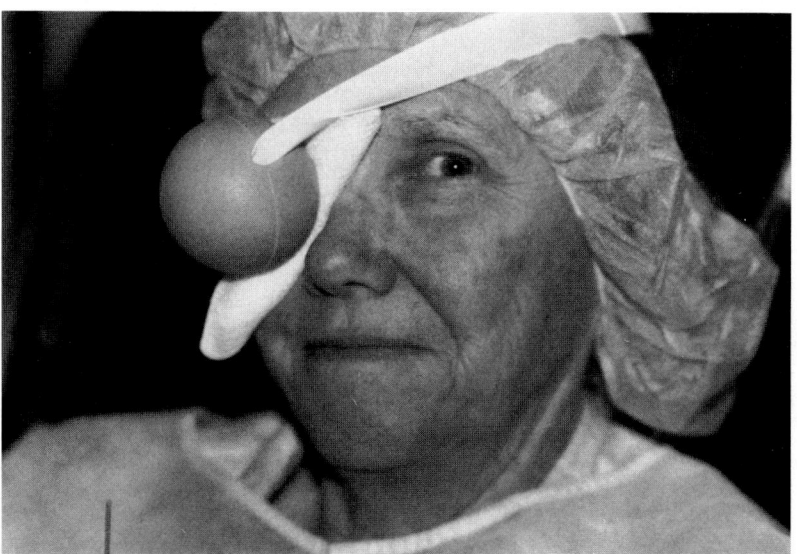

**FIGURE 9–5.** Lowering IOP with Superpinkie.

tient goes into surgery. This period may vary anywhere from 10 to 30 minutes in most ambulatory surgery centers.

## — STERILE TECHNIQUE

Relative sterility is maintained only in the immediate surgical area, with the preoperative/postoperative areas designated as "gray" as opposed to "red." The designation of "gray" means that people circulating through this area may wear street clothes without the special precautions of wearing surgical attire or gowns. The use of a "gray" area allows for intermingling of patients with family members and friends. This has greatly improved the overall atmosphere by significantly reducing the stress level associated with cataract removal.

All precautions present in any surgical suite regarding sterility and proper disposal of contaminated material (therefore designated as "red" areas) are observed in our surgical suites. Patient draping is meticulous, although the patient is allowed to wear street clothes, with a gown over them and a surgical cap and shoe covers in place (Figure 9–6).

## — INSTRUMENTATION

State of the art cataract surgery demands state of the art instrumentation such as the operating microscope, diamond blades, the phacoemulsification unit, and vitrector (see Chapter 10) (Figure 9–7). The most significant elements of modern cataract extraction such as continuous-tear capsulotomy, phacoemulsification, and self-sealing incisions are most easily initiated with a diamond blade. Recent developments in surgical wound construction have been both rapid and rewarding. The concept of "no stitch" surgery was initially bold but has resulted in the benefit of earlier visual rehabilitation for the patient. The use of diamond or other precious stone constructed blades has greatly facilitated the formation of a less traumatic wound with greater ability to self-seal.

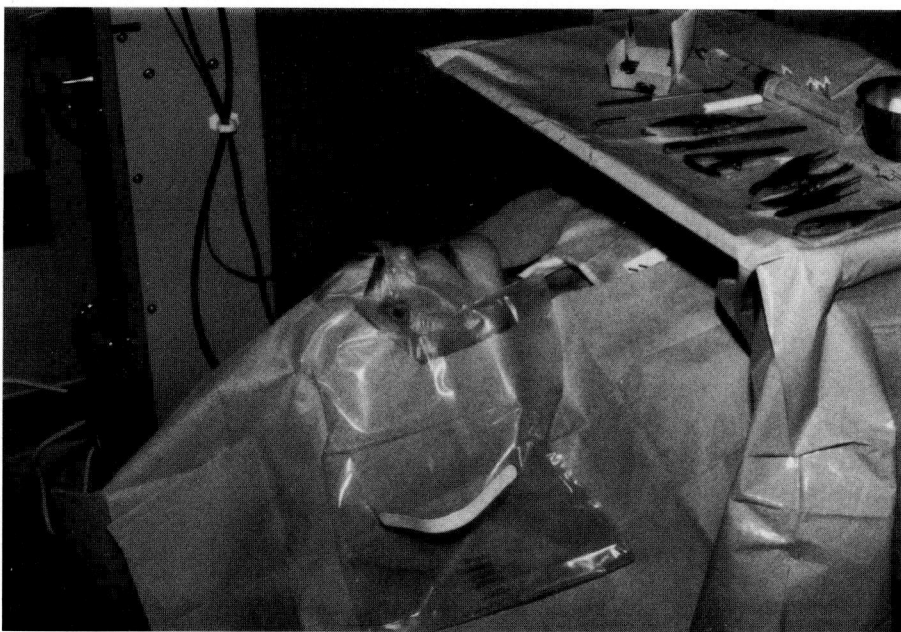

**FIGURE 9–6.** Eye draped for surgery.

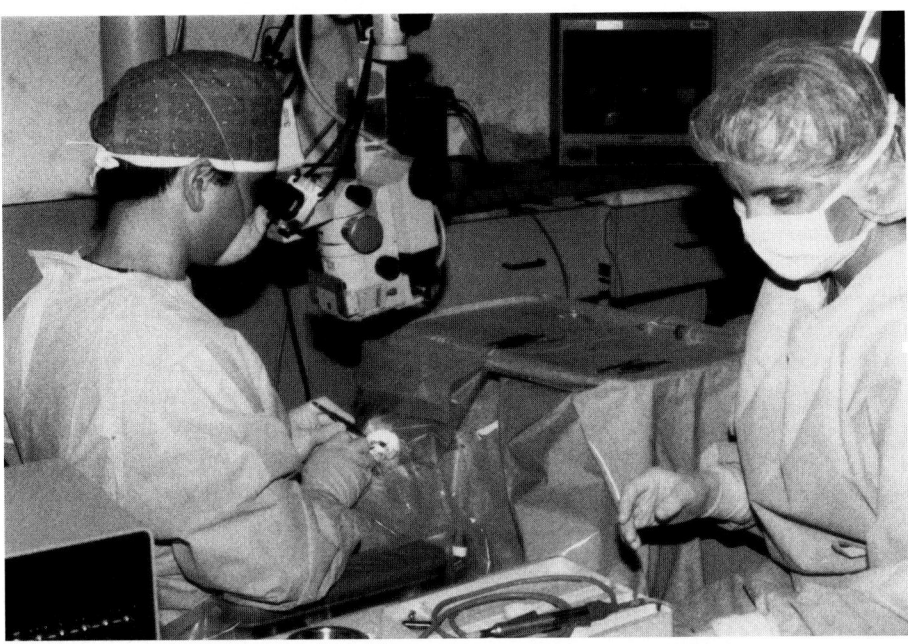

**FIGURE 9–7.** Surgical setup, as viewed from the surgeon's right, with operating microscope, surgical tray, and phacoemulsification unit prepared for use.

The capsulotomy in extracapsular cataract surgery was traditionally performed with a cystotome (cysto = sac, tome = a cutting). This was always the case when can-opener type of capsulotomy was performed. With the advent of capsulorhexis, the capsulotomy may be performed with either a cystotome or forceps. A cystotome used for capsulotomy consists generally of a needle whose tip is bent at approximately a 90-degree angle to the bevel of the needle. During the capsulotomy, infusion of balanced salt solution (BSS) is maintained.

The phacoemulsification unit is a sophisticated piece of equipment with its essential components being microprocessors. These allow for instantaneous changes in function and linear control of phacoemulsification power and suction. Vitrectomy capability has become a very significant part of managing the vitreous, specifically should the posterior capsule rupture, or for secondary implants. Again, microprocessors allow for exquisite control of the instrument functions such as cutting rate and suction. Without the ability to manage the vitreous, the surgeon would be at a great disadvantage and the surgical outcome less than satisfactory. As it is, in the event of surgical misadventure or for any other reasons, both the surgeon and the patient benefit immensely by the availability of a vitrector.

We have discussed only "significant" instrumentation for cataract extraction and intraocular lens implantation. Additionally, there are various tools used in cataract surgery, but their type and specifications vary greatly from surgeon to surgeon.

## REFERENCES

1. Jaffe NS, Jaffe MS, Jaffe GF: *Cataract Surgery and Its Complications,* 5th ed. St Louis: CV Mosby; 1990:16–18.
2. Lindquist T, Lindstrom RL: *Ophthalmic Surgery.* Chicago: Year Book Medical, 1990.
3. Wang HS: Peribulbar anesthesia for ophthalmic surgery. *J Cataract Refract Surg.* 1988;**14**:441–443.

# Operative Techniques

## CHAPTER 10

Cataract extraction techniques have undergone a revolution in the last 20 years. Intracapsular cataract extraction (ICCE) was the method of choice, specifically using cryoextraction, until the 1970s.

Harold Ridley demonstrated the feasibility of intraocular lenses in the 1940s and 1950s, but complications were great and there was a natural resistance to change. Ridley's early lenses were implanted in the posterior chamber; therefore, extracapsular cataract extraction (ECCE) including expression of the lens nucleus evolved.[1] Ridley's approach was rejected, however, and intracapsular surgery with iridocapsular intraocular lens fixation and eventually anterior chamber lenses were favored. Steve Shearing perfected the posterior chamber intraocular lens in the late 1970s, and routine ECCE again became the preferred method. Charles Kelman provided us with the innovation of a smaller wound size by developing the phacoemulsification method of cataract removal.[2]

Despite the dizzying pace of change in operative techniques, there are some basic surgical concepts that tend to remain stable. These concepts will be described in order to provide a foundation of knowledge on which an optometrist may understand and judge present and future surgical techniques.

## — OPENING INCISION* 

The incision may be described in terms of location, position, size, and type (Figures 10–1 and 10–2). (See Color Plate 10–1.) The location of the incision may be described by the clock-hour of the eye, such as 12 o'clock, 10 o'clock, 2 o'clock; or by the quadrant, such as superior, inferior, nasal or temporal; or

---

* Figures 10–1 to 10–20, refer to ECCE with IOL implantation using phacoemulsification. Figures are presented as the surgeon sees the eye with the inferior aspect of the eye at the top of the figure and superior aspect at the bottom.

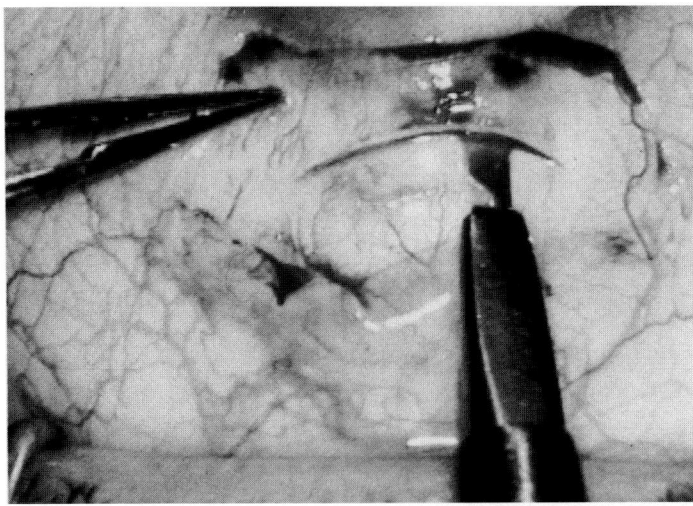

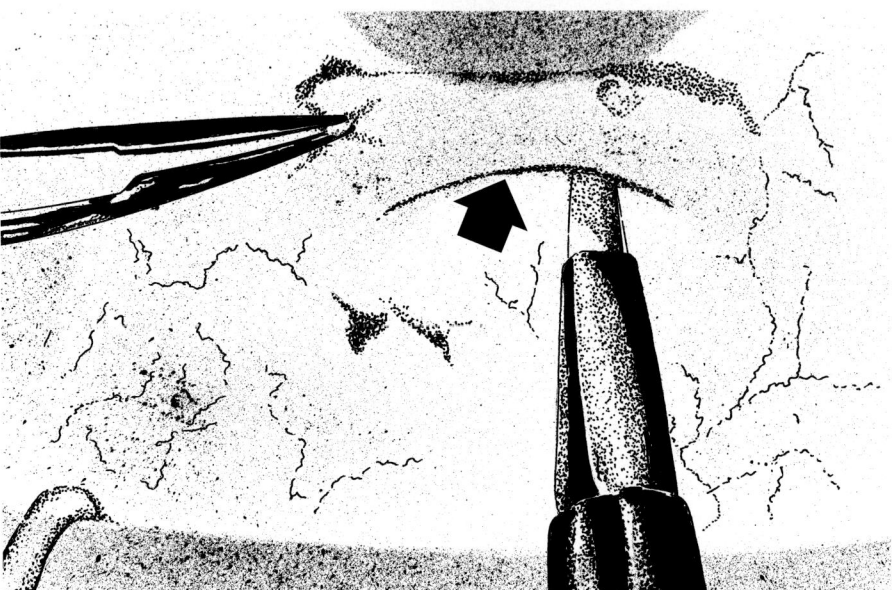

**FIGURES 10–1 AND 10–2.** Self-sealing (sutureless) opening incision through scleral tunnel into clear cornea (also called "frown" incision).

by the approach, such as medial or lateral. The superior location is used most commonly because of both tradition and its many advantages. The advantages are that the incision is hidden under the lid, gravity pulls the conjunctiva down, and perforating vessels are less exposed. Disadvantages include a more difficult access due to the superior lid, the eye may have to be rotated inferiorly, and the patient's eyebrow may be in the way. A lateral approach is advocated by some surgeons, because of the ease of access owing to better exposure. However, the lateral approach has the disadvantages of perforating vessels that are closer to the limbus intrapalpebrally and greater visibility of incised tissue and sutures postoperatively.

The position of the incision refers to the anatomic relationship of the incision to the limbus. The incision may be placed at the limbus; in which case, it is referred to as a limbal incision, or posterior to the limbus into the sclera. This is called a scleral pocket, scleral tunnel, or posterior incision. Limbal incisions are commonly used for expression of the lenticular nucleus, whereas scleral incisions are used more often for phacoemulsification. Surgeons tend to prefer one type of incision over the other; therefore, they often use all limbal or all scleral incisions no matter what type of cataract removal technique they favor.

The scleral incision has many advantages, including more comfort, less induction of astigmatism, and the reduction or elimination of sutures and hence fewer postoperative visits. It is commonly placed 1.5 to 3.0 mm posterior to the limbus. The incision may follow the curve of the limbus, which is most common, or it may mirror image the limbus, the so-called frown incision. Once the sclera is incised, usually to half depth, a lamellar incision is made toward the limbus. This is known as the tunnel or pocket through which the anterior chamber is entered.

Wound size, measured in millimeters, is determined by the method of cataract extraction and the size of the intraocular lens. Intracapsular cataract extraction by means of cryoextraction or forceps requires a large incision extending almost from 3 to 9 o'clock. Since the entire lens is removed and the lens diameter is approximately 10 mm, the incision has a 10-mm cord length, or about a 12-mm length. A dislocated physiologic lens may still have to be removed by this means.

Extracapsular cataract extraction allows for a much smaller incision. The cataract is removed by expression or phacoemulsification. Planned ECCE by expression requires an incision of 8–10 mm through which the nucleus is delivered. The nucleus has a diameter 7–9 mm. The incision therefore ends up being slightly larger than the size of the intraocular lens (IOL).

Phacoemulsification liquifies the cataract through an ultrasonic instrument. Incision size, in this case, is determined solely on the basis of the size of the IOL. Posterior chamber IOLs are either foldable or rigid. Foldable IOLs require a 3- to 4-mm wound. Rigid IOLs come in diameters of 5.0–7.0 mm and 5 mm by 6 mm oval profile, where the shorter diameter is used for insertion. Many surgeons continue to prefer rigid lenses made of polymethylmethacrylate (PMMA) owing to extensive experience with this material.

The self-sealing wound has gained popularity in the last few years. In this case, the wound involves not only the scleral pocket but a long internal flap into clear cornea. When the eye is pressurized at the conclusion of surgery, this internal flap closes and the wound seals without a suture. The biggest advantage of this wound is that there is much more rapid visual rehabilitation, comfort, and stability compared with a wound with sutures. It has been found that a wound constructed in this manner allows for insertion of IOLs up to 6.0–6.5 mm.

Future developments in cataract surgery incisions will no doubt strive to decrease wound size, create less postoperative astigmatism and hemorrhage, and allow quicker visual recovery.

## ECCE TECHNIQUE WITH PHACOEMULSIFICATION

We favor the ECCE technique by phacoemulsification. This calls for removal of a portion of the anterior capsule while leaving the posterior capsule intact. Removal of the anterior capsule by continuous-tear capsulotomy or capsulorhexis is our preferred technique. The capsulotomy is initiated with a single tear that is then carried around in a circle to meet the original tear (Figures 10–3 and 10–4) Capsulorhexis provides a strong rim of anterior capsule which resists tearing during insertion of the IOL. This ensures placement of the IOL in the capsular bag. Capsulorhexis may be performed with either a continuous flow of BSS or with the use of viscoelastics to maintain the anterior chamber (Figures

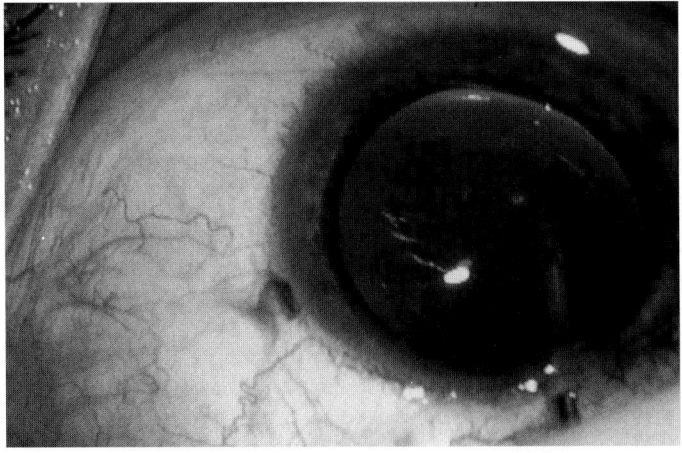

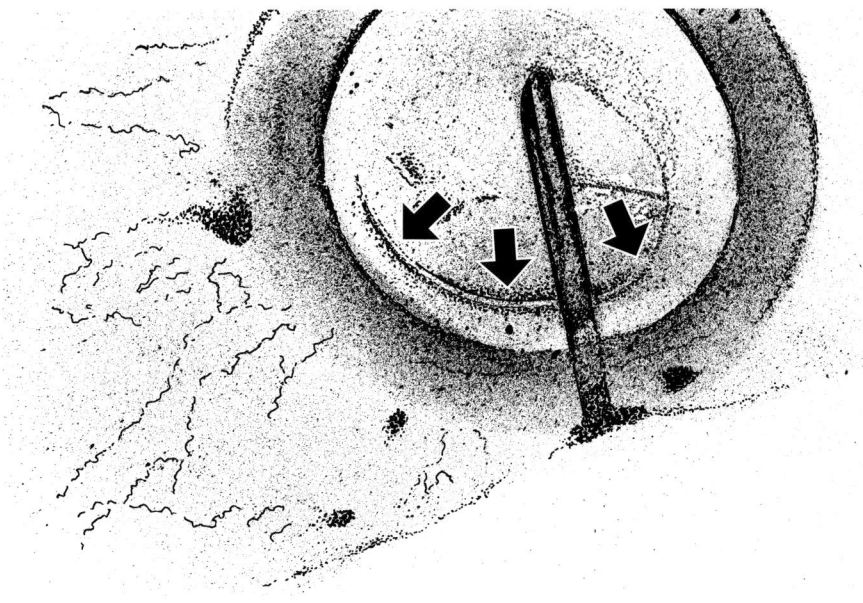

**FIGURES 10–3 AND 10–4.** Capsulorhexis (continuous tear capsulotomy).

10–5 and 10–6). With viscoelastics, many surgeons use forceps to perform the tear. The alternative to capsulorhexis is the can-opener capsulotomy. This is accomplished by connecting multiple small tears forming a circle just inside the dilated pupil border. The jagged look of this capsulotomy border gives it its name. The can-opener capsulotomy can easily tear to the periphery (or equator) of the lens capsule at the time of lens insertion. If this happens, one IOL haptic may end up in the sulcus with the other in the capsular bag. Intraocular lenses placed in this fashion have a greater likelihood of decentering toward the haptic in the sulcus.[3–5]

Some surgeons have advocated a small opening in the anterior capsule, without capsulotomy, through which phacoemulsification may be performed. This leaves the anterior capsule in place to protect the endothelium. Following phacoemulsification, the anterior capsule is then removed, cortex is cleaned away, and the IOL may be inserted.

Phacoemulsification removes the nucleus and some of the central cortex by means of ultrasonic liquefaction (Figures 10–7 and 10–8). It is more easily performed in very soft cataracts than in very dense cataracts. The length of phacoemulsification time tends to increase with the density of nuclear sclerosis.

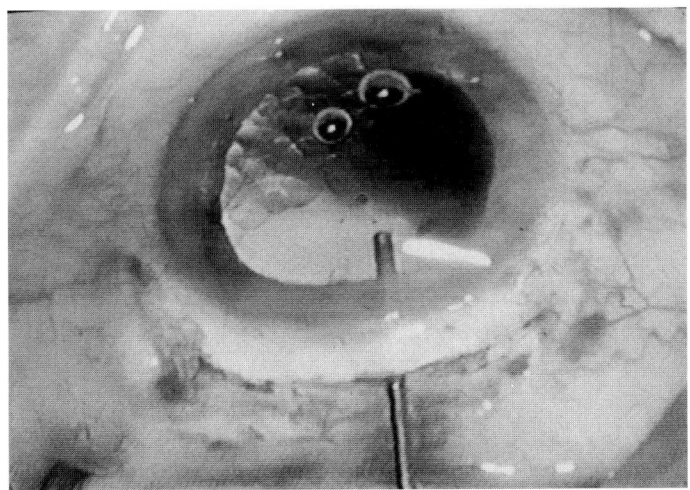
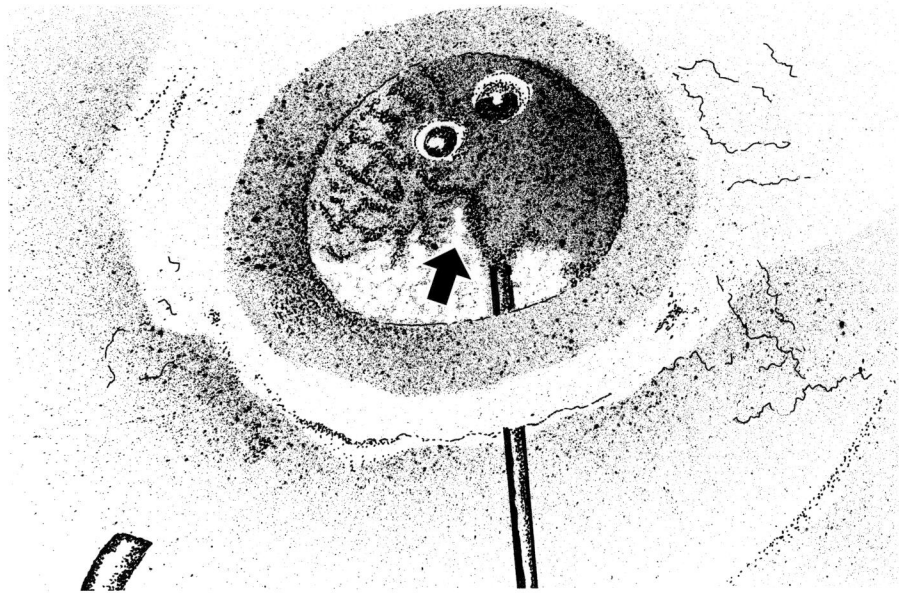

**FIGURES 10–5 AND 10–6.** Injection of viscoelastic which maintains the anterior chamber and protects the corneal endothelium during the procedure. This viscoelastic must be removed at the end of the procedure.

The longer the phacoemulsification time, the more likely there is to be damage to the corneal endothelium and therefore more postoperative corneal edema occurs. In general, phacoemulsification performed in less than two minutes in the posterior chamber plane is safe. In the case of Fuchs' endothelial dystrophy, a short phacoemulsification time becomes even more important. In these cases, the endothelium may also be cushioned by an injection of viscoelastics during the phacoemulsification.[6,7] The exact reason for the endothelial damage is unknown. However, it may be attributed to damage from the phacoemulsification energy, air bubbles or nuclear fragments hitting the endothelium, as well as flow of irrigation fluid against the endothelium. Endothelial damage is further influenced by the position of the phacoemulsification tip during the emulsification process. The more posterior the tip is placed, the less damage to the endothelium. In the case of can-opener capsulotomy, the emulsification is frequently done in a plane anterior to the iris. With capsulorhexis, the emulsification is, for the most part, done posterior to or in the plane of the iris.

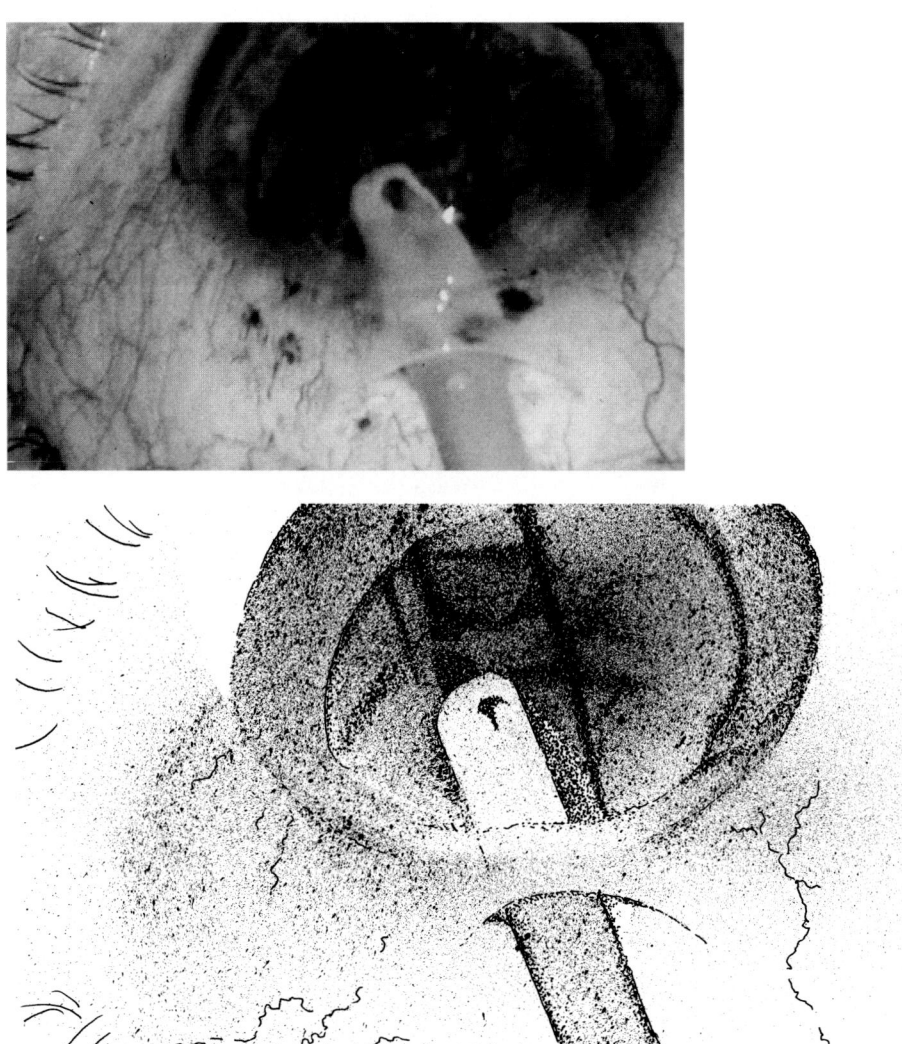

**FIGURES 10–7 AND 10–8.** Phacoemulsification of the cataractous lens nucleus.

Following phacoemulsification, there is cortical material adherent to the remaining capsule (Figures 10–9 and 10–10). This is usually removed by irrigation and aspiration. Once all the cortex is removed, the posterior capsule may require "polishing" to remove any remaining cortical fibers. Polishing of the posterior capsule is almost always necessary in posterior subcapsular cataracts (Figures 10–11 and 10–12). In fact, thickening of the posterior capsule sometimes cannot be fully removed at the time of surgery and a later Nd:YAG (neodymium:ythrium-aluminum-garnet [laser]) capsulotomy is necessary.

On completion of cortical aspiration, the incision is opened to accommodate the IOL (Figures 10–13 and 10–14). The anterior chamber depth must be maintained to avoid trauma to the endothelium. This is done via a side port infusion of balanced salt solution (BSS) or the use of viscoelastic materials. This viscoelastic must be removed at the conclusion of the surgery. When the IOL is inserted, the haptics are best placed in the capsular bag. Capsulorhexis with its firm, visible anterior leaf allows virtual certainty of "in-the-bag" placement (Figures 10–15 to 10–18). As mentioned earlier, in the case of can-opener capsulotomy, probability of tears of the capsule and poor visibility of the capsulotomy make in-the-bag placement less certain.

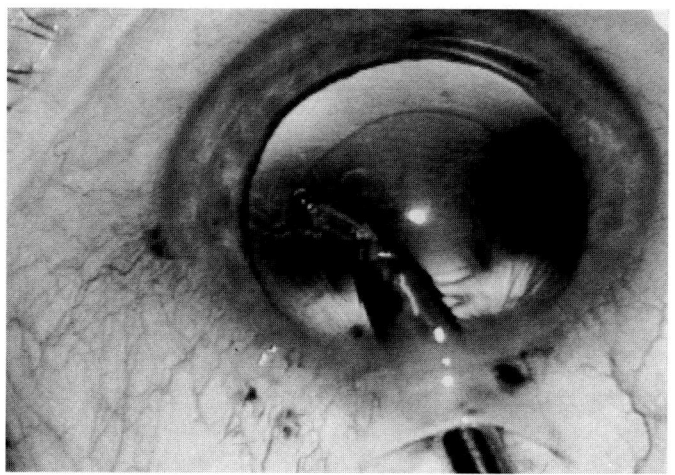

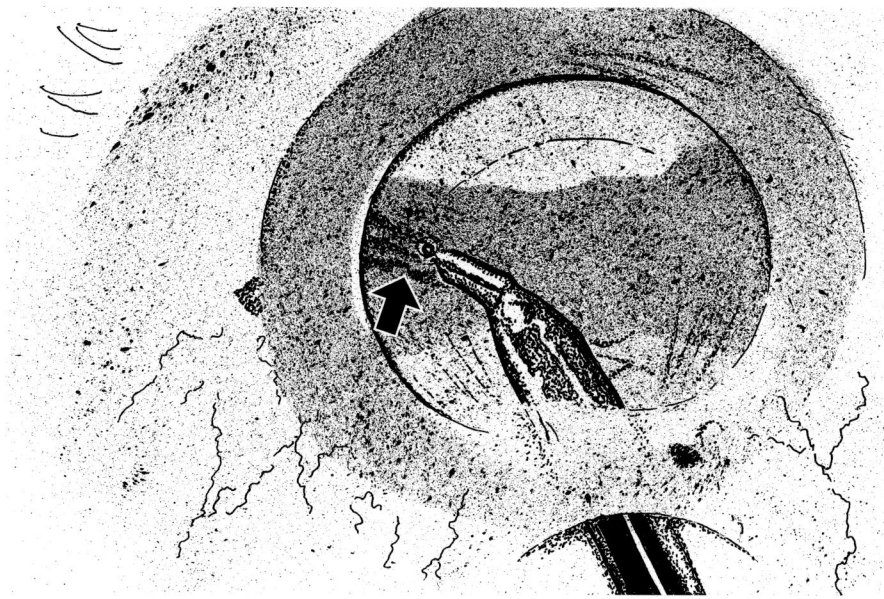

**FIGURES 10–9 AND 10–10.** Irrigation and aspiration of the residual cortical material.

On insertion of the lens implant and removal of any viscoelastic, if used, the incision is closed by either internal flap apposition and "no stitch," the use of one suture in a mattress stitch fashion, or the use of a running stitch in a bootlace fashion. The conjunctiva is then replaced over the incision site and the surgery is concluded (Figures 10–19 and 10–20).

The main advantages of ECCE by phacoemulsification are the small incision and the greater control over the intraocular environment. The small incision allows for rapid physical and visual rehabilitation of the patient. In addition, it has minimal effect on astigmatism. Because the surgeon has greater control of the intraocular environment, the intraocular pressure can be controlled during surgery. This lessens the danger of retinal detachment or choroidal hemorrhage.

The disadvantage of ECCE by phacoemulsification is the potential for damage to intraocular structures on account of the power of the phacoemulsification instrument. In all cases, some damage occurs to the corneal endothelium, with the loss of up to 15% of the endothelial cells. The amount of damage is related to the length of emulsification, the position in which the emulsification was done, and the vulnerability of the endothelium, such as presence of Fuchs'

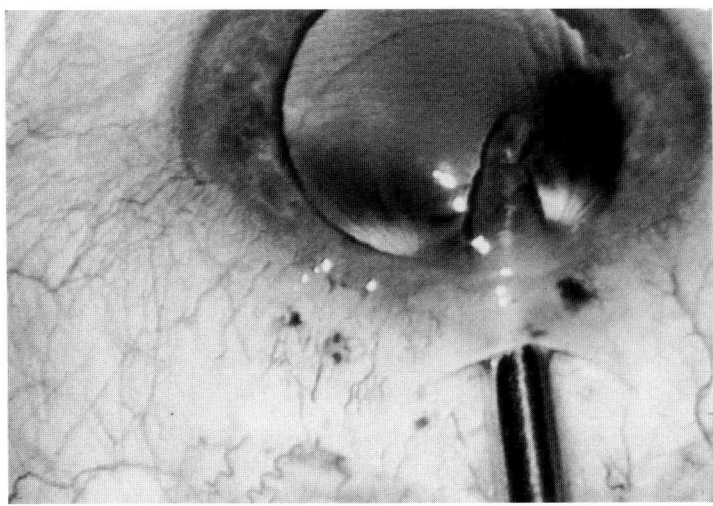

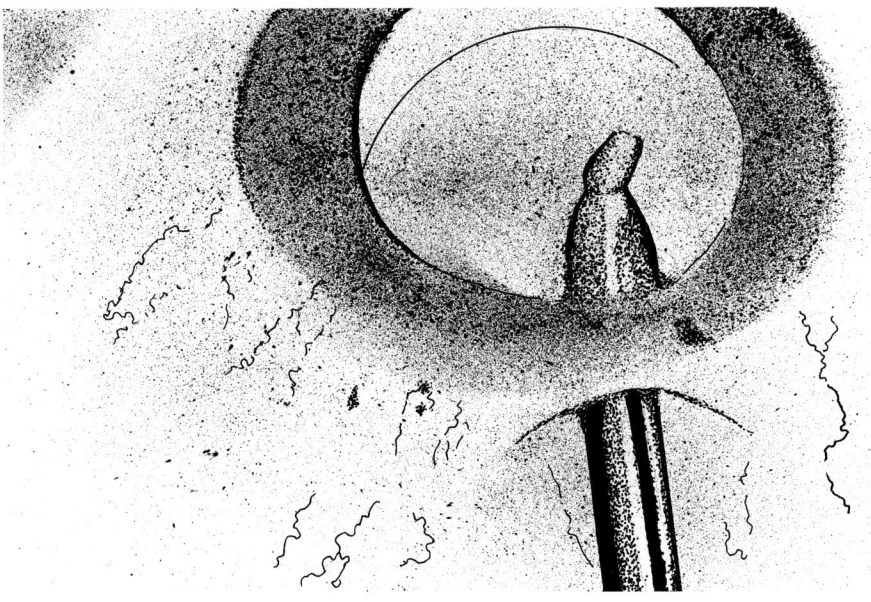

**FIGURES 10–11 AND 10–12.** "Polishing" the posterior capsule.

dystrophy. Damage to the iris is not uncommon, especially in a surgeon's early learning period of phacoemulsification. Although damage to the iris is primarily cosmetic, if it is extensive, visual aberrations may occur. Damage to the posterior capsule may create significant problems for the surgeon depending on how early in the procedure this happens and the extent of the damage (see Chapter 12). If the posterior capsule is broken and vitreous prolapses through the opening, a vitrectomy is necessitated in order to prevent the vitreous from getting in the way during the rest of the operation. Any vitreous in the anterior chamber also presents the potential for vitreous to the wound, or the "vitreous wick" syndrome, which may cause persistent cystoid macular edema (CME). Damage to the posterior capsule may also result in enough loss of structure to prevent adequate support tissue for posterior chamber placement of the IOL. In that case, an anterior chamber IOL must be substituted. If the posterior capsule break is limited, it may still be possible to place the posterior chamber lens in the bag[8] (Table 10–1).

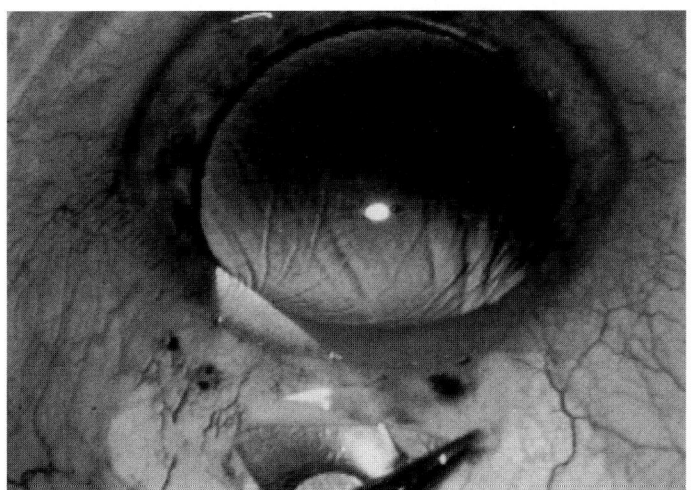
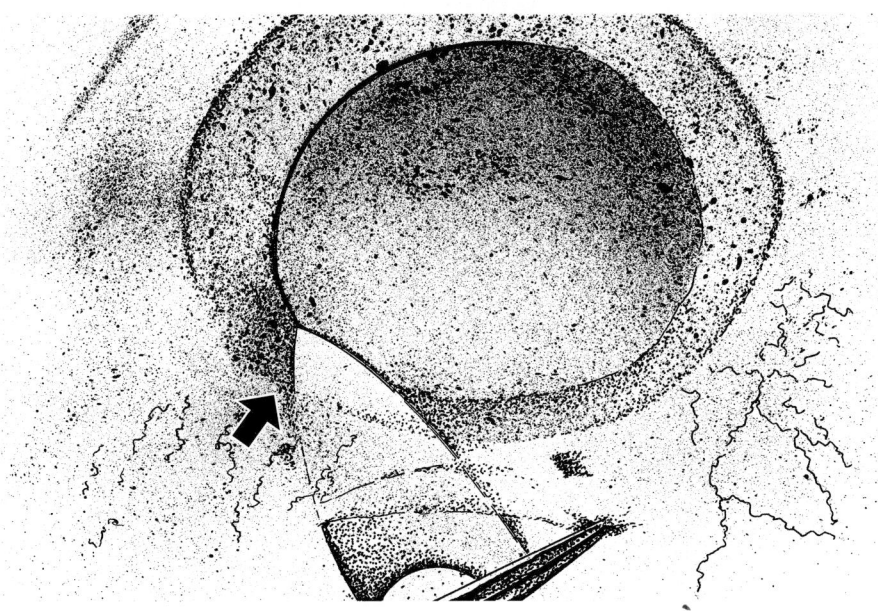

**FIGURES 10–13 AND 10–14.** Enlargement of the inner aspect of the incision to allow insertion of the posterior chamber IOL.

**TABLE 10–1. EXTRACAPSULAR CATARACT EXTRACTION CHARACTERISTICS**

| | Phacoemulsification | Nuclear Expression[a] |
|---|---|---|
| **Advantage** | Small wound size<br>  Control of intraocular environment<br>  Less astigmatism<br>May be performed through capsulorhexis | Requires less surgical skill<br>Less expensive instrumentation<br>Less potential for endothelial damage |
| **Disadvantage** | More difficult to master technique<br>More expensive instrumentation<br>Greater risk of endothelial cell loss with inexperienced surgeons | Larger wound size<br>More induced astigmatism<br>Less control of intraocular environment<br>Requires larger capsulotomy |

[a] Some surgeons now do expression through capsulorhexis and a small incision.

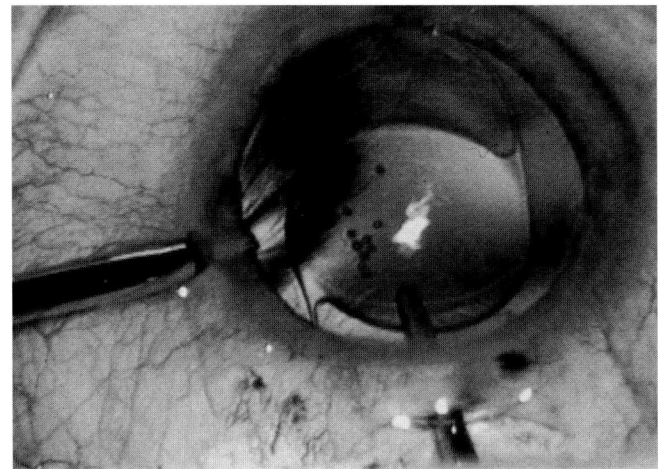

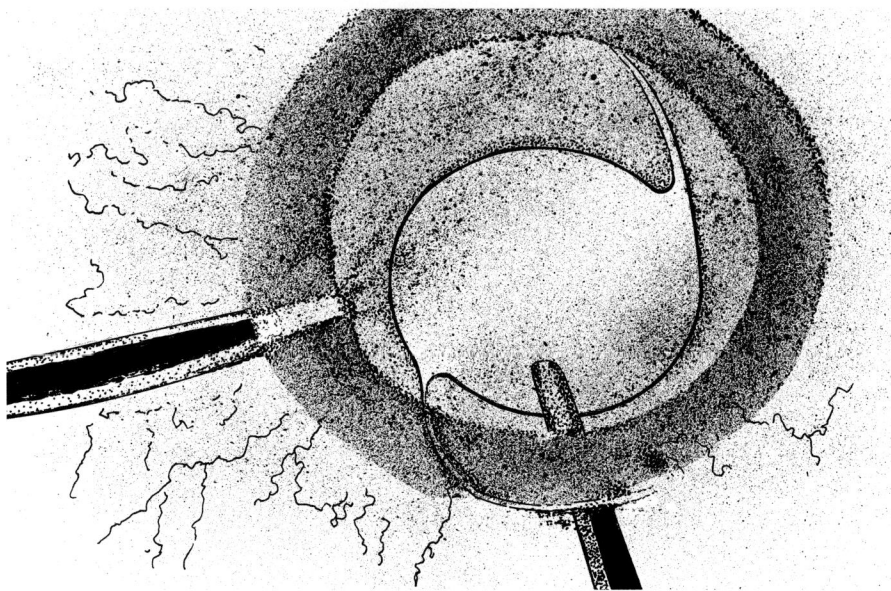

**FIGURES 10–15 AND 10–16.** Posterior chamber IOL insertion.

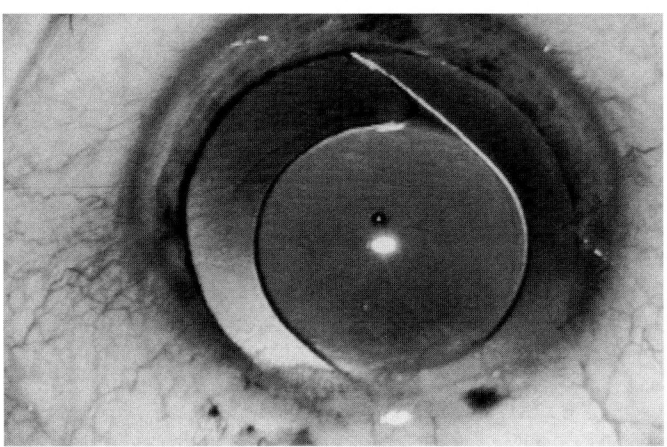

**FIGURE 10–17.** PC IOL in the capsular bag.

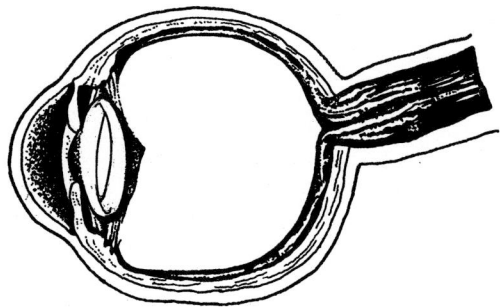

**FIGURE 10–18.** Cross section of posterior chamber IOL in the capsular bag.

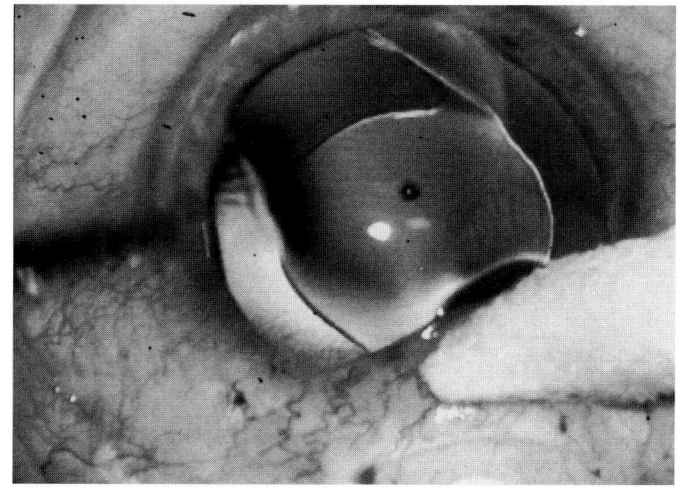

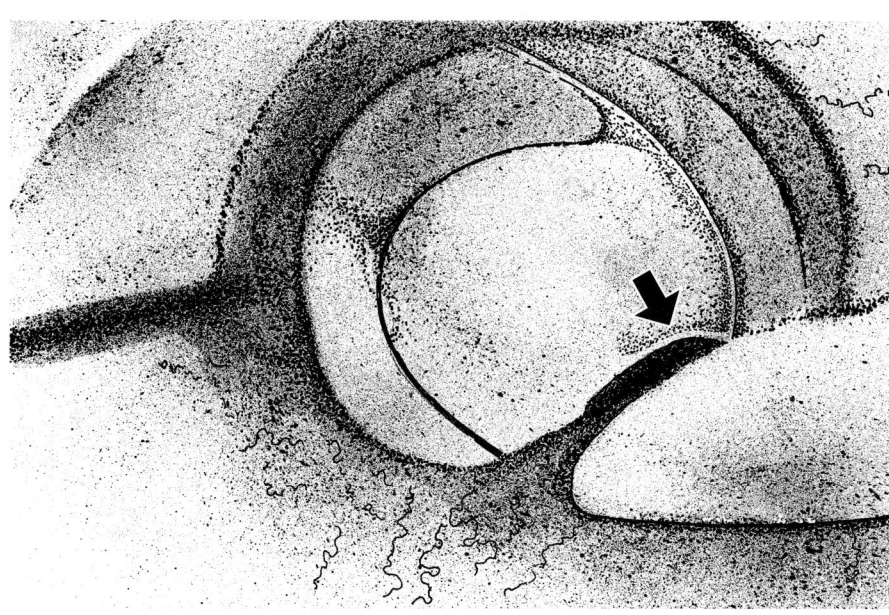

**FIGURES 10–19 AND 10–20.** Conjunctiva is replaced over the self-sealing (sutureless) incision.

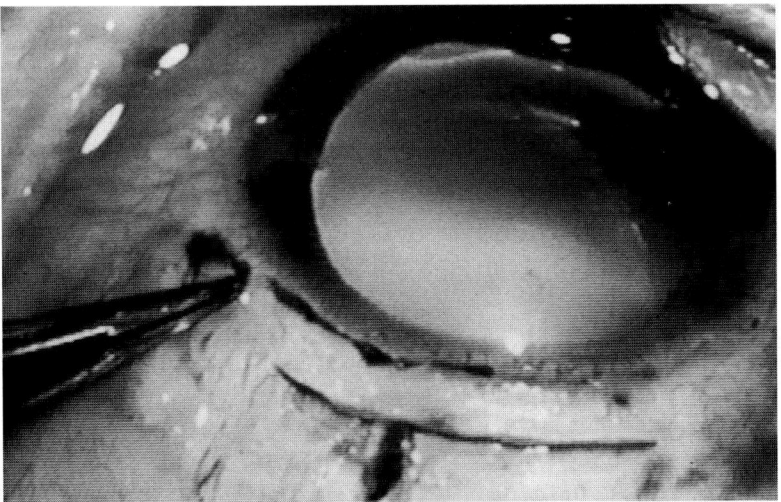

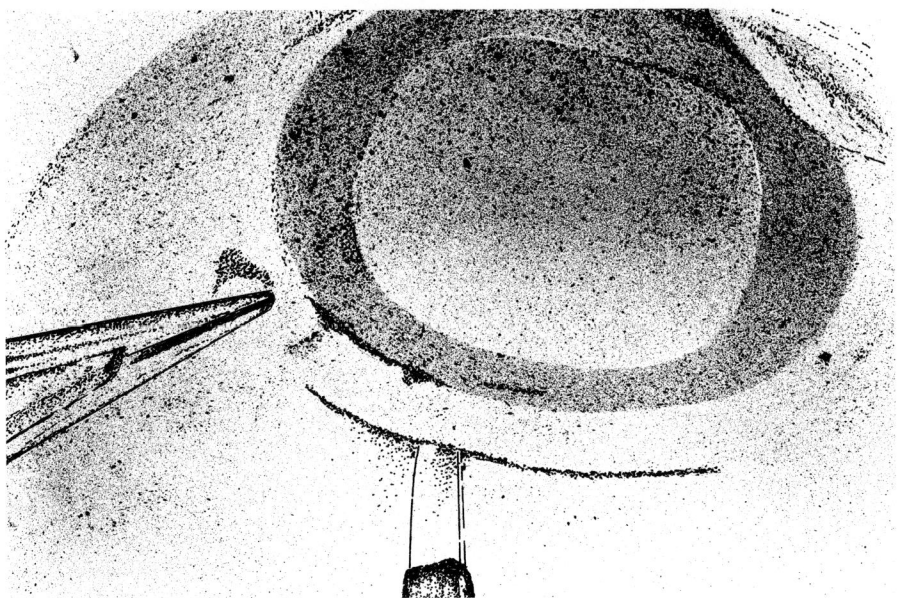

**FIGURES 10–21 AND 10–22.** Opening incision; note that this is enlarged later in the procedure to allow expression of the lens nucleus.

## ECCE TECHNIQUE WITH NUCLEAR EXPRESSION*

Some cataract surgeons use expression of the nucleus as their preferred method (Figures 10–21 to 10–26). This method is very acceptable; however, it requires a larger wound. Extracapsular cataract extraction with nuclear expression involves expressing the nucleus, which is about 7–9 mm, through the incision. Today, methods are in use where the nucleus may be fractured in half and then extracted through a smaller 6- to 7-mm incision. The can-opener type of capsulotomy is usually used, because it allows for a wide opening. Some surgeons use capsulorhexis followed by expression. They first dissect the central nucleus

---

* Figures 10–21 to 10–26 refer to ECCE with IOL implantation using nuclear expression. These figures demonstrate the steps that differ from phacoemulsification rather than the complete procedure. Figures are presented as the surgeon sees the eye with the inferior aspect of the eye at the top of the figure and the superior aspect at the bottom.

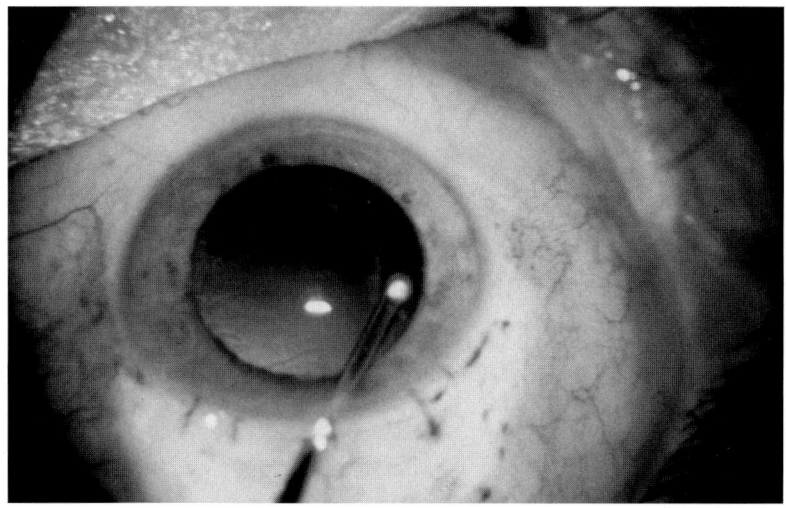

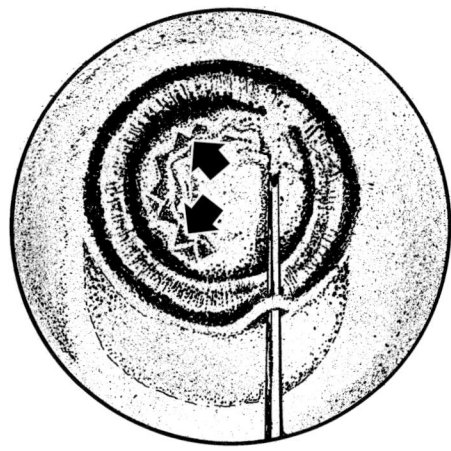

**FIGURES 10–23 AND 10–24.** Can-opener capsulotomy.

free by means of forced BSS. This is called hydrodissection. This method leaves a larger amount of cortex behind making cortical aspiration more extensive.

Following the capsulotomy, the surgeon enlarges the wound to about 8 to 10 mm. The nucleus is then loosened by irrigation and brought into the anterior chamber and out through the wound (Figures 10–25 and 10–26). As an alternative, the nucleus may be tilted anteriorly at the superior pole by depression of the eye close to the wound and pushing on the eye inferiorly, below the limbus, therefore "squirting" out the nucleus. The remaining cortex is then removed by irrigation and aspiration.

Before inserting the IOL, the wound may be narrowed with the use of sutures, and air or viscoelastic may be injected into the anterior chamber to maintain it. The IOL is then inserted, usually with an attempt to get both haptics in the capsular bag. If can-opener capsulotomy was used, it may be more difficult to place the lens in the capsular bag (see pp. 77–78). The wound is closed with interrupted or running suture(s).

The advantages of expression over phacoemulsification are few, but in advanced, hard, nuclear sclerotic cataracts, expression may result in less damage to the endothelium and iris. Further advantages of expression are simplicity of technique and less expensive instrumentation.

The primary disadvantages of expression over phacoemulsification are the size of the wound and reduced control over the intraocular environment.

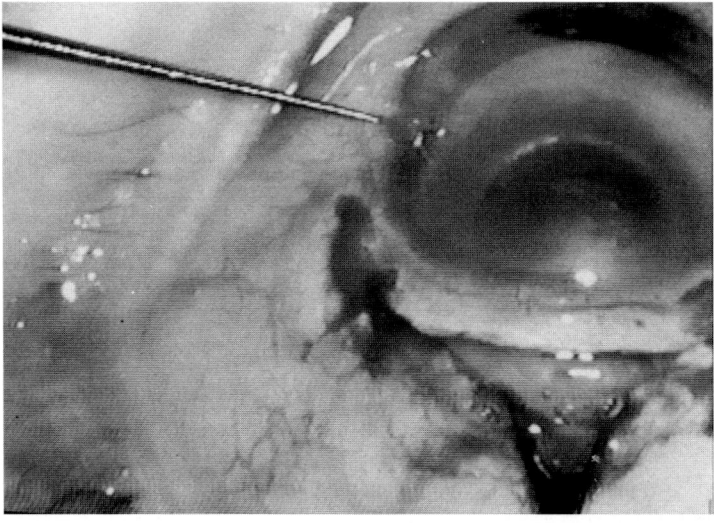

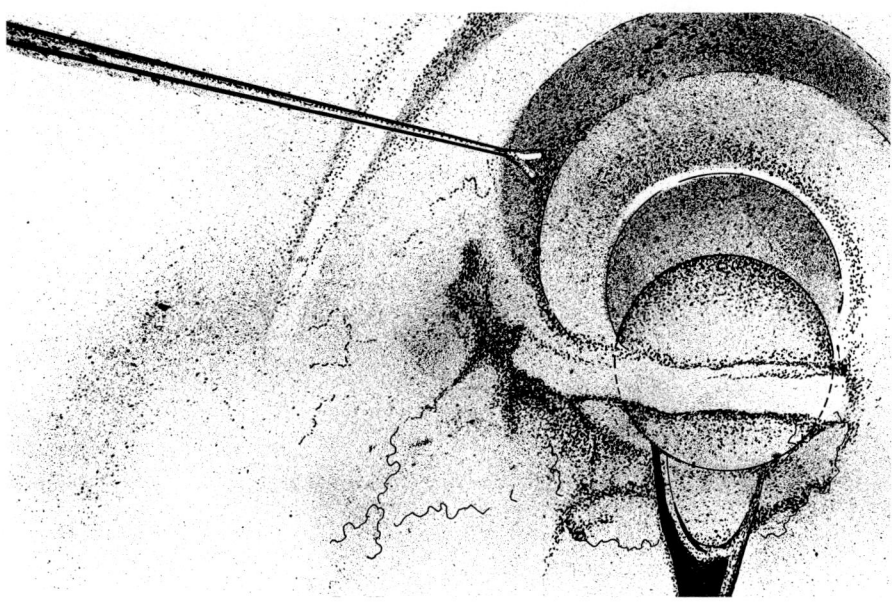

**FIGURES 10–25 AND 10–26.** Nuclear expression following enlargement of the incision.

## ICCE TECHNIQUE

Intracapsular cataract extraction is now a thing of the past except in special cases. This type of surgery may be performed on a patient with post-traumatic cataract where the zonules are damaged and there is not adequate support for a posterior chamber implant. Additionally, intracapsular surgery may be used in cases of congenital dislocation of the lens.

Intracapsular cataract extraction requires a wound that extends about 160–180 degrees (Figures 10–27 and 10–28). Once the wound is opened, alpha-chymotrypsin may be injected underneath the iris to weaken the zonules. The anterior chamber is then drained dry of aqueous, following which a cryoprobe is applied to the superior aspect of the lens and an ice ball is formed for adequate adhesion of the probe to the lens. The lens is then removed by gently rocking it from side to side while pulling it out of the eye. Care needs to be taken to do this slowly to minimize the loss of vitreous.

There are really no advantages of intracapsular cataract removal compared with extracapsular techniques except in the specific cases mentioned earlier.

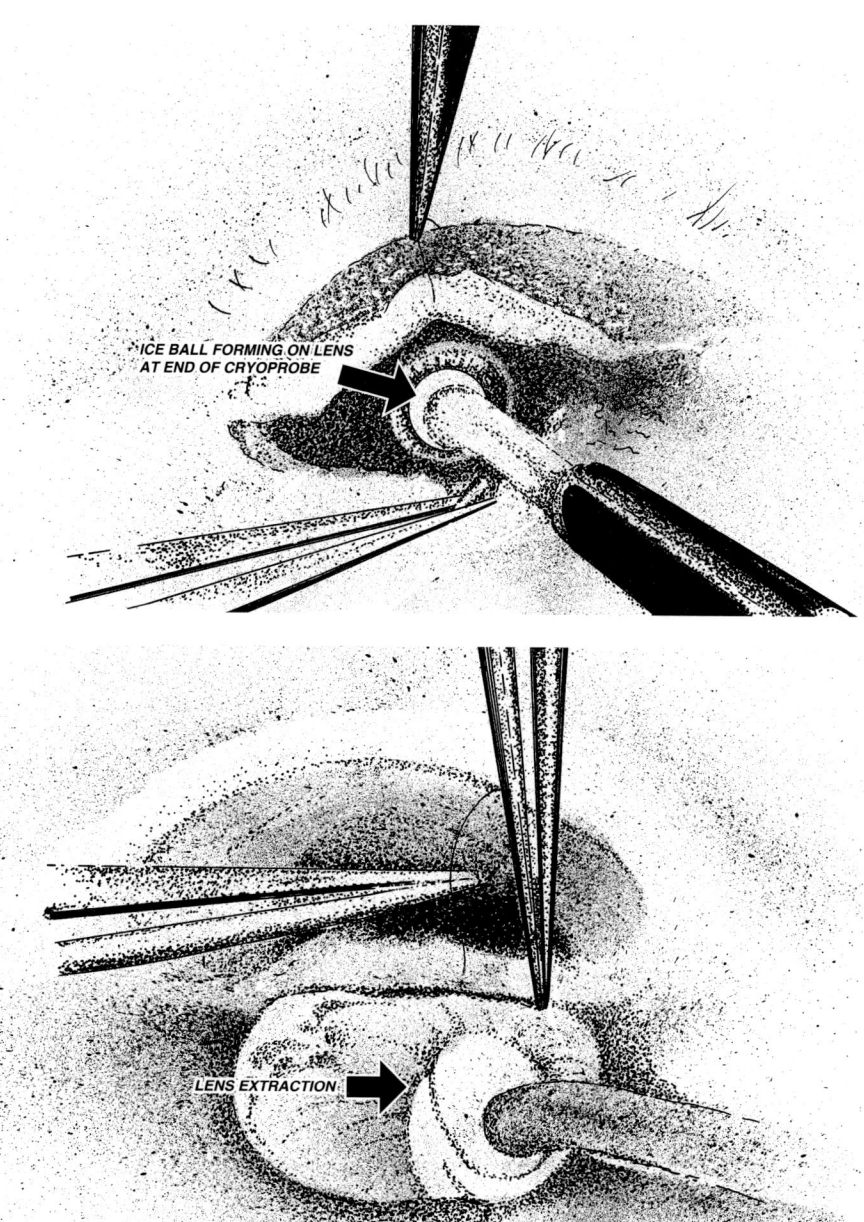

**FIGURES 10–27 AND 10–28.** ICCE whereby the lens is removed in its entirety through a 160–180 incision. Figures are presented as the surgeon sees the eye with the inferior aspect of the eye at the top of the figure and the superior aspect at the bottom.

There are major disadvantages of this technique, however. First of all, the barrier between the vitreous cavity and the anterior segment of the eye is disrupted. This disruption results in the potential for many problems such as chronic CME, loss of vitreous, vitreous wick syndrome, retinal detachment, pupillary distortion, and choroidal detachment.

## INCISIONAL CLOSURE

Proper incisional closure is a matter of balance between closing the wound tight enough to prevent leaks (watertight closure) but not too tight, thereby inducing excessive amounts of astigmatism. Surgeons hope to leave preexisting astigmatism unaffected or to improve it. Limbal incisions with interrupted sutures will generally induce astigmatism with minus cylinder axis 90 degrees from the orientation of one or more sutures (Figures 10–29 and 10–30). Fre-

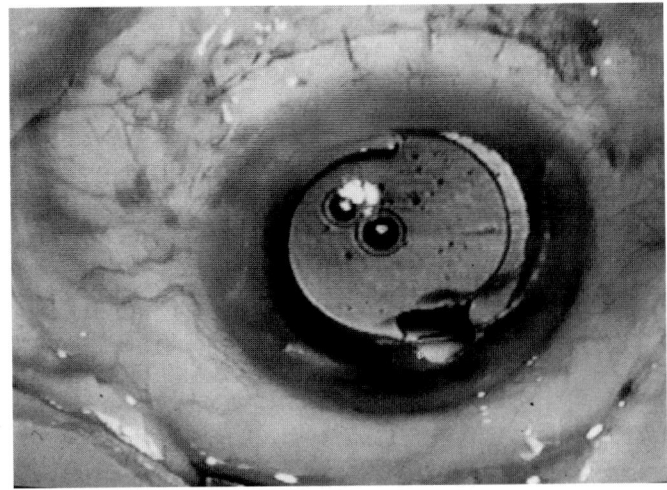

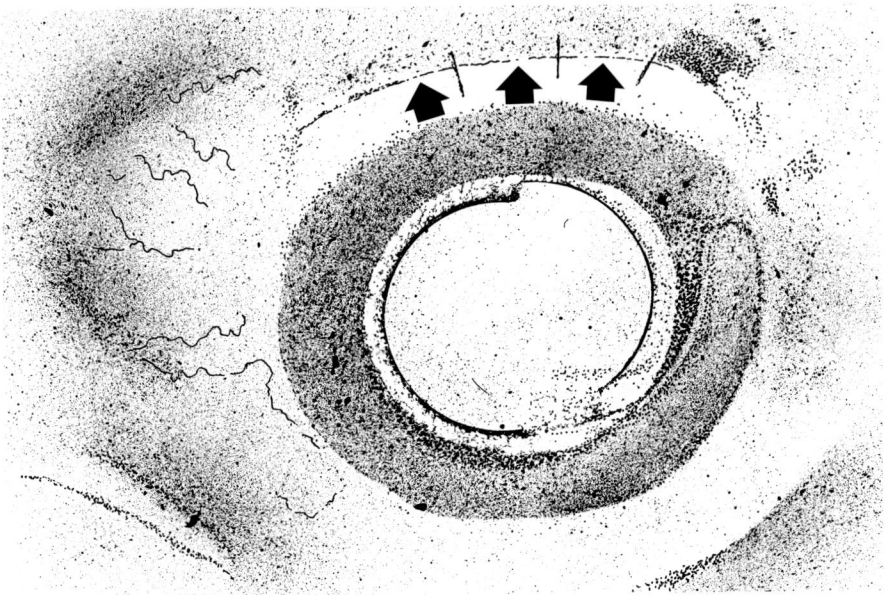

**FIGURES 10–29 AND 10–30.** Incisional closure with interrupted sutures.

quently, induced astigmatism necessitates the cutting of these sutures. Suture cutting is usually done after 6–8 weeks and one suture at a time is cut, waiting several days between to allow time for the tissue to make the proper adjustment and to determine the resultant astigmatism.

The most common sutures used in cataract wound closure are nylon, Prolene, Mersilene, and Dacron. Most surgeons use 10-0 or 11-0; however, some use 9-0 nylon. Nylon is slowly absorbable and more stretchable than the other sutures. Usually, its absorption occurs over a 2-year period. Due to the fact that nylon may unevenly absorb, it may result in suture exposure, which sometimes necessitates removal. Prolene, Mersilene, and Dacron, on the other hand, are nonabsorbable with excellent tensile strengths. Regression, which is the wound's tendency to assume its prior shape, seems to be very similar regardless of the type of suture used. Wound regression seems mostly dependent on the size of the wound (the smaller the wound the less regression) and if sutures are interrupted, continuous, or single. Limbal wounds are closed with either interrupted or continuous sutures. Scleral wounds are closed with continuous or single-stitch suturing (Figures 10–31 and 10–32). The recent scleral wounds with

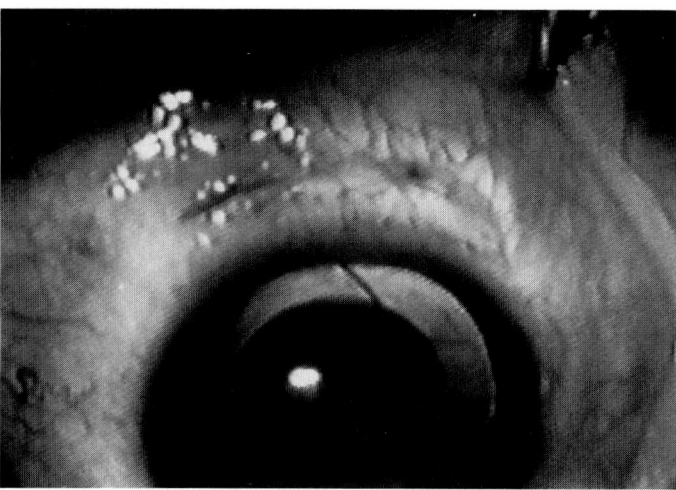

FIGURE 10–31. Running "bootlace" suture.

an internal flap into clear cornea may be left unsutured because they self-seal (Figures 10–33 and 10–34). Single-stitch and no-stitch wounds seem to create the least regression. However, because of the existence of regression, some surgeons combine cataract extraction with astigmatic keratotomy (AK).

## — CASE CONCLUSION

On completion of surgery, some cataract surgeons inject either subconjunctival steroid or steroid in combination with antibiotics. There is no proof that the use of these injections prevents postoperative endophthalmitis or lessens postoperative inflammation. Most patients receive topical applications of steroids and antibiotics plus, in some cases, pressure-lowering drops or pills (carbonic anhydrase inhibitors). A light patch is placed on the eye (Figure 10–35). Some surgeons also use oral antibiotics for a day or two postoperatively. In our setting, one drop of the antibiotic/steroid combination agent, Maxitrol (dexamethasone, neomycin sulfate, polymyxin B sulfate), and one drop of the beta-blocker, betaxolol 0.5% (Betagan) are given, unless the patient's history precludes their use. We also dispense five 250-mg capsules of cephalexin to

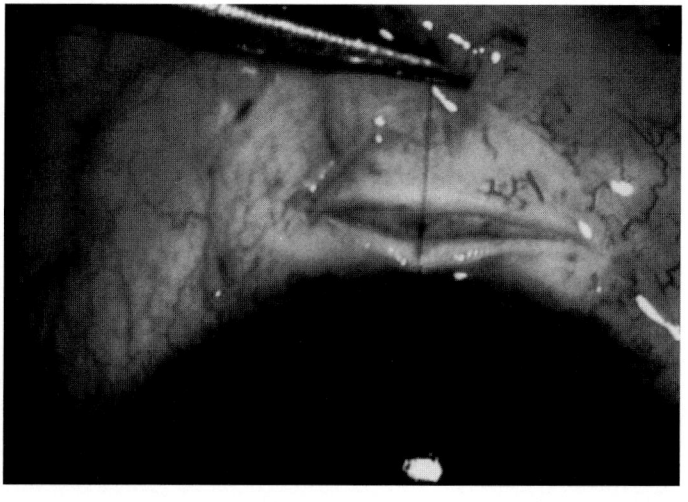

FIGURE 10–32. "One-stitch" incisional closure.

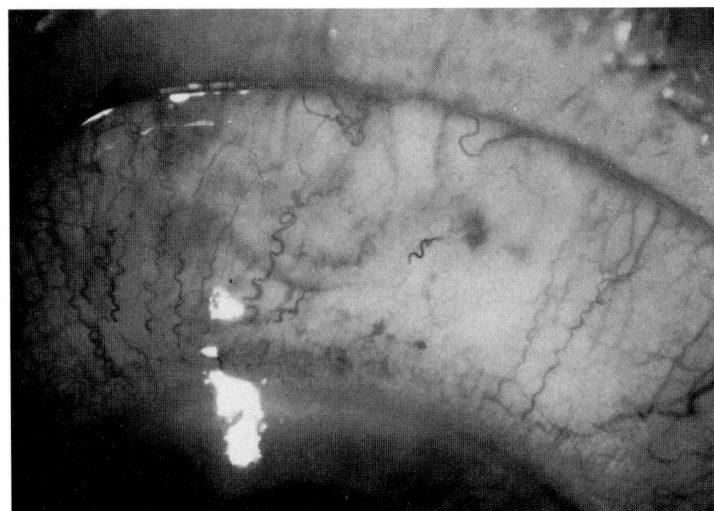

**FIGURE 10–33.** "Sutureless" or "no-stitch" wound with self-sealing corneal flap.

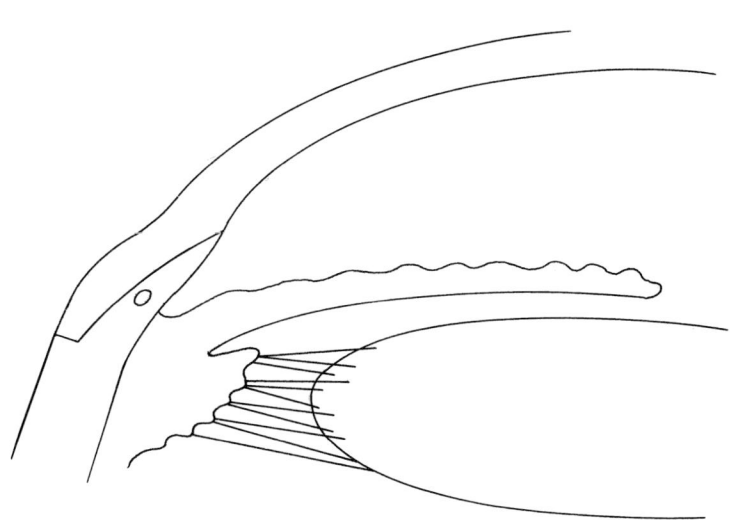

**FIGURE 10–34.** Cross section of Figure 10–33.

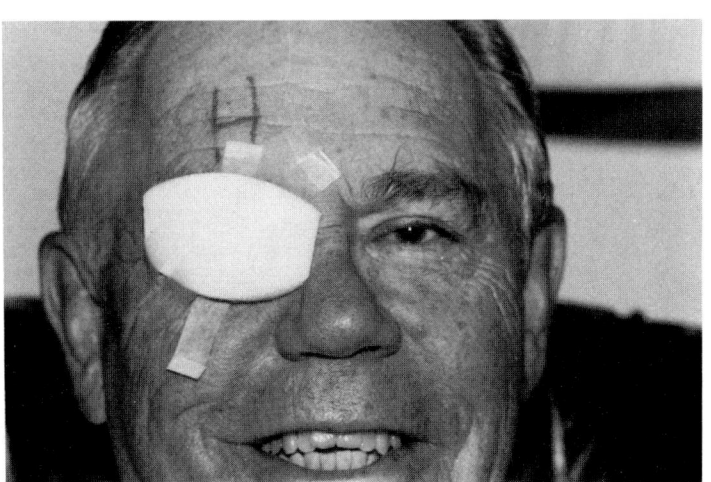

**FIGURE 10–35.** Application of a light patch immediately postoperatively.

be taken orally every 6–8 hours unless the patient reports allergies to this drug (see Appendix 7).

In our setting, the patient is called during the evening of the day of surgery to monitor his or her progress and to address questions. We have found this to be both clinically and emotionally rewarding.

## REFERENCES

1. Ridley H: Intraocular acrylic lenses. *Trans Ophthalmol Soc UK*. 1951;**71**:617–621.
2. Kelman CD: Phacoemulsification and aspiration: A new technique of cataract removal—A preliminary report. *Am J Ophthalmol*. 1967;**64**:23–35.
3. Wasserman D, Apple DJ, Castenada VE, et al: Anterior capsular tears and loop fixation of posterior chamber intraocular lenses. *Ophthalmology*. 1991;**98**:425–431.
4. Assia EI, Apple DJ, Barden A, et al: An experimental study comparing various anterior capsulotomy techniques. *Arch Ophthalmol*. 1991;**109**:642–647.
5. Assia EI, Legler UFC, Merrill C, et al: Clinicopathologic study of the effect of radial tears and loop fixation on intraocular lens decentration. *Ophthalmology*. 1993;**100**:153–158.
6. Glasser DB, Katz NR, Boyd JE, et al: Protective effects of viscous solutions in phacoemulsification and traumatic lens implantation. *Ophthalmology*. 1989;**107**:1047–1051.
7. Glasser DB, Osborn DC, Nordeen JF, Min Y: Endothelial protection and viscoelastic retention during phacoemulsification and intraocular lens implantation. *Arch Ophthalmol*. 1991;**109**:1438–1440.
8. Castenada VE, Legler UFC, Tsai JC: Posterior continuous curvilinear capsulorhexis: An experimental study with clinical applications. *Ophthalmology*. 1992;**99**:45–50.

# Special Surgical Considerations

CHAPTER

11

Often patients will present to the eye doctor with visual complaints that are not related to a "straightforward" cataract. These patients may have problems such as aphakic contact lens or spectacle intolerance, uncorrected aphakia, malpositioned intraocular lens (IOL), glaucoma, or corneal problems in addition to cataract. A patient may present with a cataract but be so myopic that no postoperative correction is indicated; namely, they are aphakically plano. There is also the consideration of whether to implant an IOL in patients with a history of iritis or other intraocular inflammatory disease. These patients require very careful consideration preoperatively because they represent a deviation from the norm. The history must be thorough, examination compulsively performed, and the patient extensively counseled regarding their situation (see Chapter 7).

## SECONDARY INTRAOCULAR LENS IMPLANTS

Secondary implantation is becoming less frequent due to the virtual disappearance of intracapsular cataract extraction (ICCE) without implantation of IOL. Eventually, secondary IOLs may be a thing of the past. In the meantime, knowledge of the procedure is helpful (see Chapter 8).

Secondary implants may be implanted either into the anterior chamber or posterior chamber. Anterior chamber implants are by far more common. Posterior chamber implants may be fixated in the posterior chamber by suturing the lens optic or haptics to the midperipheral iris or the apices of the haptics through the sclera via the ciliary sulcus.[1] If the posterior capsule is even partially intact, a posterior chamber IOL may be placed in the sulcus.[2]

Preoperative evaluation for anterior chamber IOL implantation needs to establish the health of the angle, including the presence of peripheral anterior synechiae (PAS), the presence and position of iridectomy(ies), type of iridectomy (peripheral versus sector), and whether vitreous is in the anterior chamber (see Chapter 7). The procedure for implantation of an anterior chamber IOL is similar to cataract extraction on a primary cataract. The differences in technique have to do with whether an anterior vitrectomy is indicated, orientation of the IOL, location of the wound, possible use of viscoelastic, and possible use of sutures to close the wound.

Generally, the wound made in secondary anterior chamber IOLs may be centered at the 12-o'clock position, which is the traditional site of entry for cataract surgery. Should the patient have a significant amount of postoperative astigmatism from the first surgery, the surgeon may elect to move the entry wound to be able to alter that astigmatism.[3] The wound may be constructed to be self-sealing, although this might depend on the amount of scarring from the previous surgery.

Whether or not to do vitrectomy is a highly individual decision made by the surgeon. Generally, the presence of vitreous in the anterior chamber requires an anterior vitrectomy to avoid "snagging" the vitreous with the IOL haptic or to prevent prolapse of the vitreous through the wound. Vitreous strands may also deform the pupil. In addition, a vitrectomy may help avoid vitreous traction and subsequent postoperative chronic cystoid macular edema (CME) (Figures 11–1 and 11–2).

Vitrectomy requires extra steps, extra planning, and sometimes results in specific postoperative and intraoperative complications. Vitreous traction during the vitrectomy is capable of tugging on the retina and choroid. This may

**FIGURES 11–1 AND 11–2.** Anterior vitrectomy in an aphakic eye, prior to placing an IOL.

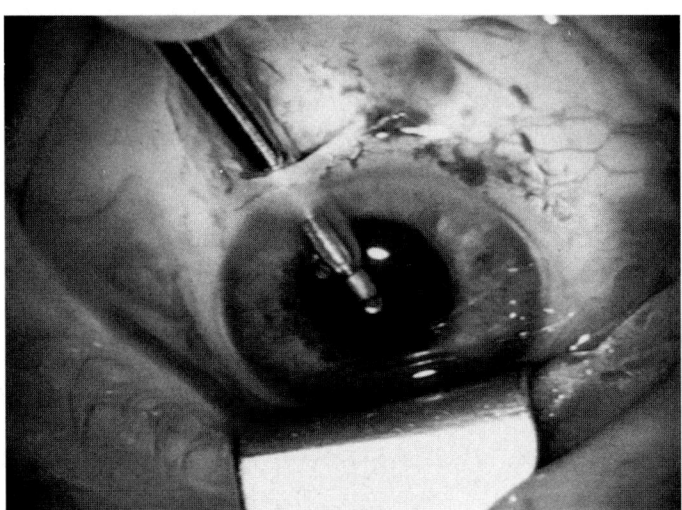

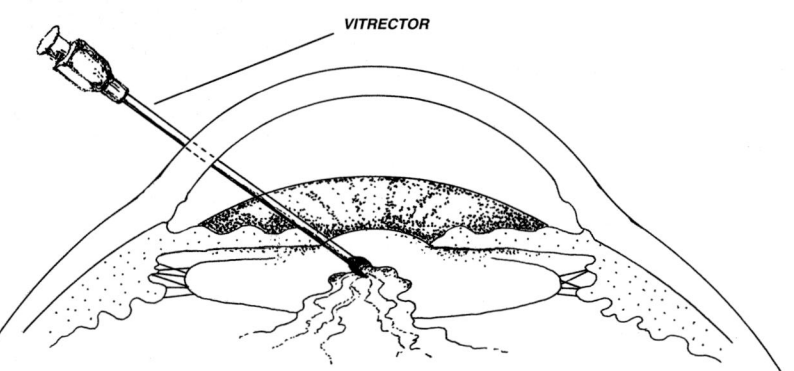

result in retinal detachment or choroidal hemorrhaging. If not already present, an iridectomy is usually performed with a vitrectomy, which may result in bleeding as well as a misshaped pupil. Additionally, the vitreous may protrude through the wound at the time of surgery, but not be visible to the surgeon. Postoperatively, this can result in a wound leak, risk of endophthalmitis, or chronic CME.

Following the vitrectomy, the surgeon either injects air or viscoelastic to maintain the anterior chamber. This may also be done by constant infusion of balanced salt solution (BSS) from a side port. Viscoelastic is the most protective way of maintaining the anterior chamber, but it does require removal by irrigation and aspiration to prevent postoperative problems such as high intraocular pressure and iritis.

The next step is to insert the IOL. Most surgeons use a flexible IOL because it has been shown to be the most trouble free of the anterior chamber IOLs. The IOL that is inserted through the wound into the anterior chamber has three- or four-point fixation[4] (Figures 11–3 and 11–4). Most surgeons will then rotate the IOL to orient the haptics as far away as possible from an iridectomy, angle fibrosis, or other anterior segment abnormality. This usually means that the haptics are oriented horizontally, since iridectomies are generally found in the superior quadrant.

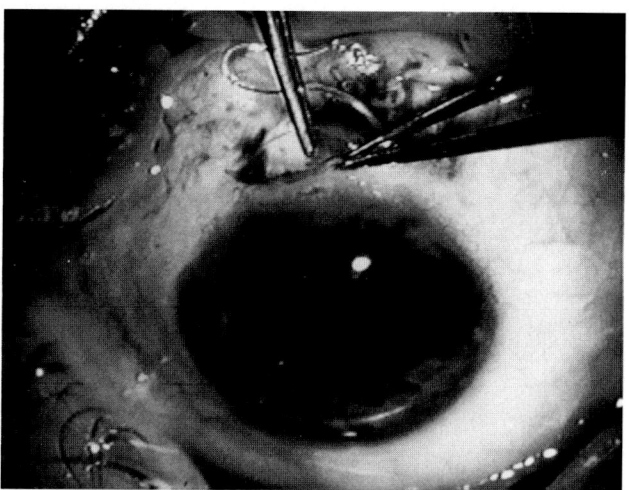
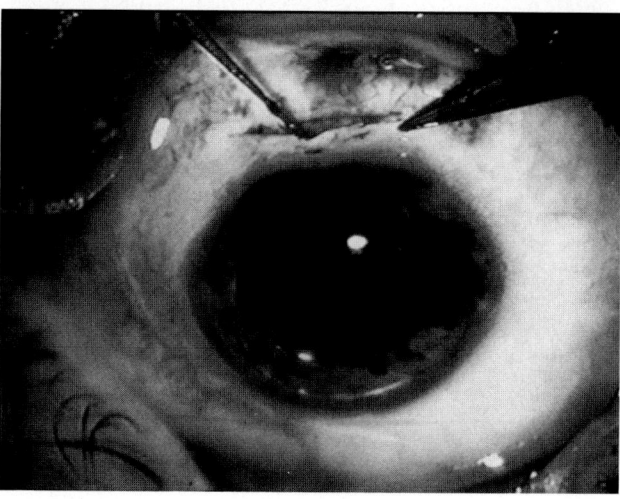

**FIGURES 11–3 AND 11–4.** Insertion of secondary anterior chamber IOL into an aphakic eye.

Following insertion of the IOL, viscoelastic, if used, is removed, pressure is reestablished in the eye, and wound integrity is inspected to ensure watertightness in sutureless wounds. The eye is also inspected once it is pressurized to make certain that there is no pupillary block. Should there be pupillary block, then further vitrectomy or another iridectomy may be performed.

The advantages of secondary implants over aphakic spectacles are well known. The secondary IOL creates a normal image size and field of vision not possible with aphakic spectacles.[4] The advantage of secondary implants over contact lenses is that the risk of contact lens–induced corneal pathology is avoided. The care and management of contact lenses becomes increasingly more difficult for elderly patients; therefore, contact lens handling problems can be solved with secondary IOLs.

The greatest disadvantages of secondary IOL implantations have to do with the risks related to undergoing surgery. These are very similar to the risks of primary cataract surgery, with the addition of problems related to vitreous prolapse and vitrectomy. Intraoperative corneal complications are rare in secondary IOL surgery.

Long-term problems with anterior chamber IOLs are related to the fact that the haptics rest against the angle structures. These may be divided into problems from inflammation, rise in intraocular pressure, and hemorrhaging (see Chapters 14–16). Chronic or recurrent iritis is one of the more annoying long-term problems with secondary implants. Constant contact between the iris and IOL may be the cause of this inflammatory response requiring chronic anti-inflammatory therapy. Sizing is very important in secondary implants. Implants that are too large or too small may be sources of irritation. An implant that is too large results in progressive erosion of the iris and angle adhesions. Recurrent microhyphema or gross hyphema may result. This was observed so frequently with early rigid implants that it was termed uveitis, glaucoma, hyphema (UGH) syndrome. Explantation of the implant was usually necessary. An implant that is too small may result in excessive pseudophacodonesis. If severe, it has been called the windshield wiper syndrome. Excessive movement of an anterior chamber IOL results in iritis and possible movement of the haptics into iridectomies with resultant problems such as decreased vision from a decentered lens, chronic iritis, and CME.

## CATARACT EXTRACTION WITHOUT IOL

There are three situations where a cataract may be removed without implanting an IOL at the time of surgery: The patient may have a history of chronic iritis, the refractive status of the patient may be such that the desired IOL power is near plano, or the patient may not want an IOL.

Debate over implantation of an IOL in a patient with chronic iritis still exists. Most clinicians in private practice, and especially those who do many cataract surgeries, will implant an IOL in a patient with quiescent chronic iritis (see Chapter 7). Since most of the IOL is covered by the capsule, the technique of doing continuous tear anterior capsulotomy (capsulorhexis) as opposed to can-opener capsulotomy greatly reduces the risk of postoperative inflammation related to exposure of the IOL surface to circulating antibodies. Surface-modified IOLs may make this issue moot someday, but the reality is that it is a judgment call as to whether iritis patients should have lenses implanted at the present time. When an IOL is implanted in an iritis patient, additional preoperative, intraoperative, and postoperative steroids may be recommended by the surgeon.

In the case of a highly myopic eye, a reasonable course of action would be not to implant an IOL. However, most surgeons prefer to put in an IOL after cataract removal to "stabilize the system." The presence of an IOL in an eye after cataract removal helps to maintain the integrity of the iris-lens diaphragm, which makes the vitreous more stable and possibly lessens the risk of retinal detachment and other problems from vitreous instability. This especially holds true if the patient needs a capsulotomy at a future date. Without an IOL in place, vitreous prolapse is a possibility following capsulotomy. Plano IOLs are available on special order for this purpose.

A surgeon may elect not to implant an IOL during a cataract extraction with a surgical "misadventure." This is a very individual decision that calls into play many factors at the time of the actual surgery. Hence, it is difficult to sit in judgment or comment on those situations.

Occasionally, a patient may wish not to have an implant when their cataract is removed. This is becoming less common. Efforts should be made to educate the patient fully of the postoperative situation if no IOL is implanted.

## EXPLANTATION OF IOLS

Several thousand IOL explantations are performed in the United States every year. With improved surgical techniques and improved IOL technology, this is becoming much less common. The majority of explantations are done on anterior chamber implants. The most common complications necessitating anterior chamber explantation are corneal decompensation (pseudophakic bullous keratopathy), angle closure with attendant pressure rise, hemorrhaging, dislocations, opacification of the media, persistent iritis or CME, persistent pain, and extrusion.[5] The reasons for anterior chamber IOL having these associated problems are a combination of design faults, manufacturing imperfections, associated pathology, and surgical technique.

Explantation of posterior chamber IOLs is far less common than anterior chamber IOL removal. However, problems with posterior chamber IOLs still exist. The major reasons for removing posterior chamber IOLs are dislocation, dioptric errors, and hemorrhaging.

When lens removal is necessary due to inflammation and its sequelae, lens malposition, or incorrect dioptric power, extreme care must be exercised.[5] The implant may be attached to iris, angle recess tissue, ciliary body, and/or lens capsule. The surgical technique requires careful dissection of these attachments to avoid excessive hemorrhage, iridodialysis, and cyclodialysis. The IOL optic may have to be removed separately from the haptics. The haptics may be removed in sections to extract them from their surrounding tissue fibrosis (Figure 11–5). In some cases of posterior chamber lens explantation, some portion of the loops may be left in place if it is not a source of further tissue damage.

The risks and benefits of lens explantation must be weighed carefully by the surgeon and with the patient. Both must feel that the potential intraoperative and postoperative complications are worth risking to remove the problems of the implant in question. Finally, a second decision as to whether the eye can tolerate a replacement IOL (exchange) must be made. In each case, this decision is individual and based on extent of already present tissue damage, coexistence of other eye disease, and patient wishes.

## COMBINED PROCEDURES

A combination of procedures in ophthalmology are named in terms of the number of conditions corrected at one time. For example, a triple procedure may involve penetrating keratoplasty, cataract extraction, and IOL implantation. Over the years, the philosophy of doing these procedures has changed from

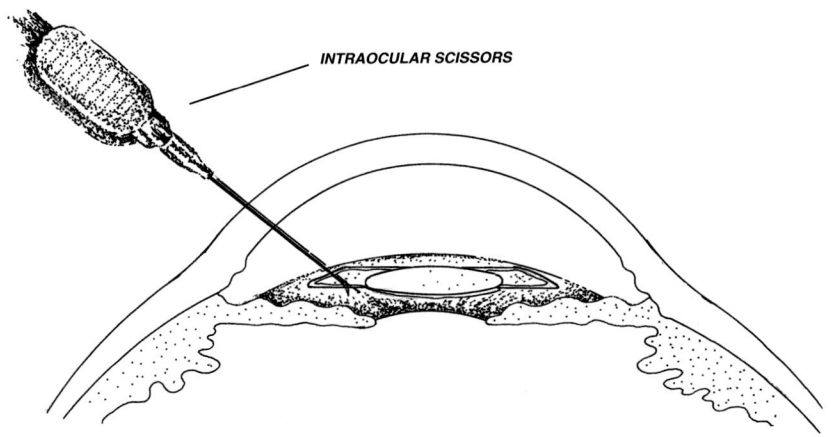

FIGURE 11–5. Cutting anterior chamber IOL haptics from the anterior chamber angle to allow IOL explantation.

avoiding them, for the most part, to becoming quite accepted at present. Improved technology, increased experience, and widespread communications of outcomes are responsible for the change in attitude.

## Trabeculectomy with Cataract Extraction and IOL Implantation

Combining cataract surgery with a trabeculectomy would seem to be a natural surgical maneuver whereby intraocular pressure could be controlled in the immediate as well as long-term postoperative period, along with providing improved vision from cataract removal (Figure 11–6). (See Color Plate 11–1.) However, there has been a fair amount of resistance to this idea over the years. This may have been an outgrowth of the fact that early IOLs (irido-capsular fixated lenses and anterior chamber IOLs) were frequently associated with glaucoma complications, specifically the UGH syndrome.

Nevertheless, surgeons are coming to the conclusion that successfully combining lens implantation with trabeculectomy is possible.[6-8] There is presently no majority opinion on the exact technique to use, but more surgeons are reporting the benefits of using capsulorhexis and phacoemulsification as the method of choice for cataract extraction when combining the two procedures.[9] The reason for this is because can-opener capsulotomy is associated with about

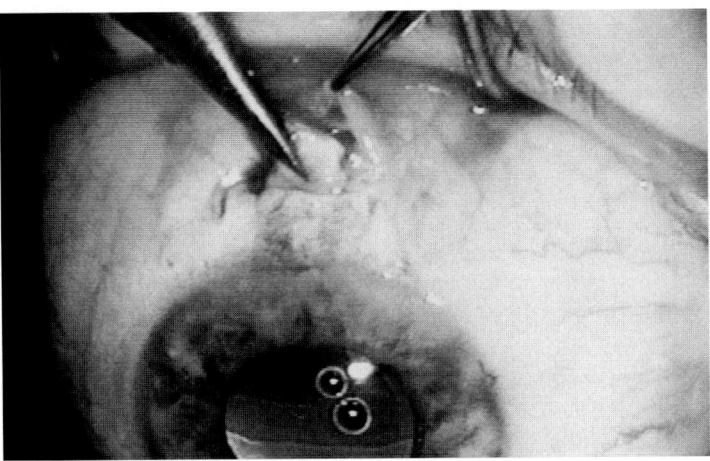

FIGURE 11–6. Combined ECCE, IOL implantation, and trabeculectomy.

70% chance of one or both of the IOL haptics resting in the sulcus. A posterior chamber lens in the sulcus may result in a tuck of the iris, pigment dispersion, erosion into an artery, forward displacement of the IOL, and intrusion of the angle, as well as pupillary block. Capsulorhexis is not associated with any of these difficulties; therefore, it makes intuitive sense to combine trabeculectomy with the continuous-tear capsulotomy to avoid all of these difficulties. In addition, when an IOL is placed in the capsular bag following capsulorhexis, the IOL is anatomically further from the iris allowing the angle to widen. Finally, the small incision used in phacoemulsification aids watertight conjunctival closure, decreases risk of suprachoroidal hemorrhage, and may make repeat trabeculectomy surgery easier, if necessary, at a later date.

The surgical technique involved is very similar to a standard cataract extraction by phacoemulsification and posterior lens implantation described in Chapter 10. Following insertion of the implant, a block of trabeculum is excised beneath the already present scleral flap. The scleral flap is then closed with two sutures that may be released postoperatively by argon laser if more filtration is necessary. Following removal of any viscoelastic, if used, the filter is tested for adequacy and the conjunctival flap is closed to watertightness.

The most obvious advantages of combining the procedures of trabeculectomy with cataract extraction and IOL implantation have to do with avoiding the risks associated with two separate procedures, the immediate increased visibility of the fundus following cataract extraction, and short- and long-term intraocular pressure control with fewer or no antiglaucoma medications.

The major disadvantage of combining these procedures is the required technical expertise. The greatest difficulties arise from the trabeculectomy. The success rate of trabeculectomy is not entirely encouraging and this is all the more true in the hands of a surgeon who routinely does not perform many trabeculectomies. The difficulties include how tightly to suture the scleral flap, postoperative pressure problems, and hyphemas. Following the surgery, close follow-up is necessary to determine if postoperative medications need adjusting, sutures need release, or antimetabolite injections are necessary to control the intraocular pressure and maintain a functioning filtering bleb.

## Penetrating Keratoplasty with Cataract Extraction and IOL Implantation

Penetrating keratoplasty (PK) is sometimes combined with cataract extraction and IOL implantation since PK alone has a tendency to worsen an already existing cataract (Figure 11–7). The majority of patients who need PK need it because of pseudophakic bullous keratopathy (PBK) or keratoconus. Those needing a combined PK with cataract extraction and IOL have decompensated or scarred corneas secondary to Fuchs' endothelial dystrophy, keratoconus, Chandler's syndrome, or trauma.[10] Most penetrating keratoplasties today are performed by corneal specialists. Usually the cataract is removed with the "opensky" technique; that is, when the corneal button has been removed, the cataract is removed by expression followed by removing the cortex by aspiration[11] (see Figures 11–7 and 11–8). The lens implant is inserted by suturing it in the posterior chamber, placing it in the capsular bag, or placing an anterior chamber IOL.[12] Then the new corneal tissue is attached.

It should be noted that variations of this technique are utilized for PK combined with IOL exchange and also PK combined with secondary IOL placement.[13]

Advantages of combined PK with cataract extraction and IOL implantation seem to be convenience, reduced risks and costs of one procedure, reduced risk to the graft, and quicker recovery of visual acuity.[14] Disadvantages are re-

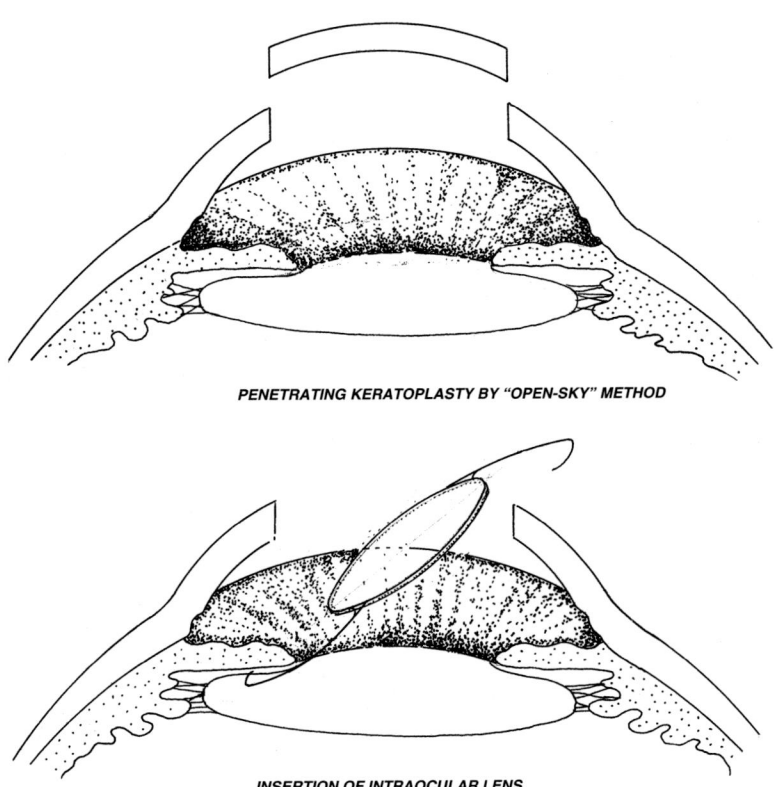

**FIGURES 11-7 AND 11-8.** Combined ECCE, IOL implantation, and penetrating keratoplasty by "open-sky" method.

ported to be possible worse unaided acuity, greater astigmatism, and anisometropia.[15]

## — THE TRAUMATIC CATARACT —

Removal of a traumatic cataract may be complicated by zonular ruptures and angle recession. Extensive zonular loss may prevent the use of phacoemulsification. In that situation, either expression or intracapsular surgery may be performed (Figure 11-9). The extent of zonular integrity determines whether a pos-

**FIGURE 11-9.** Traumatic cataract removal by ICCE.

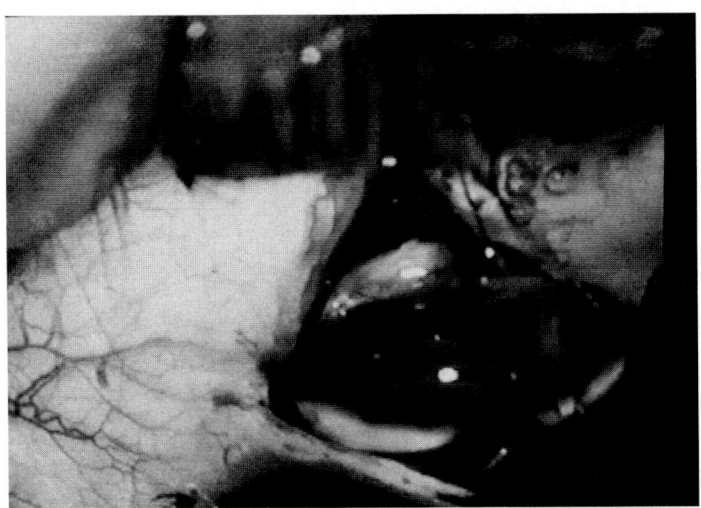

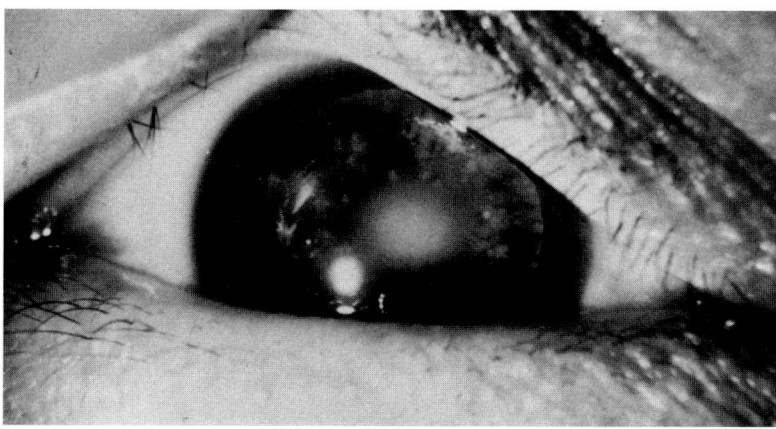

**FIGURE 11–10.** Subluxated lens.

terior chamber IOL may be placed.[2] If there is not enough structural integrity to the posterior capsule to support an IOL, the use of an anterior chamber or posterior chamber IOL sutured to the sclera may be necessary.[1,3] With significant angle recession, especially in the presence of already elevated intraocular pressure, the implantation of an anterior chamber IOL may be contraindicated because of the risk to intraocular pressure control.

## CONGENITAL LENS DISLOCATIONS

Congenital diseases, such as collagen disorders, that affect zonular integrity resulting in dislocation of the lens are rare. However, if present, dislocation usually worsens throughout life (Figure 11–10). Complete dislocation may be treated with refractive care alone, whereas partial dislocation is more of a problem due to variability in the location of the lens. In the case of partial dislocation, Nd:YAG (neodymium:yttrium-aluminum-garnet) laser has been used to further disrupt the remaining zonules and thereby dislocate the lens out of the visual axis.

Surgically removing the lens may be approached either from the anterior or posterior aspect. The posterior approach allows more control on account of constant infusion of fluid during the procedure. The anterior approach requires the use of ICCE, since the zonules are not strong enough to allow either expression or phacoemulsification. Intracapsular cataract extraction of a dislocated lens not only diminishes control of the intraocular environment but also may be complicated by the presence of vitreous prolapse. When vitreous interferes with the cryoextraction process, a vitrectomy must be performed. This may result in further dislocation of the lens into the vitreous cavity.

Removal of congenitally dislocated lenses is usually not accompanied by implantation of IOLs. These patients are mostly young, so a lens implant is not advised. An IOL may be considered in some circumstances as the patient matures.

## REFERENCES

1. Stark WJ, Gottsch JD, Goodman DF, et al: Posterior chamber intraocular lens implantation in the absence of capsular support. *Arch Ophthalmol.* 1989;**107**:1078–1083.
2. Smiddy WE, Avery R: Posterior chamber IOL implantation with suboptimal posterior capsular support. *Ophthalmic Surg.* 1991;**22**:16–19.

3. Balyeat HD: Secondary lens implantation. In Cangelosi GC (ed): *Advances in Cataract Surgery: New Orleans Academy of Ophthalmology*. Thorofare, NJ: Slack; 1990:147–156.
4. Jaffe NS, Jaffe MS, Jaffe GF: *Cataract Surgery and Its Complications*, 5th ed. St Louis: CV Mosby; 1990:140–145,200.
5. Apple DJ, Mamalis N, Olson RJ, Kincaid MC: *Intraocular Lenses: Evolution, Designs, Complications and Pathology*. Baltimore: Williams & Wilkins; 1989;80–90,387–402.
6. Simmons ST, Litoff D, Nichols DA, et al: Extracapsular cataract extraction and posterior chamber intraocular lens implantation combined with trabeculectomy in patients with glaucoma. *Am J Ophthalmol.* 1987;**104**:465–470.
7. Krupin T, Feitl ME, Bishop KI: Postoperative intraocular pressure rise in open-angle glaucoma patients after cataract or combined cataract filtration surgery. *Ophthalmology.* 1989;**96**:579–584.
8. Longstaff S, Wormald RPL, Mazover A, Hitchings RA: Glaucoma triple procedures: Efficacy of intraocular pressure control and visual outcome. *Ophthalmic Surg.* 1990;**21**:786–793.
9. Samuelson TW, Lindstrom RL: Combined glaucoma filtration surgery and phacoemulsification. *Semin Ophthalmol.* 1992;**17**:279–285.
10. Sanford DK, Klesges LM, Wood TO: Simultaneous penetrating keratoplasty, extracapsular cataract extraction, and intraocular lens implantation. *J Cataract Refract Surg.* 1991;**17**:824–829.
11. Kaufman HE: Combined keratoplasty and cataract extraction. *Am J Ophthalmol.* 1974;**77**:824–829.
12. Groden LR: Continuous tear capsulotomy and phacoemulsification cataract extraction combined with penetrating keratoplasty. *Refract Corneal Surg.* 1990;6:458–459.
13. Hassan TS, Soong HK, Sugar A, Meyer RF: Implantation of Kelman-style, open-loop anterior chamber lenses during keratoplasty for aphakic and pseudophakic bullous keratopathy. *Ophthalmology.* 1991;**98**:875–880.
14. Binder PS: Intraocular lens implantation after penetrating keratoplasty. *Refract Corneal Surg.* 1989;**5**:224–230.
15. Geggel HS: Intraocular lens implantation after penetrating keratoplasty: Improved unaided visual acuity, astigmatism, and safety in patients with combined corneal disease and cataract. *Ophthalmology.* 1990;**97**:1460–1467.

# Intraoperative Complications

## CHAPTER 12

Were it not for intraoperative complications, the experience of performing cataract surgery would indeed be a delight all the time. Complications unfortunately are the nemesis of every surgeon regardless of expertise. Increasing surgical experience usually translates to decreasing intraoperative complications. The fewer the intraoperative complications, the less stormy the postoperative course. Certain postoperative complications may or may not be the direct result of problems during surgery. For example, endophthalmitis may occur even with flawless surgery. Technique-dependent postoperative problems include intraocular lens (IOL) decentration/dislocations, iris damage/pupil deformation, vitreous changes, corneal problems, and inadvertent bleb formation. Retinal problems such as cystoid macular edema (CME) and retinal detachment (RD) may or may not be technique dependent.

## RETROBULBAR HEMORRHAGE

Retrobulbar anesthesia is performed by introducing the needle into the muscle cone and depositing anesthetic. Owing to the vascularity of this space, there is an increased risk of piercing a blood vessel and causing retrobulbar hemorrhage (Figure 12–1). In addition, complications such as optic nerve injury, globe perforations, central retinal artery occlusion, intravascular injection of embolic material, and central nervous system effect may be encountered with retrobulbar anesthesia.[1-3] Recent changes in local anesthesia for cataract removal include the switch from retrobulbar injection to peribulbar injection, thereby decreasing the risk of retrobulbar hemorrhage. Peribulbar anesthesia usually deposits anesthetic in the less vascularized inferior-lateral compartment of the orbit, but any extraconal space may be used. Additional anesthetic may be injected in the inferior medial space or superior to the globe. We have found the peribulbar approach to be much safer. Since beginning its use in 1989 we have

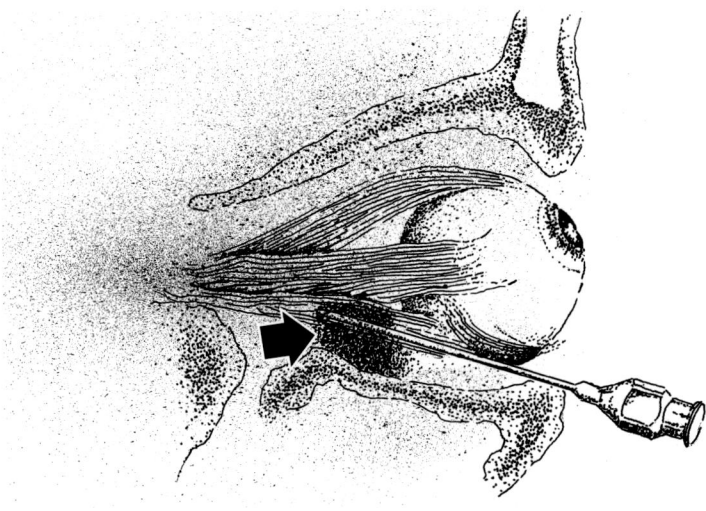

FIGURE 12-1. Intraoperative retrobulbar hemorrhage.

had no cases of optic atrophy, globe perforations, nor blindness secondary to peribulbar anesthesia.

Retrobulbar hemorrhages vary in severity. Mild to moderate hemorrhage is not of grave concern, and in fact, surgery may often be completed without incident.[1] A retrobulbar hemorrhage results in increased orbital volume, which causes increased intraocular pressure. At the time of surgery, this translates to anterior displacement of the iris-lens diaphragm (posterior pressure). The increased posterior pressure increases the risk of posterior capsule rupture and vitreous loss. If these occur, it may be necessary to implant an anterior chamber lens.

A severe retrobulbar hemorrhage, with significant displacement of the globe anteriorly (proptosis) is of great concern, and usually surgery is delayed for a period of time. With severe hemorrhage, the intraocular pressure will be significantly elevated, with danger to the optic nerve. To relieve the intraocular pressure, a lateral canthotomy may be performed (Figure 12-2). If the intraocular pressure is not lowered to a safe level, then a drainage procedure may have to be performed. A serious sequela of retrobulbar hemorrhage is damage to the optic nerve with subsequent optic atrophy. Sometimes the loss

FIGURE 12-2. Lateral canthotomy.

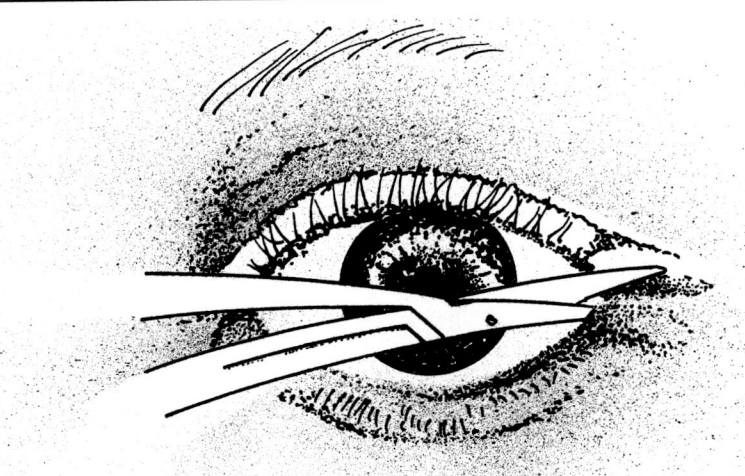

of vision may be complete; in which case, the eye would manifest an amaurotic pupil.

## CHOROIDAL HEMORRHAGE

Choroidal hemorrhages are rare with present-day cataract surgery, especially with small-incision phacoemulsification. The excellent control of the intraocular environment with small incisions has contributed greatly to the reduction of this unfortunate complication. Choroidal hemorrhages vary in severity from being hardly noticeable to being so severe that complete expulsion of the intraocular contents occurs. The risk of choroidal hemorrhage is dependent on associated ocular disease, systemic factors, and surgical technique.[4] Choroidal hemorrhages are most common in patients with preoperative glaucoma, especially if the postoperative pressure is low. Choroidal sclerosis is thought to be a factor in choroidal hemorrhage. Systemic hypertension is a factor in the risk of choroidal hemorrhage as well. The higher the systolic blood pressure at the time of surgery, the more likely the patient is to bleed. Finally, the more complicated the surgery, the longer the procedure, and the more tissue disruption that occurs, the greater the chance for hemorrhage.

## POSTERIOR CAPSULAR TEARS/ VITREOUS LOSS

Fear of damage to the posterior capsule during the process of phacoemulsification represents one of the greatest barriers to its acceptance by surgeons. Many factors contribute to, or increase the likelihood of, posterior capsule rupture. These include physician experience and expertise, density of the cataract, posterior segment pressure, strength of the posterior capsule, and mechanical factors. Physician experience and expertise are usually directly proportional; the more the experience overall, the greater the expertise. Capsulorhexis in the presence of a posterior capsular tear has the advantage over can-opener capsulotomy in that even though the posterior capsular integrity is compromised, there is an intact anterior capsule ring (or tire) to allow for posterior chamber implantation. In that case, the implant would be placed in the sulcus as opposed to the bag.

The density of cataract, especially nuclear sclerosis, contributes greatly to the chance of breaking the capsule. With increasing density, the posterior capsule is broken more often. However, the surgeon with greater expertise may perform phacoemulsification on denser cataracts with less structural damage to the eye. In extremely dense nuclear sclerotic cataracts, nuclear expression may be done rather than phacoemulsification to avoid damage to the posterior capsule.

Vitreous loss secondary to broken posterior capsule is one of the most common intraoperative complications during phacoemulsification (Figure 12–3). If the posterior capsule breaks, vitrectomy may have to be done to reduce the risk of vitreous traction, incarceration into the wound, and their associated complications (see Chapters 14 to 16).

## ZONULAR RUPTURE

Rupture of the zonules occurs occasionally even in nontraumatic cataracts. This may occur anywhere, but is more common superiorly from phacoemulsifica-

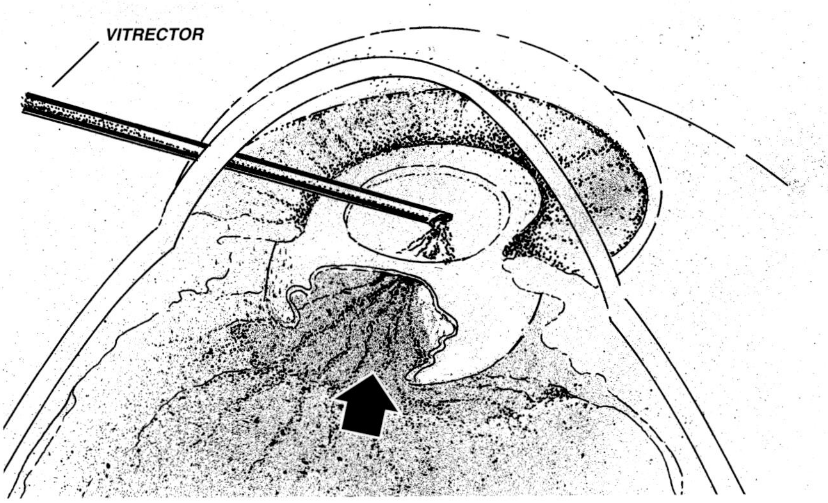

**FIGURE 12–3.** Vitreous loss following capsular bag rupture during phacoemulsification.

tion and inferiorly from the suction of expression of the nucleus. Minimal disruption of zonules does not preclude implantation of a posterior chamber lens in the capsular bag,[5] but extensive damage requires placement of an anterior chamber or sutured posterior chamber IOL.

## DESCEMET'S DETACHMENT

Descemet's membrane may be torn and detached during cataract extraction. Small amounts of detached Descemet's membrane are not uncommon and do not interfere with the postoperative recovery of vision. Moderate or more severe detachments of Descemet's membrane may be repaired by injection of air into the anterior chamber, which is then left to absorb unaided postoperatively. Viscoelastics left to absorb, a combination of air and viscoelastics, or suturing also may be used to repair Descemet's detachments (Figure 12–4).

Should a large portion of Descemet's membrane be lost, postoperative acuity may be affected due to residual corneal edema.

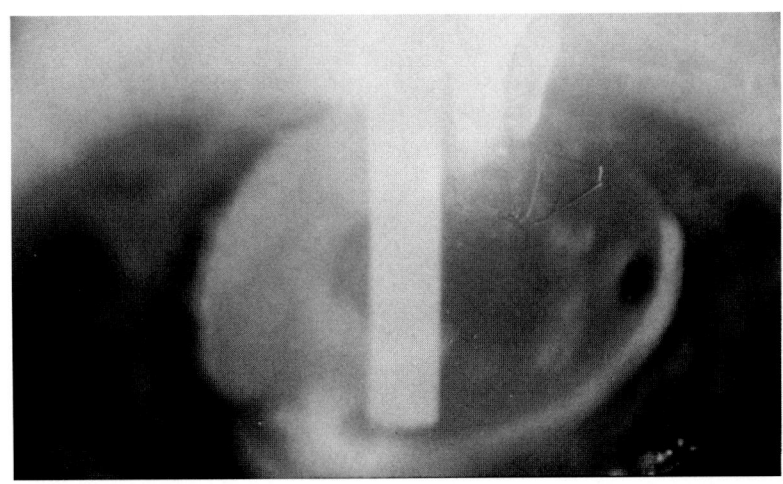

**FIGURE 12–4.** Descemet's detachment.

## REFERENCES

1. Goldsmith MO: Occlusion of the central retinal artery following retrobulbar hemorrhage. *Ophthalmologica*. 1967;**153**:191–196.
2. Klein ML, Jampol LM, Condon PI, et al: Central retinal artery occlusion without retrobulbar hemorrhage after retrobulbar anesthesia. *Am J Ophthalmol*. 1982;**93**:573–577.
3. Mieler WF, Bennett SR, Platt LW, Roenig LW: Localized retinal detachment with combined central retinal artery and vein occlusion after retrobulbar anesthesia. *Retina*. 1990:**10**:278–283.
4. Beyer CF, Peymon GA, Hill JM: Expulsive choroidal hemorrhage in rabbits: A histopathologic study. *Arch Ophthalmol*. 1989;**107:**1648–1653.
5. Smiddy WE, Avery R: Posterior chamber intraocular lens implantation with suboptimal posterior capsular support. *Ophthalmic Surg*. 1991;**22**:16–19.

# Postoperative Care

## SECTION IV

# Uncomplicated Course, Visits, and Procedures

CHAPTER 13

The normal inflammatory signs and symptoms that accompany cataract surgery have a wide spectrum of presentations that dissipate quickly during the postoperative course. Although there are as many distinct variations in the examining sequence of postoperative patients as there are doctors, there remain certain procedures and examining schemes they all share.[1-4] In our clinics, uncomplicated postoperative patients are typically seen at 1 day, 1 week, approximately 3 weeks if signs or symptoms dictate, and 5 weeks. A dilated fundus examination is recommended for at least one of these visits. We also recommend an examination within 6–12 months and yearly thereafter. (See Appendix 3.)

## FIRST VISIT—DAY 1

The patch is removed if not already done so by the patient. The timing of patch removal is a function of the duration of the anesthetic used during the surgery. In our setting, we have the patient remove the patch at bedtime, when the eye has had some return of sensation, motility, and lid function. The patch also may be left on until the morning of the first day examination. A history is taken to find out how comfortable the patient was during the night (Table 13–1). If there are any lingering questions about the surgery, the postoperative medications, or instructions, these are identified at this time.

### Symptoms

The patient undergoing an uneventful surgery is usually quite comfortable on the first day. There is often a report of mild foreign body sensation, itching, mild tearing, or a complaint of redness, glare, photophobia, and occasionally an increase in floaters. Any report of pain should be carefully investigated. Most patients reporting pain have a corneal abrasion. These patients usually describe

**TABLE 13–1. EXAMINATION RECOMMENDATIONS: FIRST VISIT**

History: comfort, vision
Visual acuity: unaided and pinhole if worse than 20/80
Pupils
Biomicroscopy
Intraocular pressure
Fundus examination if unexplained vision loss

being more comfortable by the time of the examination compared with during the night unless the abrasion is quite large. Any residual discomfort is usually relieved by topical anesthetic instilled during the examination. In patients with severe pain that kept them awake during the night, a possible intraocular pressure spike or endophthalmitis must be ruled out by careful examination (see Chapter 14).

Diplopia may occur and is transient and lasts up to a day or two in most patients. Rarely, it may be intermittent for several weeks. Reassurance is the best therapy, and the patient should be encouraged to restrict activities until the diplopia resolves.

Occasionally, a patient may report mild local neuralgia along the face and top of the head secondary to anesthesia. In addition, it is not uncommon for patients to report a peripheral "arc" or "crescent" of light. This is commonly due to residual pupillary dilation and reflections off the edge of the intraocular lens (IOL). This should be differentiated from the signs and symptoms of vitreoretinal traction.

Patient reactions range from being pleasantly surprised to very disappointed by their visual acuity on the day #1 examination. Assuming normal examination findings, those with poor vision need to be reassured that this is not a prediction of their eventual visual outcome.

## Signs

### Visual Acuity

Unaided visual acuity may be quite variable due to immediate postoperative inflammation. Pinhole acuity, when taken, is a much more accurate estimate of the eventual postoperative acuity, as it is not as affected by corneal edema and anterior chamber inflammation. If the visual acuity is poor but all other day #1 signs and symptoms are within normal limits, the patient should be reassured that this is not unexpected.

In our setting, expected day #1 visual acuity ranges from 20/20 to 20/100. Most patients with an expected 20/20 final visual acuity are in the range of 20/30 to 20/60.

### Intraocular Pressure

Intraocular pressure may be taken before or after the doctor inspects the eye depending on preference. Noncontact tonometry may be the technique of choice until a wound leak is ruled out by biomicroscopy. Many doctors wish to view the eye prior to fluorescein instillation to judge anterior chamber inflammation accurately. On the first day of an uneventful postoperative course, the intraocular pressure may range from the mid single digits to the mid 20s. Patients with higher pressures are candidates for hypotensive therapy (see

Chapter 14) and lower pressures may indicate a wound leak, ciliary body shutdown, and/or choroidal detachment (see Chapter 14).

### Lids

A small amount of ptosis, often 1–2 mm, is not uncommon. Ptosis of greater than 2 mm is found in some cases and will usually resolve over a period of days to weeks. Surgery may be indicated in those cases of incomplete resolution after 3–6 months (see Chapters 15 to 16).

Ecchymosis is seen occasionally depending on the amount of periocular hemorrhage secondary to local anesthetic injection. This often resolves within a 2-week period or less. (See Color Plate 13–1.)

## Biomicroscopy (Table 13–2; Figures 13–1 and 13–2)

### Conjunctiva

Injection is very common, even to severe degrees, in uncomplicated cases.

Subconjunctival hemorrhage is usually most severe over the incision but may be circumcorneal. The hemorrhagic component will typically disappear in less than 2 weeks and conjunctival vessel injection may persist over the wound area for approximately a month. Conjunctival edema is often mild but may be moderate to severe and cause tissue dissection This edema usually disappears in a few days but may reoccur or persist due to topical medication reaction.

### Cornea

The cornea epithelium is examined for abrasions, which range from superficial erosions to large full-thickness defects. Many patients reporting minor to moderate foreign body sensation on the night of the surgery are found to have a resolving corneal abrasion (Figure 13–3). These patients may be treated with the normal postoperative medications and need not be patched, as they will completely reepithelialize before the first postoperative day is complete.

The corneal epithelium may show a small amount of edema that quickly resolves. There may be epithelial microcystic edema if there is moderate to severe stromal edema with or without high intraocular pressure. The corneal stroma may show small amounts of edema in the uncomplicated course that will dissipate in a few days. Descemet's folds, or striae, are often seen on a day #1 examination and resolve quickly in most cases. In our experience, superior corneal edema that occurs from the limbus to the mid cornea may be found in scleral tunnel incisions with "no-stitch" surgery due to localized endothelial trauma.

**TABLE 13–2. BIOMICROSCOPY: POSTOPERATIVE EXAMINATION**

Cornea
Anterior chamber reaction and depth
Iris and pupil
Intraocular lens
Capsule
Wound
Stereoscopic vitreoretinal examination

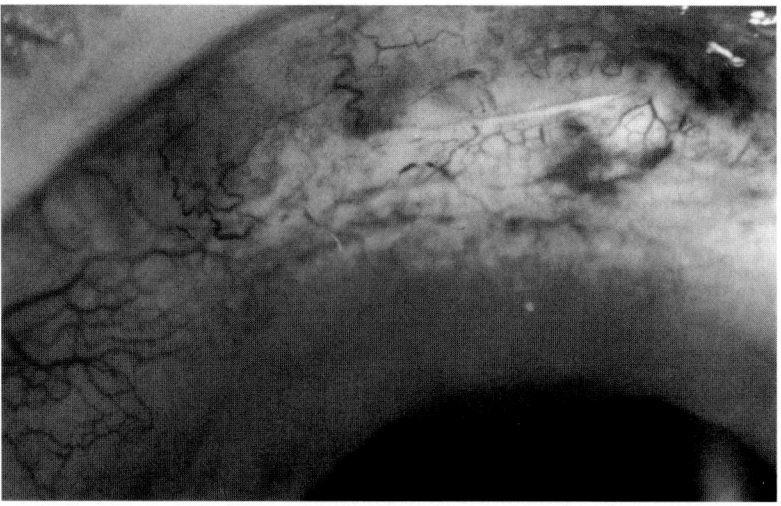

FIGURE 13–1. One day—cornea. Note superior corneal edema.

### Anterior Chamber

The anterior chamber is examined for cells and flare and recorded on the scale of 1+ to 4+ (see Chapter 4). A grading of 1+ to 3+ cells and 1+ flare is common after surgery. The majority of patients will have a 1+ to 2+ cellular response. The presence of red blood cells (hyphema) or layered inflammatory cells (hypopyon) should be ruled out. There may be iris pigment floating in the anterior chamber. Often, it is hard to distinguish between newly released pigment and circulating red blood cells or inflammatory cells. (See Color Plate 13–2.)

Hyphema, either diffuse or layered, is seen occasionally, and it is of moderate concern unless severe. However, minor hyphemas will slow visual recovery. More severe hyphemas may be associated with elevated intraocular pressure (see Chapter 15). Larger hyphemas may take 2–4 weeks to resolve adequately for good visual acuity. Corneal blood staining is rarely seen after significant hyphema.

The anterior chamber may rarely contain capsular debris or cortical fragments of varying sizes. These are not usually of concern. They often settle inferiorly and may attach to the posterior corneal surface and typically resorb within a few weeks.

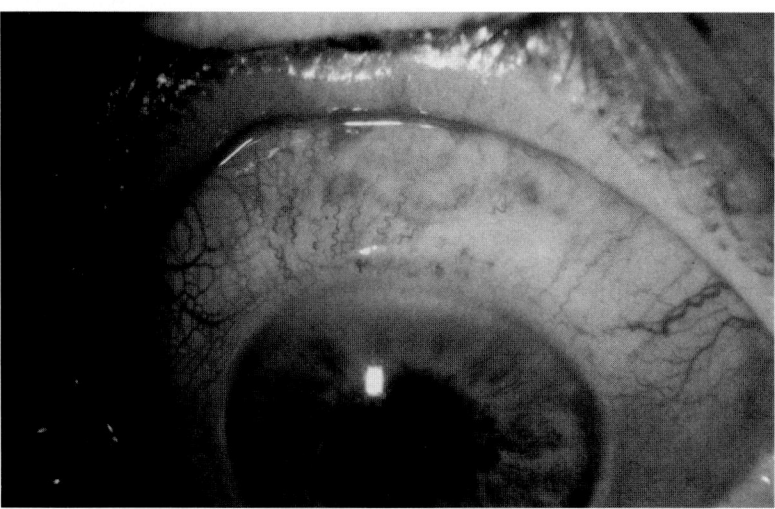

FIGURE 13–2. One day—wound.

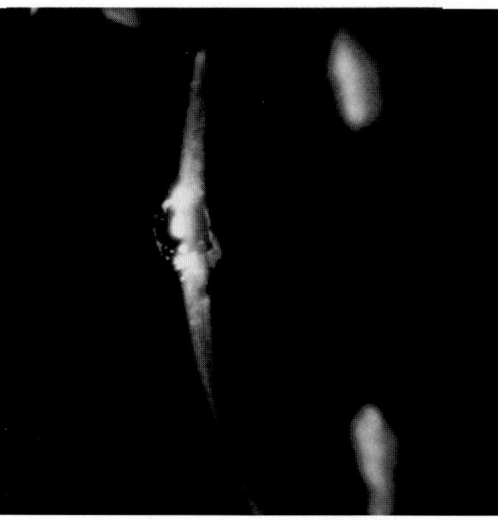

**FIGURE 13–3.** One day—corneal abrasion.

The anterior chamber is examined for the presence of vitreous that may accompany a broken posterior capsule. The depth and integrity of the anterior chamber is noted. A shallow anterior chamber is suspicious for wound leak or hypotony.

### Wound

The wound is inspected to ensure proper apposition and to rule out iris incarceration or the "vitreous wick syndrome" (see Chapters 12 and 14). The external aspect of the wound may appear to gape on a day #1 examination with scleral tunnel no-stitch surgery. This is quite normal. It is especially evident if the overlying conjunctiva is retracted. Posterior scleral incisions may often be obscured by overlying subconjunctival hemorrhage.

There may be a 2+ to 3+ conjunctival injection over the wound. In a wound with sutures, the sutures should be well placed with equal width along the course of the wound. With fluorescein, a normal finding would be green fluorescent pooling around the sutures or in the wound area. A Seidel test may be performed to check for wound leaks. In an uncomplicated course, the Seidel test is usually negative (see Chapter 14 for Seidel test technique).

### Intraocular Lens and Capsule

The intraocular lens (IOL) should be centered within the pupillary area; however, mild decentrations of less than 1 mm usually are not of great concern. A decentered lens usually indicates a lens with one haptic in the capsular bag and one haptic in the ciliary sulcus (see Chapter 15). Any tilt of the lens should also be noted.

The position of anterior chamber lens haptics should be noted by clock-hour for future reference in case rotation occurs.

The posterior capsule should be clear and without breaks. There may be some residual capsular wrinkles that typically dissipate over the course of 1–2 weeks.

### Vitreous

The vitreous is normally clear after surgery, although there may be some mild inflammatory debris in cases of iridocyclitis. If a new posterior vitreous detachment is seen after surgery, vitreal hemorrhage or retinal tear should be ruled out.

### Retina

The fundus should be completely examined during the postoperative course but need not be examined on the first day unless the patient is having new symptoms of vitreoretinal traction and/or significant loss of vision (see Chapter 14). Often, a retinal examination is obscured during the first day if the cornea has significant edema. When the cornea and/or anterior chamber are clear enough to allow examination, posterior vitreous detachment, new retinal tears, phototoxicity of the retina secondary to the operating microscopic light, or any optic neuropathy secondary to the surgery should be ruled out.

### Pupil

The pupil should be round and centered. A peaked pupil may be a sign of iris incarceration to the wound or vitreous to the wound area from a break in the posterior capsule. A round pupil following instillation of one to two drops of pilocarpine rules out these two possible complications. The pupillary border may show small nicks that are probably secondary to phacoemulsification strikes during surgery.

### Visual Fields

Confrontation visual fields may be performed, but formal fields are not routinely performed unless the patient complains of unexplained acute vision loss or has a suspicious optic nerve finding.

## Patient Treatment and Counseling

A review of the postoperative instructions and medications is undertaken, and new medications are added. Postoperative medications are prescribed as directed by the surgeon. Although medications vary, most will include a prophylactic topical antibiotic and anti-inflammatory agents or a drug that combines the two. Sometimes a dilating/cycloplegic agent is added. Our patients receive four capsules of cephalexin (Keflex), 250 mg, taken by mouth, over the first postoperative day and they are given dexamethasone, neomycin sulfate, polymyxin B sulfate combination (Maxitrol) drops to be used four times daily for 14–21 days. Patients are advised to call or return if symptoms worsen. Emergency call numbers are reviewed. (See Appendix 7.) In the case of large corneal abrasions accompanied by significant pain, they may be pressure patched with an antibiotic or combination antibiotic/steroid ointment for 24 hours or the patient may be given a bandage lens. Low water–content soft therapeutic or collagen lenses may be used for this purpose. If the anterior chamber reaction is mild, the doctor may decide to withhold topical steroid use in patients with large corneal abrasions until the epithelium is healed. The doctor may also elect to use topical cycloplegics or to substitute nonsteroidal anti-inflammatories (ie, suprofen 1% [Profenal] or diclofenac 0.1% [Voltaren]) in the place of topical steroids along with antibiotics until the corneal epithelium is intact.

## — SECOND VISIT—3–14 DAYS —

The second visit is usually at 1 week (see Table 13–3). A recommended examination sequence includes visual acuity, both aided and unaided; intraocu-

**TABLE 13-3. EXAMINATION RECOMMENDATIONS: SECOND AND THIRD VISITS**

History: comfort, vision
Visual acuity: unaided and pinhole
Pupils
Keratometry
Refraction (optional)
Biomicroscopy (see Table 13-2)
Intraocular pressure
Vitreoretinal examination (optional)
Visual fields (optional)

lar pressure; biomicroscopic evaluation of corneal status, anterior chamber status, IOL position, integrity of the capsule, pupil position and function; and wound integrity. Visual fields may be performed on this visit, as well as examination of the vitreous and fundus if not done previously or if symptoms warrant.

## Symptoms

It would be unexpected for the patient to report more symptoms at this visit than he or she did at the day #1 examination. Any patient noting that they are less comfortable than they were on the day #1 examination with increasing ocular pain and/or visual loss should be thoroughly examined, and an examination by the surgeon should be considered.

## Signs

### Visual Acuity

Visual acuity is typically equal or improved from the day #1 visit, and in cases where the visual acuity is still poor, pinhole or refraction should be performed. Patients with corneal incisions and interrupted sutures usually have higher amounts of induced corneal with-the-rule astigmatism (minus cylinder axis 180) than patients with scleral tunnel incisions with one-stitch or no-stitch surgery.

### Pupil Examination

The pupil should be positioned normally and the pupillary function normal.

### Intraocular Pressure

Intraocular pressure should be normalized from the day #1 examination.

### Biomicroscopy (Figures 13-4 and 13-5).

The cornea should be clearing with a few stria or endothelial folds remaining. The anterior chamber should be deep and well formed. There should be reduced cells and flare from the day #1 visit. The intraocular lens should be clean and well positioned. The capsule should be clear with decreased wrinkling

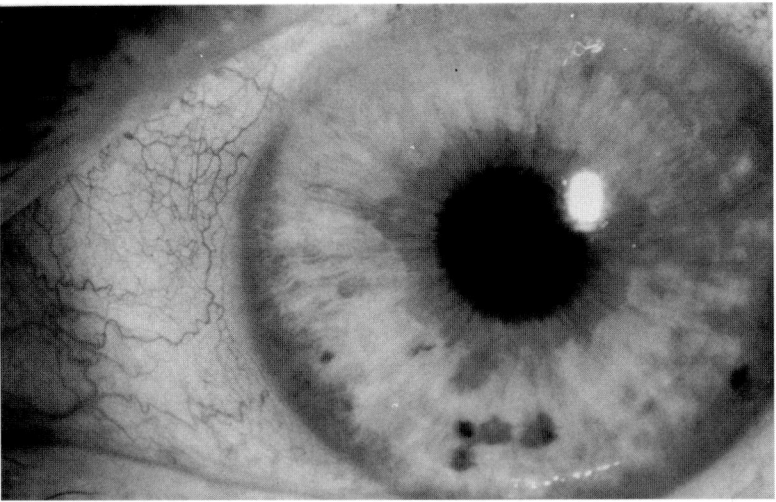

**FIGURE 13–4.** One week—cornea.

(Figure 13–6). The wound is typically intact with clearing conjunctiva over it. However, subconjunctival hemorrhage and edema are still common at the 1-week examination. Conjunctival injection may dissipate and then increase again as a result of reaction to topical medications (medicamentosa), especially with antibiotics such as aminoglycosides.

If a dilated fundus examination is undertaken at this visit, the retinal findings should be equal to the preoperative appearance.

## Patient Treatment and Counseling

The postoperative instructions and use of medications are reviewed. Usually there is a continuation of combination antibiotic and anti-inflammatory drops used four times a day. In cases where the expected postoperative visual acuity has been met with no evidence of infection, the antibiotic drops may be discontinued and steroid drops alone may be continued or tapered. At this visit, patients showing signs of medicamentosa or drug toxicity may also be changed to a steroid only.

**FIGURE 13–5.** One week—wound.

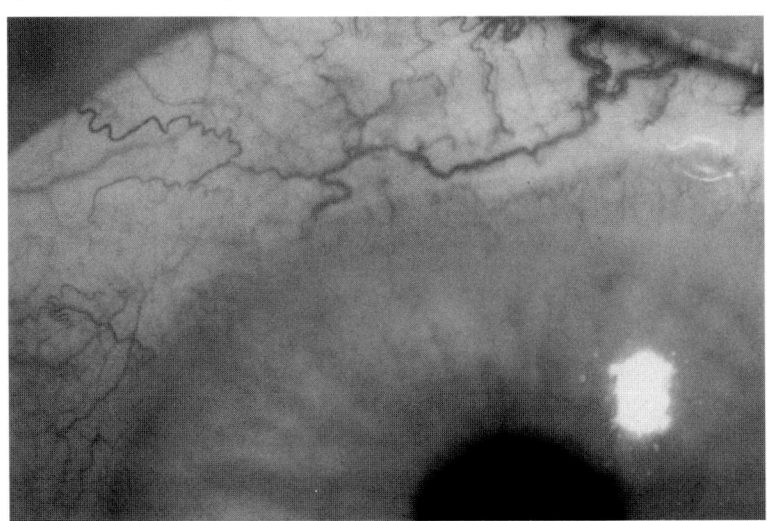

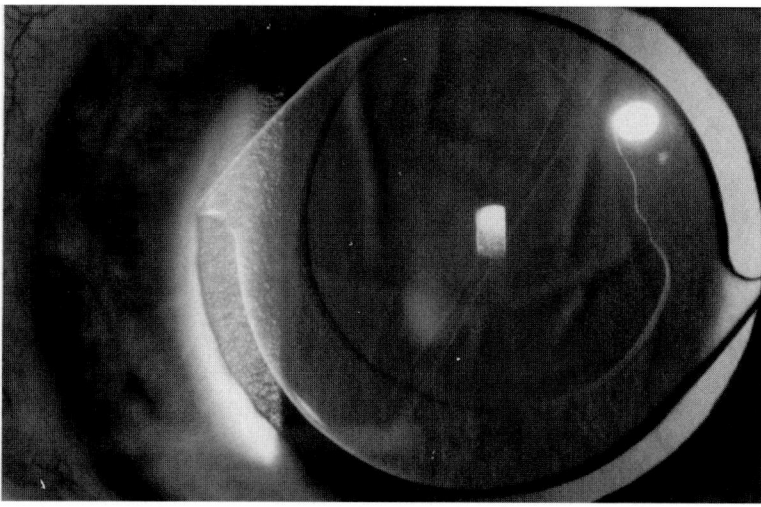

*FIGURE 13–6.* First week—posterior capsular wrinkling.

## THIRD VISIT—2–4 WEEKS

### Signs and Symptoms (see Table 13–3)

The patient should be relatively asymptomatic at this visit, with the exception of refractive error complaints. Visual acuity on the third visit should be close to the preoperative potential levels. Refraction may show with-the-rule corneal astigmatism that is often reduced from earlier testing. Pupillary function should be normal. Intraocular pressure is normalized. Careful biomicroscopy should be performed noting status of cornea, anterior chamber, IOL, pupil, capsule, and wound (Figures 13–7 and 13–8). The cornea is typically clear. Anterior chamber is deep and well formed without cell or flare. The IOL is clean and well centered and the capsule clear. The wound should be intact with decreased conjunctival injection over the wound area. Dilated fundus examination should be performed if symptoms warrant and the fundus and vitreous findings should be stable. If not done previously, visual fields may be considered at this time.

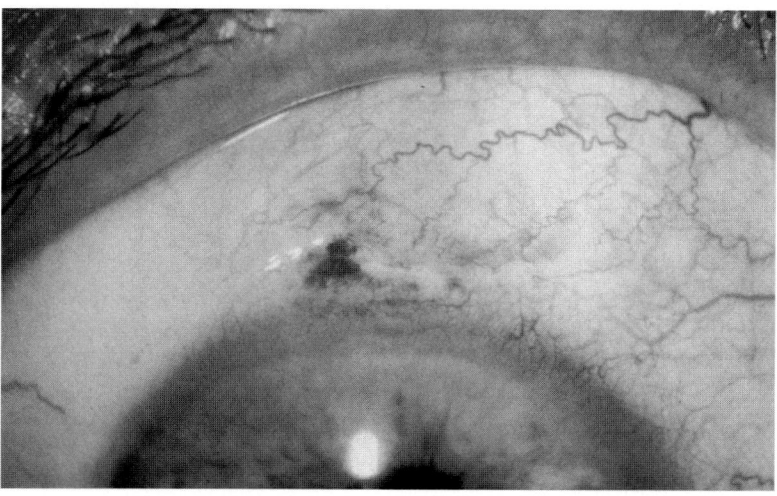

*FIGURE 13–7.* Three weeks—cornea. Note clear superior cornea.

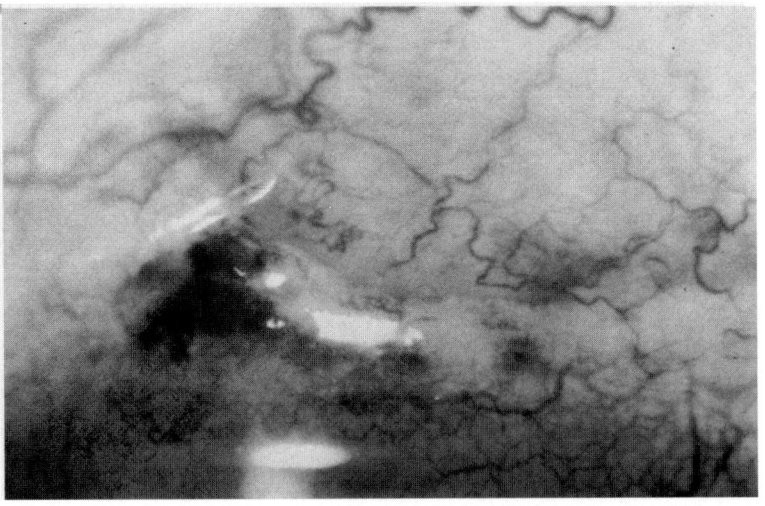

**FIGURE 13–8.** Three weeks—wound.

## Patient Treatment and Counseling

If there are any resolving signs or symptoms of inflammation either conjunctival or anterior chamber, anti-inflammatory drops should be continued.

## FOURTH VISIT—5-8 WEEKS

This visit is typically 5–6 weeks after surgery (Table 13–4). Visual acuity, unaided and refracted, is recorded. Measurement of intraocular pressure is performed as well as biomicroscopy, which should evaluate the cornea, anterior chamber, IOL and capsular status, and wound. Visual fields and dilated fundus examinations may be considered if not performed on previous examinations or if indicated by symptoms.

### Signs and Symptoms

The patient should be relatively asymptomatic at this visit, with the exception of uncorrected refractive error complaints. The cornea, IOL, and anterior chamber should be clear and quiet. The wound may have mild conjunctival injection but is very close to preoperative appearance (Figures 13–9 and 13–10).

**TABLE 13–4. EXAMINATION RECOMMENDATIONS: FOURTH VISIT**

History: comfort, vision
Visual acuity: unaided and pinhole
Pupils
Keratometry
Refraction for spectacle prescription
Biomicroscopy (see Table 13–2)
Intraocular pressure
Vitreoretinal exam (dilated)
Visual fields (optional)

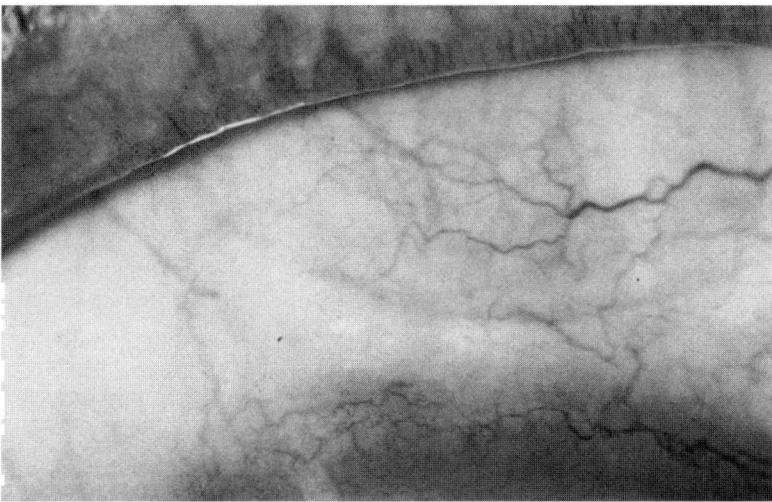

*FIGURE 13–9. Five weeks—wound.*

## Patient Treatment and Counseling

Patients with corneal incisions and interrupted sutures showing induced corneal astigmatism may be candidates for tight suture cutting to reduce spectacle cylinder. The cylinder correction, when placed in the plus cylinder form, often has the axis coinciding with the location of the tight suture. Sutures should be cut according to the individual surgeon's preference.

If the patient's refraction is stable and suture cutting is not necessary, a spectacle prescription may be given. Recommendations and/or limitations of the patient's vision are reviewed. For example, the need for bifocals and/or other limitations secondary to preexisting ocular disease, such as macular degeneration, are reviewed. The patient should have discontinued postoperative medications. The patient is instructed to return if any decrease in vision is noticed or if any new symptoms arise. Specifically, if sutures are present, they may become exposed at a later date causing itching, foreign body sensation, and a papillary response on the superior palpebral conjunctiva. Advise the

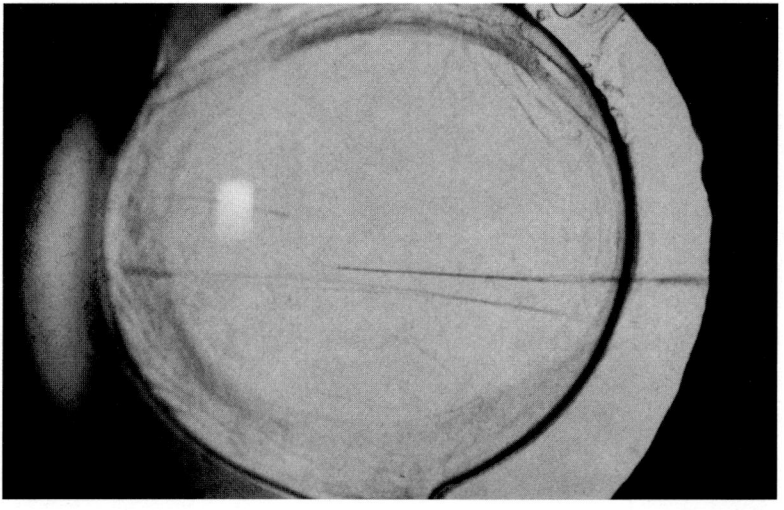

*FIGURE 13–10. Five weeks—posterior capsular wrinkling.*

patient to return to the clinic for suture removal if these symptoms occur. In addition, posterior capsular opacification symptoms and treatment should be reviewed. The next examination should be scheduled in 6 months to 1 year. (See Color Plate 13–3.)

## REFERENCES

1. Weinstein GW: Cataract surgery. In Tasman W (ed): *Duane's Clinical Ophthalmology,* Vol 5. Philadelphia: JB Lippincott. Harper & Row; 1991:41–42.
2. Jaffe NS, Jaffe MS, Jaffe GF: *Cataract Surgery and Its Complications,* 5th ed. St Louis: CV Mosby; 1990:334–337.
3. Perkins RS, Olson RJ: A new look at postoperative instructions following cataract extraction. *Ophthalmic Surg.* 1991;**22**:66–68.
4. O'Day DM, Adams AJ, Cassem EH, et al: *Cataract in Adults: Management of Functional Impairment.* Clinical Practice Guideline Number 4. US DHHS, PHS, Agency for Health Care Policy & Research; 1993:21.

# Early, 1- to 14-Day (Emergent) Complications

**CHAPTER 14**

## OCULAR HYPERTENSION

Early postoperative elevated intraocular pressure (IOP) following cataract surgery may occur in glaucomatous or nonglaucomatous eyes. One generally avoids using the term *glaucoma* to describe this elevation if it is brief and does not damage the optic nerve or result in visual field compromise. In most cases, the postoperative IOP rise is transient and may or may not require treatment depending on many factors: the degree of elevation, preexistence of glaucoma, or associated findings such as corneal edema. If the IOP is chronically elevated, then treatment is more likely.

Transient postoperative pressure rise is very common following cataract surgery by any technique[1-5] and possibly occurs in all eyes. Gross et al[2] found that within the first 3 hours of surgery, 59% of patients undergoing extracapsular cataract extraction developed an IOP of 25 mm Hg or greater. Patients who have had their cataracts removed by phacoemulsification had slightly less pressure elevations than those with nuclear expression.[2] When viscoelastics are used during surgery, there is an increased risk of pressure elevation.[3] The placement of the incision also is a factor in the development of early pressure spikes. Corneal incisions have been associated with lower postoperative IOPs than limbal sutured incisions presumably due to increased angle distortion from a tightly sutured wound.[4] Patients with preexisting glaucoma are also more apt to have elevated IOP following cataract surgery regardless of technique.[5]

### Open Angle

#### Background
As with any surgical procedure, it is best to prepare the patient psychologically for the occurrence of postoperative sequelae such as transient IOP rises. This is best done through written and verbal informed consent. (See Appendix 6.)

Following cataract surgery, lens particles, inflammatory debris, intraoperative substances, red blood cells, vitreous, and pigment may obstruct the trabecular pores resulting in a transient pressure elevation.[6] Pigment, red blood cells, or lens particles are most commonly responsible for the elevation (see Figure 14–1). Although some liberation of these substances will occur in almost every patient, it is generally well tolerated by those individuals with a healthy trabecular meshwork. When the amount of particles dispersed exceeds the capacity of the trabecular pores to clear, then a pressure elevation may occur. However, in our experience, the degree of pressure elevation does not always correspond to the amount of debris liberated. Some patients with a large hyphema may have normal IOP, whereas others with a minimal diffuse hyphema and a quiet eye may show a marked elevation. Patients with pupils that dilate poorly are at greater risk of having pigment dispersion and inflammatory debris due to trauma to the iris during surgery. Glaucomatous eyes are certainly more susceptible, since their outflow mechanism is already compromised. Fortunately, in most cases, the IOP rise is only temporary and seldom results in visual loss. The exception is the patient with severe glaucoma whose optic nerve may be susceptible to even a short-term elevation of pressure.

Viscoelastics have been shown by many investigators to cause an IOP elevation if not removed at the time of surgery.[3,7] The elevation is due to a direct obstruction of the trabecular meshwork by the viscoelastic molecules. Those viscoelastics that have shorter molecular chains may be at less risk of causing a pressure elevation.[7] Many investigators have reported that the adverse effects of increased IOP can be minimized by removing the viscoelastic at the time of surgery and administering acetazolamide (Diamox).[3,7] One contrasting study, however, has shown that the postoperative IOP in patients who have not had the viscoelastic (sodium hyaluronate) removed at the time of surgery, is similar to those in whom the viscoelastic has been aspirated.[8]

The inflammation from surgery may cause a trabeculitis resulting in an obstruction secondary to the trabecular edema. The trabecular meshwork can also be distorted by tight sutures, particularly if a limbal-based incision is used. Rothkoff et al found that 23% of patients with limbal-based incision developed an early postoperative pressure elevation versus none with a corneal-based incision.[4]

Other causes of early postoperative pressure elevation include the use of alpha-chymotrypsin, when used during intracapsular cataract extractions, and vitreous debris if a vitrectomy has been performed.[6,9] Topical steroids usually will not cause a pressure response for 2–3 weeks; however, instances of IOP elevations have been reported within days.[6] Steroid response should be kept in mind during the early postoperative period if there is no other explanation for the pressure elevation.

### Clinical Presentation and Assessment

Postoperative management decisions will often depend on the findings encountered during the preoperative evaluation; therefore, it is prudent to review prior examination records, including ocular history, the appearance of the optic disc, IOP measurements, as well as visual fields prior to deciding how to manage an early pressure rise.

Postoperatively, small IOP spikes are usually well tolerated by patients; however, large spikes can induce corneal edema resulting in blurry vision. The patient in such cases may also complain of pain and/or an ipsilateral headache.

#### Slit Lamp Examination

The conjunctiva and episclera may or may not be injected. The cornea may be edematous due to the pressure elevation, inflammation, or surgical trauma (Fig-

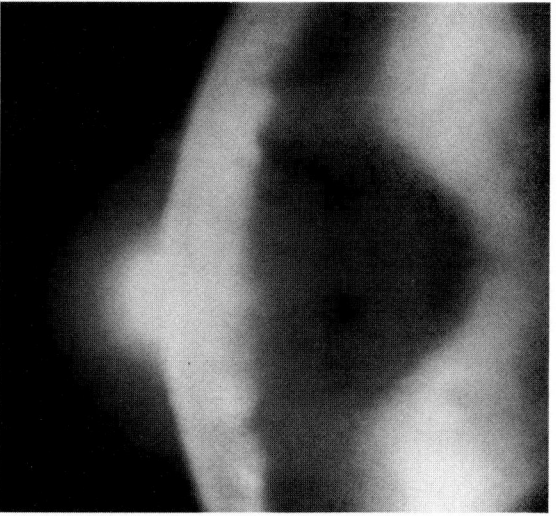

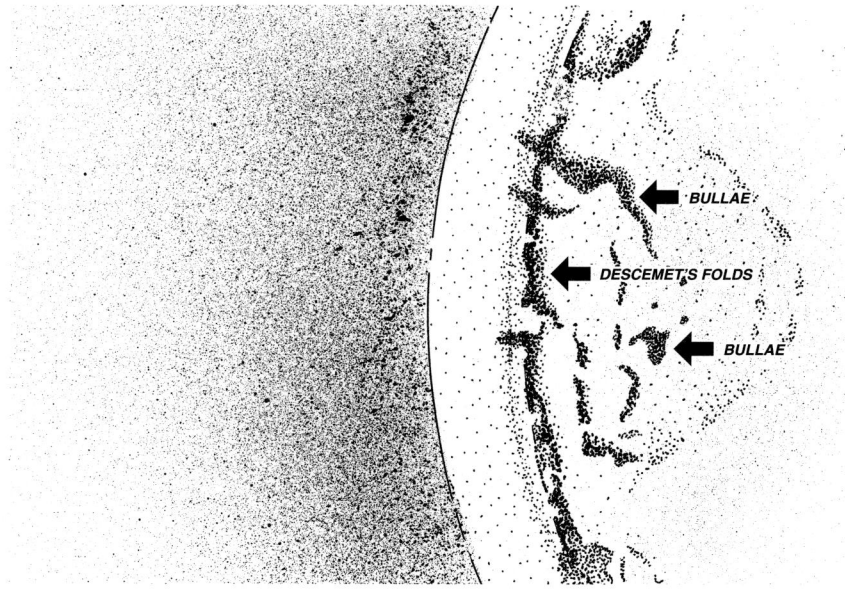

**FIGURES 14–1 AND 14–2.** Corneal edema 1 day following cataract surgery secondary to endothelial trauma from extended phacoemulsification time. Note diffuse epithelial microcytic edema, bullae, stromal thickening, and Descemet's folds.

ures 14–1 and 14–2). One should particularly suspect increased IOP if microcystic epithelial edema without significant stromal edema is encountered. As with all cases of ocular hypertension, it is imperative to determine if the mechanism of pressure elevation is due to an open or closed angle. Therefore, one should carefully assess the depth of the anterior chamber both centrally and peripherally. Gonioscopy should be performed if the IOP remains persistently elevated or if the angle appears narrowed. The inferior aspect of the anterior chamber should be carefully examined for a layering of red blood cells (hyphema) (Figure 14–3) or retained lens material. The anterior chamber may sometimes contain numerous diffuse red blood cells that do not layer. Excessive cells, flare, or inflammatory membranes are notable findings.

The type and position of the intraocular lens (IOL) should be noted. Anterior chamber IOLs are more prone to be associated with ocular hypertension due to their contact with the angle. This contact may result in obstruction of outflow due to peripheral anterior synechiae formation and may also exacerbate the inflammatory response.[9,10] Vaulted posterior chamber IOLs that are placed in the ciliary sulcus also are at greater risk of forming peripheral ante-

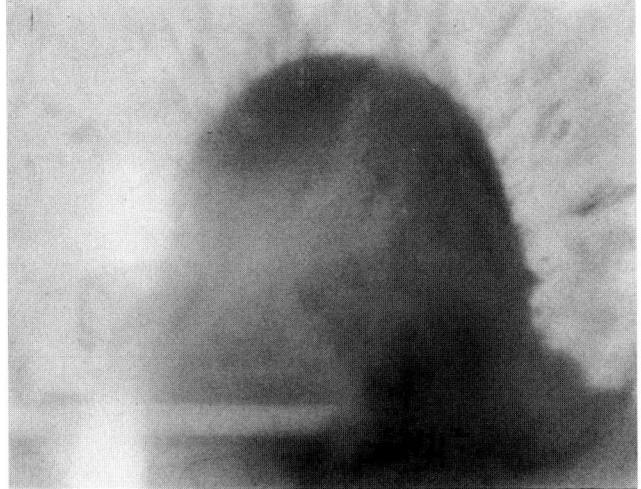

**FIGURE 14–3.** A clot hyphema observed at the 1-day postoperative visit. The IOP measured 36 mm Hg with count fingers vision. The IOP and vision were normal by day 3 using a topical beta-blocker.

rior synechiae than when placed in the capsular bag.[11] The integrity of the posterior capsule seems to influence the incidence of glaucoma.[9] If the posterior capsule has been broken, the eye should be carefully examined for residual vitreous in the anterior chamber and wound.

Significant iris findings include trauma secondary to phacoemulsification that may result in increased IOP due to a mechanical blockage of the trabecular meshwork by iris particles. In patients with shallow or closed angles, the presence or absence of an iridectomy should be noted. In addition, regardless of IOP, any patient with an anterior chamber IOL must be examined for the presence of a patent peripheral iridectomy.

The IOP should be tested using an applanation tonometer. Various noncontact "air-puff" tonometers are useful for screening purposes[12]; however, numerous studies have shown them to be inaccurate outside the range of normal IOPs.[13,14] If excessive corneal edema is found, the Goldmann applanation tonometer may also be inaccurate. Other tonometer devices such as the Tonopen (Mentor, Inc, Norwell, MA) may be the instrument of choice when Goldmann tonometry readings cannot be obtained due to corneal distortion.

Information regarding the fundus should be gleaned from the preoperative examination, particularly looking for risk factors such as diabetes or pre-existing glaucoma. In the presence of a shallow anterior chamber, the pupil should be dilated to rule out choroidal detachments.

### Differential Diagnosis

The differential diagnosis for early open-angle ocular hypertension includes pseudophakic angle closure, which is discussed later in this chapter.

### Treatment

The management of an early postoperative IOP rise will depend on the degree of elevation, the patient's symptoms, associated clinical findings such as corneal edema, and probably, most importantly, the status of the optic nerve. Those individuals with severe glaucomatous damage may be susceptible to even brief periods of elevations.

If the optic nerve is healthy, no treatment is generally indicated unless the IOP is 30 mm Hg or above (Table 14–1). In the case of pressures of 30–35 mm Hg with a healthy optic nerve, and given there are no contraindications, a single drop of a beta-blocker is typically placed in the eye and the pressure is retested. In individuals with IOPs of 35 mm Hg or greater, we administer a sin-

### TABLE 14-1. TREATMENT OPTIONS: EARLY POSTOPERATIVE HYPERTENSION

| | No Preexisting Glaucoma |
|---|---|
| **Intraocular Pressure (mm Hg)** | **Treatment** |
| 30–35 | Beta-blocker, one to two drops (in office); follow-up in 2–3 days. |
| 35–45 | Add acetazolamide (Diamox) 250 mg by mouth, once. Recheck IOP within 24 h. |
| 45–55 | Add apraclonidine 1% (Iopidine) in office, two drops 20 min apart; check IOP in 1 h. Recheck IOP within 4 h. |
| 55+ | Add oral 50% glycerin (Osmoglyn) 2 oz over ice; if diabetic, use 45% w/v solution isosorbide (Ismotic). Keep patient until pressure is below 35 mm Hg. Recheck IOP within 4 h. |

gle drop of beta-blocker plus 250 mg of acetazolomide (Diamox) by mouth and recheck the IOP within 24 hours. In some cases, depending on the clinical findings, we ask the patient to remain in the clinic until we measure a lowering of the pressure. With higher IOPs or if the patient is nonresponsive medically, some surgeons have advocated gentle depression of the auxiliary incision with the beveled end of a sterile needle to release aqueous from the anterior chamber.[15] The examiner should keep in mind that this carries a risk of temporary hypotony due to excessive release of aqueous or of endophthalmitis due to the introduction of microbes into the anterior chamber. This procedure should probably be avoided in patients with a postoperative hyphema due to the risk of increasing the hemorrhaging from the abrupt lowering of the IOP. Additionally, we have had good success in lowering postoperative pressures with 1% apraclonidine HCl (Iopidine). This alpha-adrenergic agonist is commonly used following laser procedures of the anterior segment[16] and has also been shown to be effective in controlling postoperative pressure spikes in glaucomatous patients following cycloplegia.[17] Its effect on reducing pressure spikes following cataract surgery is greatest in patients who are administered the drug prior to surgery rather than immediately afterward.[18] It has also been found to be effective in reducing pressure spikes following combined cataract and glaucoma operations.[19] The mechanism of action of apraclonidine is by improving outflow. Its effect has been found to be additive to other glaucoma medications.[20] Oral hyperosmotics should be used as a last line of defense due to the reported side effects that range from mild nausea to cardiac arrhythmias.[21] In diabetics, isosorbide solution is the preferred hyperosmotic of choice.

In glaucomatous patients, the IOP should be more aggressively treated and followed. The patient should be instructed to resume using their glaucoma medications with the exception of the epinephrine compounds, which may induce pseudophakic macular edema. Although miotics are typically avoided in the presence of inflammatory disease, this is generally resumed in the glaucomatous postoperative cataract patient, since they may experience abrupt elevations of their IOP if the miotic is withheld. In patients with compromised outflow function, the pilocarpine helps clear debris and red blood cells by opening the trabecular pores.

In glaucomatous postoperative pressure elevations, standard topical corticosteroid therapy should be administered, which may even help to lower the IOP by suppressing the trabecular inflammation. Nonsteroidal anti-inflammatory drugs may be of benefit in treating patients with a prior history of steroid response. Diclofenac 0.1% (Voltaren) has been specifically approved for postoperative inflammation and its efficacy in treating inflammation is currently being compared with various steroidal anti-inflammatory drugs. A recent study has shown that diclofenac sodium ophthalmic solution used in the preoperative period neither increases nor decreases the IOP.[22]

## Closed Angle with Pupillary Block

Aphakic or pseudophakic pupillary block is an infrequent but potentially serious complication that may occur in the early to late postoperative periods. Factors that influence the risk of pseudophakic pupillary block include the type and position of the IOL and the occurrence of vitreous loss (Figures 14–4 to 14–7).

### Background

One risk factor for the development of pupillary block is the IOL type. Iris-fixated and anterior chamber lenses are much more frequently associated with pupillary block than are posterior chamber lenses due to their proximity and/or contact with the pupil margin. Surgeons may minimize the risk of angle clo-

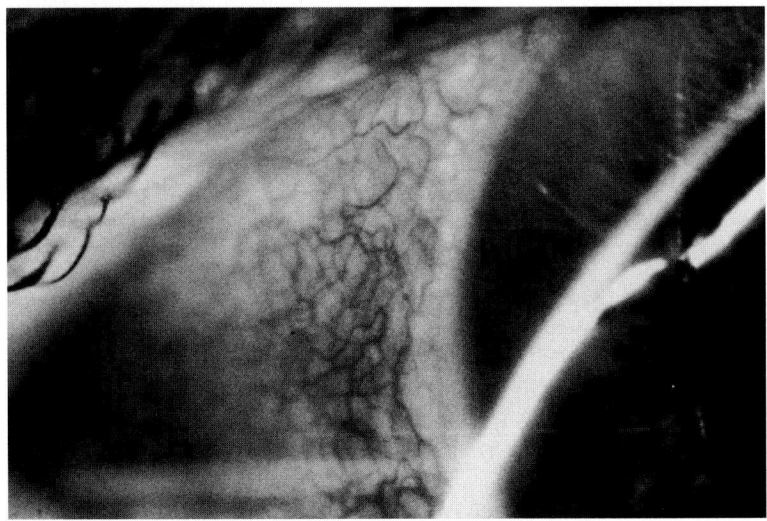

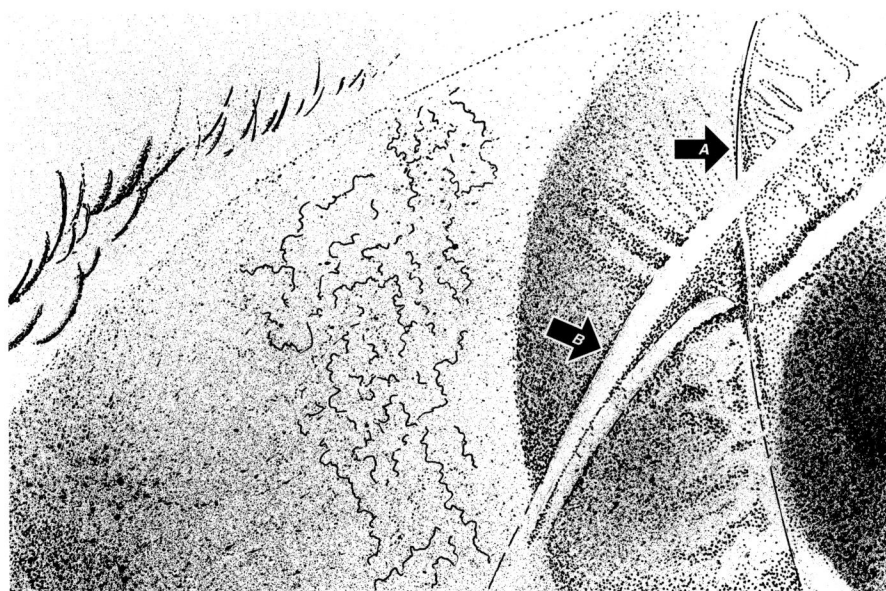

**FIGURES 14–4 AND 14–5.** Pseudophakic pupillary block due to obstruction of an iridectomy by the haptics of a Choyce-style anterior chamber IOL (A). Note peripheral iris bombé along the edge of the implant (B).

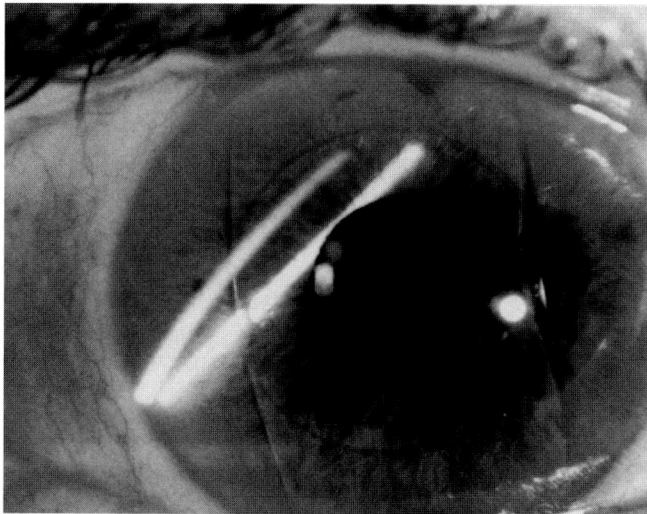

FIGURE 14–6. Pseudophakic pupillary block following laser iridotomy.

sure when inserting an anterior chamber lens by performing a peripheral iridectomy. Fortunately, cataract surgeons are no longer implanting iris-fixated lenses and generally reserve anterior chamber lenses for secondary implants and when the lack of capsular support prohibits insertion of a posterior chamber IOL. Although reports have implicated posterior chamber IOLs as causing pseudophakic pupillary block,[23–25] in our practice, it is an extremely rare entity. It primarily occurs when the posterior capsule has been broken and results in vitreous prolapse into the anterior chamber or when the IOL is placed in the sulcus rather than in the bag.[24] Sulcus fixation places the IOL closer to the iris plane, which increases the likelihood of pupillary block. We have not seen pupillary block from a posterior chamber IOL inserted properly in the capsular bag following capsulorhexis.

The mechanism of pupillary block in the pseudophakic eye is similar to that in the phakic eye. The pupillary margin contacts the IOL and obstructs the

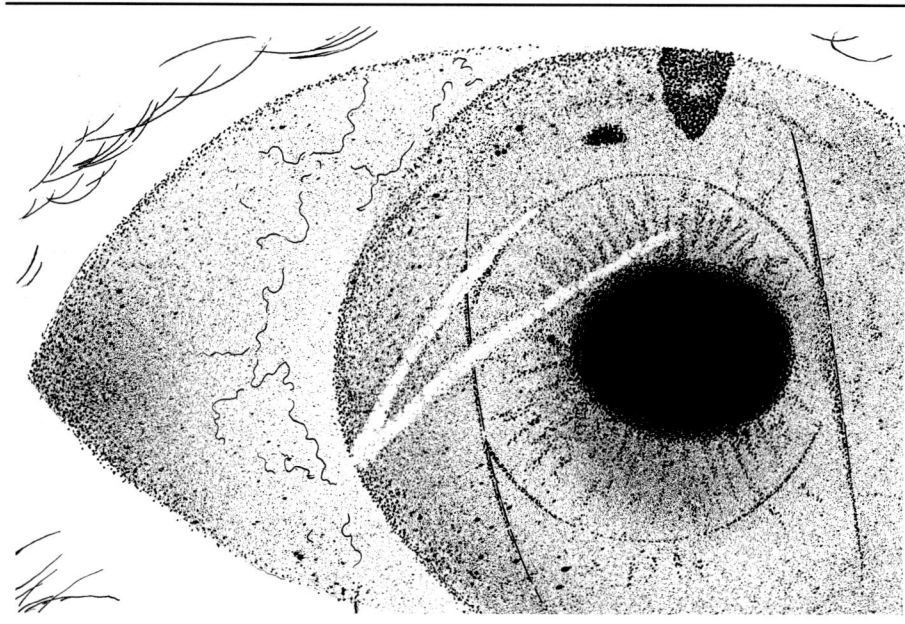

FIGURE 14–7. Pseudophakic pupillary block following laser iridotomy; note deepening of peripheral anterior chamber.

proper flow of aqueous from the posterior chamber to the anterior chamber. Due to the elevated pressure in the posterior chamber, the peripheral iris is pushed forward and obstructs the anterior chamber angle. In aphakic eyes, the vitreous may block the pupil in a similar fashion.[23] In pseudophakic eyes following a torn capsule, vitreous may prolapse through the pupil inducing pupillary block. For this reason, many surgeons perform a peripheral iridectomy in any patient in whom the posterior capsule is broken or when inserting an anterior chamber IOL.

### *Clinical Presentation and Assessment*

Patients with pseudophakic pupillary block typically present with pain and blurred vision; however, some cases may be asymptomatic.[26] Many patients will have elevated pressures, but if the closure has been chronic, the IOP may be normal or low due to ciliary body shutdown.[23,26]

On slit lamp examination, the conjunctiva is usually injected, the cornea edematous, and a mild anterior chamber reaction is noted. The diagnosis is ascertained by observing iris contact with the IOL or vitreous face associated with a bombé of the peripheral iris. The central chamber is typically deeper than the periphery, which is in contrast to malignant glaucoma in which the central and peripheral chambers are uniformly shallow. An iridotomy or iridectomy is usually not observed, but if it is present, it is obstructed by the intraocular lens haptic or vitreous.

### *Differential Diagnosis*

The differential diagnosis includes retained lens fragments behind the iris, malignant glaucoma, and choroidal detachment. Typically with choroidal detachment, the IOP is quite low. (Malignant glaucoma is discussed below.)

### *Treatment*

If the IOP is elevated significantly, assuming no contraindications, the patient should be administered a beta-blocker topically and 250–500 mg of acetazolamide (Diamox) orally to inhibit aqueous secretion. If the IOP remains elevated, assuming no contraindications, an oral hyperosmotic may be administered. If laser therapy cannot be immediately performed, administer a short-acting mydriatic drop (tropicamide 1%) in an attempt to dilate the pupil beyond the outer edge of the IOL.[26] (This is in contrast to phakic angle closure, which is treated by miotic drops.) Once the attack is under control, an iridotomy should be performed with the Nd:YAG (neodymium:ytterium-aluminum-garnet) or argon laser. Prior to performing an iridotomy, the dilation may need to be reversed with dapiprazole and/or pilocarpine[26] (Table 14–2).

## Malignant Glaucoma

### *Background*

Malignant glaucoma is a rare group of diseases thought to occur due to a vitreous-ciliary or lens-ciliary block mechanism (Figure 14–8). This is most commonly found following ocular surgery when aqueous becomes misdirected behind the vitreous; then the vitreous pushes the iris and physiologic lens or IOL forward obstructing the angle and possibly touching the cornea.[6,9]

### *Clinical Presentation and Assessment*

Clinically, the IOP is found to be elevated. The cornea is edematous and, most notably, the anterior chamber is uniformly shallow axially as well as peripher-

## TABLE 14–2. TREATMENT OPTIONS: PSEUDOPHAKIC PUPILLARY BLOCK

**Should Be Done**

For control of IOP (mm Hg):

| | |
|---|---|
| 25–35 | One drop of beta-blocker and/or 1% apraclonidine HCl (Iopidine); repeat if necessary in 20 min |
| 35–45 | Add 250 mg acetazolamide (Diamox) by mouth |
| >45 | Add oral 50% glycerin, or 45% w/v solution isosorbide (Ismotic) if diabetic; administer per body weight |

Laser iridotomy (if dilated, may need to reverse dilation with pilocarpine HCL or dapiprazole HCL prior to laser treatment)

If laser iridotomy cannot be performed immediately, instill one drop of tropicamide 1%; repeat if necessary in 20 min

**May Be Done**

With permanent anterior synechia, iridectomy with trabeculectomy may be indicated.

---

ally. In some cases, the physiologic lens or IOL may be in contact with the cornea.

### Differential Diagnosis

Malignant glaucoma must be differentiated from angle-closure glaucoma, which has been previously discussed.

### Treatment and Prognosis

Shields[6] recommends that the proper medical management of this condition should include a mydriatic-cycloplegic agent, beta-blocker, carbonic anhydrase inhibitor, and hyperosmotic agent. After the attack is under control, the patient is maintained on a mydriatic-cycloplegic to prevent recurrent episodes.[6]

Various surgical procedures have been recommended in cases that are nonresponsive medically. These include lensectomy, pars plana vitrectomy, and posterior sclerotomy with air injection and Nd:YAG photodisruption of the anterior vitreous.[6]

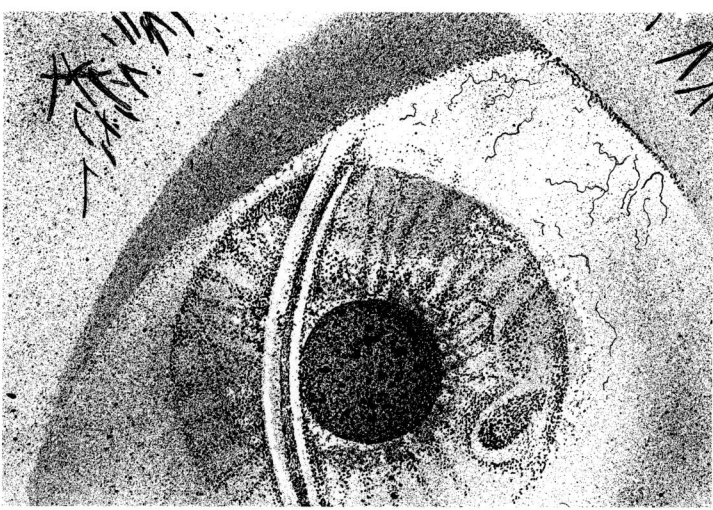

**FIGURE 14–8.** Malignant glaucoma; note the uniform shallowing of the anterior chamber.

## WOUND LEAK WITH SHALLOW ANTERIOR CHAMBER

Fortunately, a postoperative eye presenting with a shallow anterior chamber and low IOP is a rare occurrence. The presence of a flat anterior chamber is usually associated with a wound leak or a choroidal detachment that dictates further examination and treatment (Table 14–3).

### Background

Wound leaks most often occur on account of improper surgical technique, poor wound healing, or trauma.[27] There are also cases where they occur in a well-executed surgery without obvious complication or suggestive history (see discussion of choroidal detachment in Chapter 15).

**TABLE 14–3. MANAGEMENT OF FLAT ANTERIOR CHAMBER: A FLOW CHART**

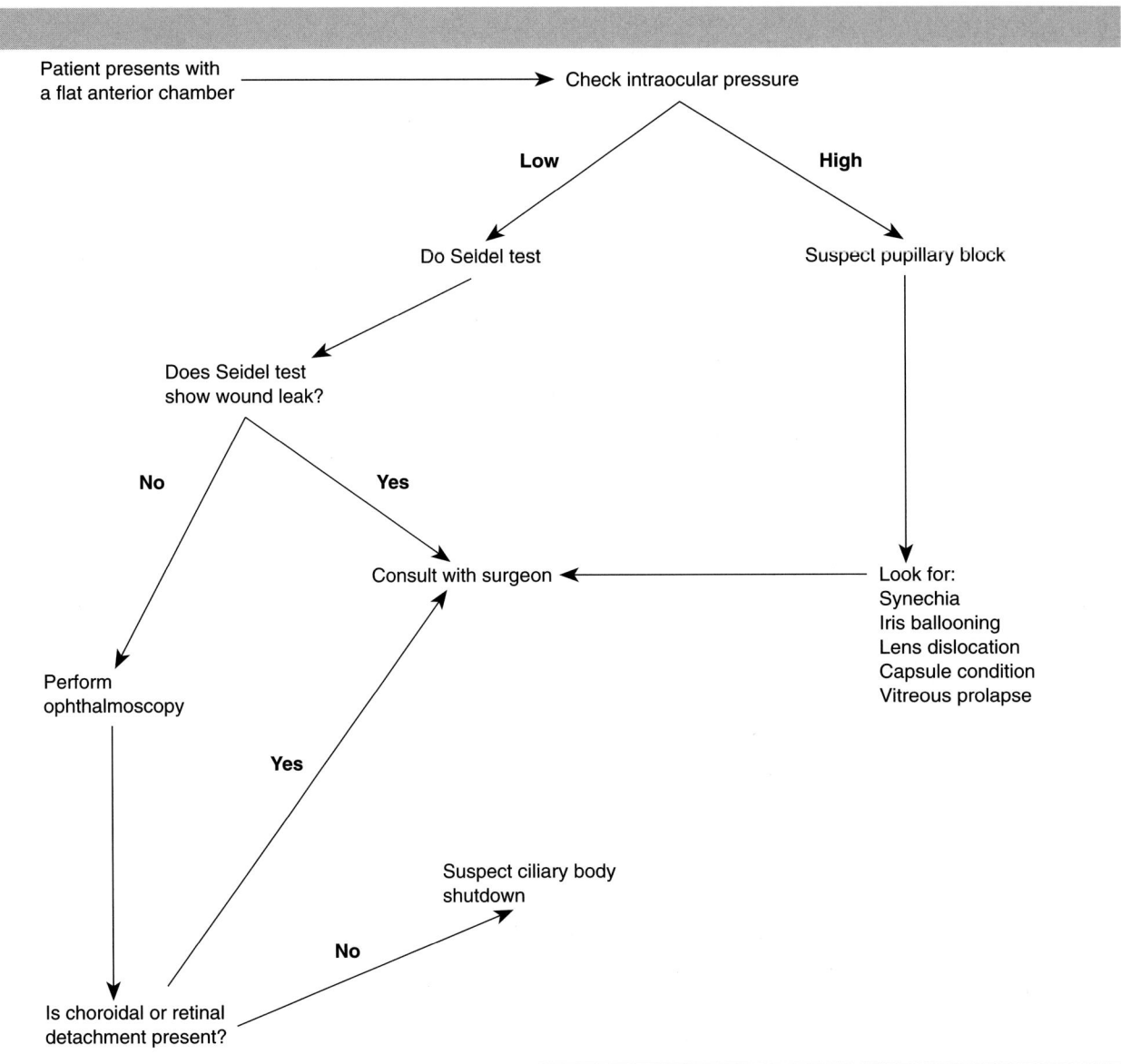

## Clinical Presentation and Assessment

The patient presenting with a wound leak and shallow anterior chamber may or may not report pain. Slit lamp examination should be performed to differentiate between a shallow and a flat chamber. A shallow chamber will appear to be deeper centrally than peripherally, whereas a flat chamber will be uniformly shallow with iris and IOL touch to the corneal endothelium (Figures 14–9 and 14–10). The cornea may exhibit moderate to severe endothelial folds that are often aligned more vertically than the multidirectional ones seen on the normal one day examination. In addition, following the instillation of fluorescein, a waffled staining may appear on the corneal surface due to ocular hypotony (Figures 14–11 and 14–12). The area of the leak may show a wound gape or a suspicious area of poor healing around a suture entry site. The conjunctiva over the wound, if present, may be thickened with a soft, boggy appearance, and there may be subconjunctival hemorrhage.

When a shallow or flat anterior chamber is observed, ocular hypotony is expected. However, the examiner should measure the IOP to rule out pupil-

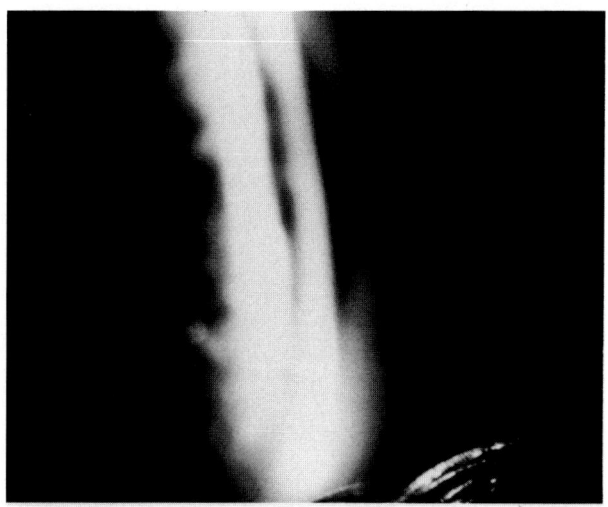

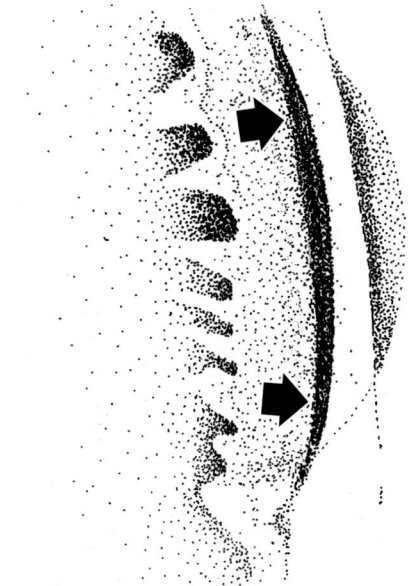

**FIGURES 14–9 AND 14–10.** Shallow anterior chamber from a wound leak (arrows).

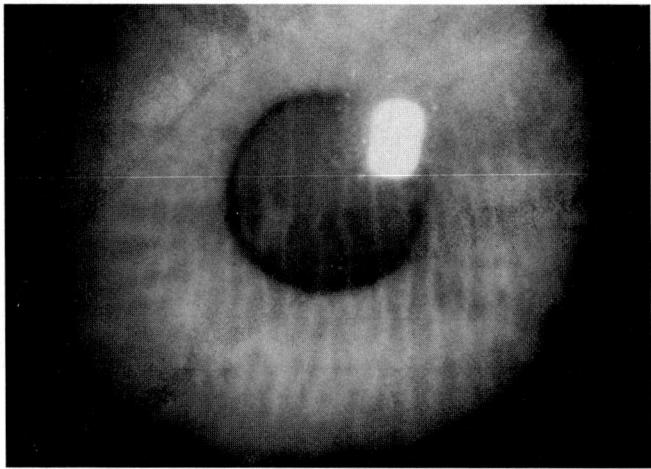

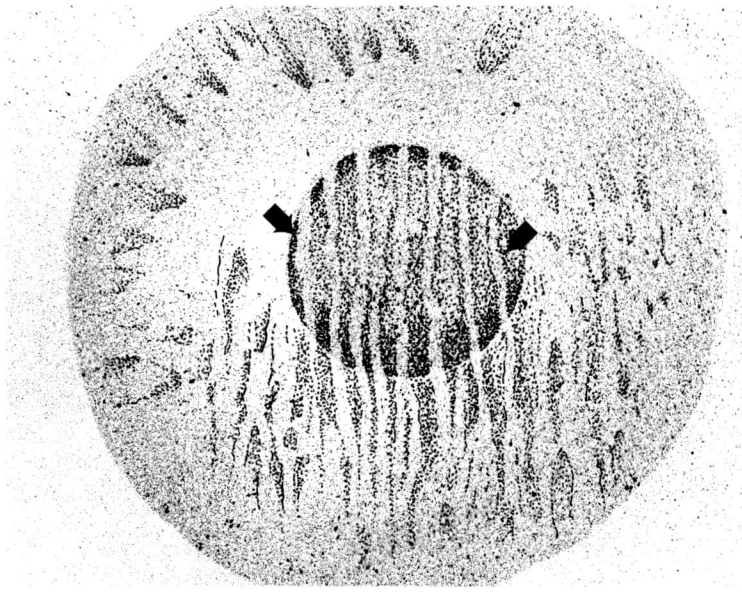

**FIGURES 14–11 AND 14–12.** A waffled fluorescein pattern characteristic of ocular hypotony (arrows).

lary block, which may present with a shallow anterior chamber without wound leak and normal to high IOPs (see discussion of pupillary block in Chapter 14). We recommend using a Goldmann applanation tonometer to measure the IOP. Although all tonometers are inaccurate at low IOPs, in our experience, a noncontact tonometer such as an air-puff tonometer, has been especially inaccurate.

The wound should be examined with fluorescein sodium to determine if a leak is present (Seidel's sign) (Figures 14–13 and 14–14). This is done by wetting a fluorescein strip with sterile saline, using a commercial preparation of topical fluorescein anesthetic, or using a single unit dose of fluorescein sodium 2% preparation. In all cases, it is most prudent to avoid contamination by using only saline or fluorescein that is fresh and sterile. The fluorescein sodium is instilled with the eye in the straight-ahead or downward position. The lid is held securely against the superior orbital rim and taking care to avoid applying any pressure to the globe. The wound edge is inspected through the slit lamp with a cobalt filter. The doctor looks for a small continuous cascade of aqueous with a bright green border originating at a leak, whereas fluorescein on the ocular surface appears more yellow-green.

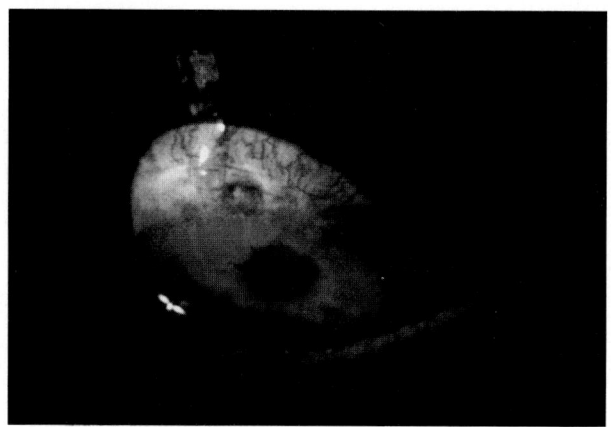
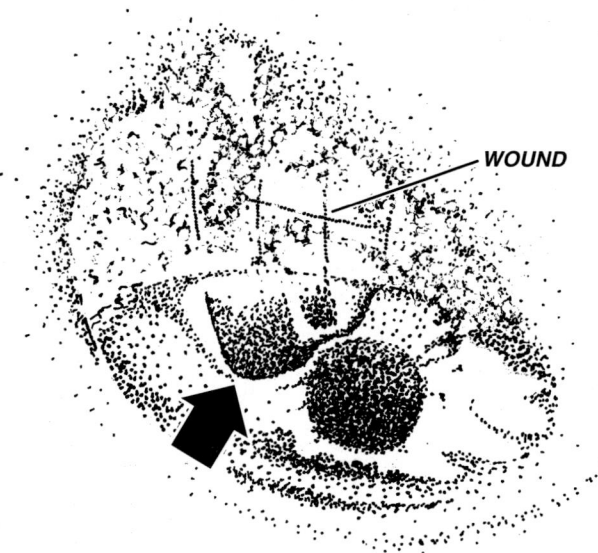

**FIGURES 14–13 AND 14–14.** *A positive Seidel test from cataract incision. Note the cascading stream of aqueous with bright green fluorescence on its border (arrow).*

In cases where there is a very small, slow-flowing leak, one may see the disappearance of fluorescein around the area of the wound or a specific suture. It may be viewed only after multiple instillations of fluorescein or when the globe is gently massaged. Only gentle massage is advocated and any other manipulation of the globe should be left to the surgeon.

When possible, the eye should be dilated and choroidal detachment ruled out.

## Differential Diagnosis

The differential diagnosis for wound leak includes pupillary block, malignant glaucoma, and choroidal detachment.

## Treatment

Wound leak with a flat anterior chamber sets the stage for anterior synechia, glaucoma, recurrent inflammation, intraocular infection, and/or long-standing choroidal detachment. Therefore, on identification of a wound leak, a consultation with the surgeon is mandatory. Treatment must be swift and it is suggested that the anterior chamber be reformed immediately to decrease the incidence of serious sequelae[27] (Table 14–4).

**TABLE 14-4. TREATMENT OPTIONS: WOUND LEAK WITH SHALLOW ANTERIOR CHAMBER AND WITH FLAT CHAMBER**

**Wound Leak with Shallow Anterior Chamber**

Consult with surgeon, who may choose to return the patient to surgery immediately
Rule out choroidal detachment
*Or*
 Atropine 1.0%, one drop
 Ciprofloxacin 0.3%, two drops
 Prednisolone acetate 1%, one drop if moderate inflammation
 Cephalexin, 250 mg, by mouth, four times per day
 Pressure patch may be applied for 24 h
 Shield at night
 Consider surgery if no response after 48 h

**Wound Leak with Flat Chamber**

Immediate consultation and return to surgery for repair

---

In cases where the anterior chamber is shallow secondary to a wound leak within a few days of surgery, the surgeon must immediately be consulted. The surgeon may choose to operate again to reform the anterior chamber and suture the wound. As an alternative, the eye may be pressure patched with dilation and followed in the hope that the wound healing will seal the leak and the anterior chamber will reform.[28] In addition, one may give the patient an oral hypotensive such as Diamox in the hope that decreasing aqueous production and slowed aqueous percolation through the wound will allow the wound to heal. In a posterior scleral tunnel incision, decreasing aqueous secretion may be counterproductive, as aqueous flow helps achieve a wound seal of the corneal flap. If pressure patching with dilation, with or without ocular hypotensives, fails, the anterior chamber may have to be reformed with air or a viscous agent such as sodium hyaluronate (Healon). If the leak is localized, the patient may be returned to surgery and the area of the leak repaired. If choroidal detachment is present, additional treatment may be necessary (see Chapter 15).

## ENDOPHTHALMITIS

Probably the most feared complication during the postoperative course is infectious endophthalmitis. Although this is a rare complication, its potentially devastating effect warrants our thorough understanding and recognition of its early signs and symptoms. (See Color Plate 14–1).

### Background

The incidence of infectious endophthalmitis is reported to be as high as 0.5% following cataract surgery.[29] At the Barnes Hospital, Washington University, St. Louis, MO, 1 out of 800 (0.125%) patients undergoing cataract surgery developed culture-proven endophthalmitis.[30] Recently, Javitt et al reviewed records of 338,141 Medicare beneficiaries over 65 years of age, and found that 0.17 % of patients undergoing intracapsular cataract extraction and 0.12% undergoing phacoemulsification or extracapsular cataract extraction were rehospitalized with the diagnosis of endophthalmitis during the year of 1984.[31] Although this possibly does not represent the true incidence of endophthalmitis using current techniques in an ambulatory setting, it nevertheless represents the largest population study to date. In our own surgical experience, 8 of 35,000 patients undergoing cataract extraction by phacoemulsification developed infectious endophthalmitis (0.023%).

Endophthalmitis results from a direct invasion by microbes into the anterior chamber and posterior segment either at the time of surgery or during the postoperative follow-up. Specific causes of the intraoperative infection have previously been traced to contaminated IOLs,[32] viscoelastics, and invasion by microbes that are in the normal flora of the patient and/or surgical personnel.[33] Patients who have implants with polypropylene haptics are probably at a greater risk of infection, since that material has been shown to bind bacteria with greater affinity.[34] Considering the large number of bacteria that are normally found around the ocular adnexa, it is remarkable that more intraoperative infections do not occur. It is commonly thought that the eye is able to tolerate a small number of pathogens. However, when the number exceeds the immune system's capacity to defend, an infectious endophthalmitis results. Late endophthalmitis may result from microbial invasion during the postoperative period if there is wound dehiscence, or from an infected filtering bleb if a combined cataract extraction and trabeculectomy is performed.[35] The use of 5-fluorouracil in trabeculectomies has been shown to increase the risk of infection.[36] Endophthalmitis has been reported to be associated with sutureless scleral tunnel incisions, presumably secondary to a scleral abscess.[37,38] In our experience, we have seen 3 cases of endophthalmitis out of over 10,000 cataract surgeries with sutureless scleral tunnel incisions.

The most common organisms responsible for postcataract surgery infections treated at Bascom Palmer Eye Institute, Miami, FL, from 1974 through 1983 were *Staphylococcus epidermidis* (38%), *Staphylococcus aureus* (21%), *Streptococcus* species (11%), gram-negative species (16%), *Propionibacterium acnes* (5%), fungi (8%), and *Corynebacterium* (1%).[39] The clinical presentation and prognosis is directly related to the pathogenicity of the offending organism. Streptococcal and gram-negative species are much more aggressive than *Staphylococcus aureus* and *S. epidermidis*.[30,39–44]

Delayed-onset endophthalmitis is now a well-recognized entity.[45–47] Bohigian and Olk found that one-half of cases with endophthalmitis studied presented several or more days following surgery.[30] The delayed onset occurs with organisms of low virulence and may also occur when the bacteria become sequestered between the capsule and the IOL.[45–47] In cases of localized endophthalmitis, the classic picture may not occur until an Nd:YAG capsulotomy disperses the organisms. *Propionibacterium acnes* is a well-recognized cause of delayed-onset localized endophthalmitis.[45]

## Clinical Presentation and Assessment

Classically, patients who present during the postoperative course with pain, reduced vision, increased IOP, lid edema, severe anterior chamber reaction, vitreous inflammation, and hypopyon within 72 hours of surgery have infectious endophthalmitis until proven otherwise (Table 14–5 and Figure 14–15). The gram-negative (*Pseudomonas*) and *Streptococcus* species are more likely to present in this aggressive fashion.[40]

The doctor should realize, however, that the presentation of endophthalmitis is quite variable and the classic signs and symptoms may not be present at the onset of infectious endophthalmitis. A more subtle presentation may occur, particularly with coagulase-negative staphylococcal infections, most no-

**TABLE 14–5. ENDOPHTHALMITIS: CAUSATIVE ORGANISMS**

| Organism (in order of frequency) | Onset | Presentation of Signs and Symptoms | Visual Prognosis |
| --- | --- | --- | --- |
| Staphylococcal epidermidis | Days to weeks | Mild to moderate | Good to poor |
| Staphylococcal aureus | Days to weeks | Mild to moderate | Fair to poor |
| Gram-negative species | 1–4 days | Severe | Poor |
| Streptococcal species | 1–4 days | Severe | Poor |
| *Propionibacterium acnes* | Weeks to months | Indolent | Good to poor |

tably *Staphylococcus epidermidis*[43,44] (Figure 14–16). These patients may present without hypopyon and without severe pain anytime from days to weeks following cataract surgery. Often this is misdiagnosed as a sterile inflammatory reaction or phacoanaphylactic uveitis and treated with topical corticosteroids.[43,44] Initially with topical steroids, an improvement may be noted, only to worsen again as the steroids are tapered.

Another presentation is one of a delayed-onset endophthalmitis, secondary to *Propionibacterium acnes*. Due to its ability to become sequestered, a smoldering iritis and vitritis results that may last for months or even years until it is correctly diagnosed. The infection is often exacerbated following an Nd:YAG posterior capsulotomy that disperses the organisms into the vitreous and accelerates the inflammatory component.[45] The patient with chronic unexplained vitritis and iritis following cataract surgery should be suspected of having a *Propionibacterium* infection. A careful inspection of the posterior capsule should be performed through the dilated pupil to observe for a whitish plaque of capsular infiltrate which is highly suggestive of a localized colony of *Propionibacterium acnes*.[45,47]

Any patient who presents in the postoperative period with inflammatory signs out of proportion to what would be expected should be suspected of having endophthalmitis. An evaluation to rule out endophthalmitis versus sterile inflammation should be performed as follows.

### History

Patients with infections that are of high pathogenicity have a rapid onset of progressive pain and loss of vision over a 24-hour period. The pain may be so severe as to awaken the patient at night. Often these patients request pain med-

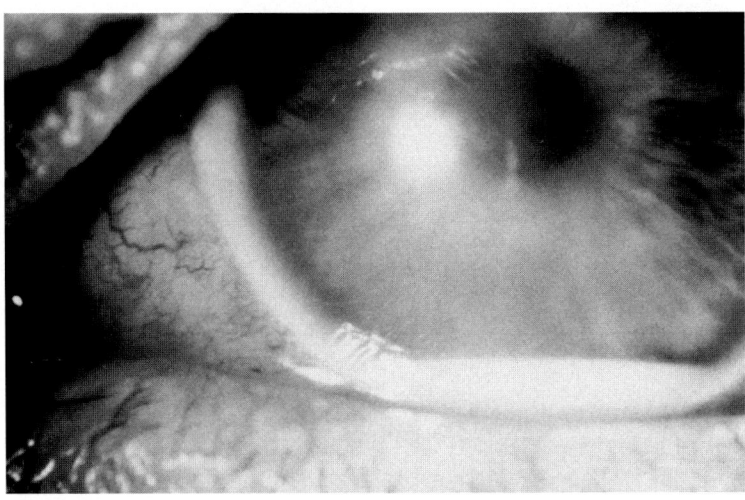

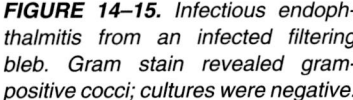

*FIGURE 14–15.* Infectious endophthalmitis from an infected filtering bleb. Gram stain revealed gram-positive cocci; cultures were negative.

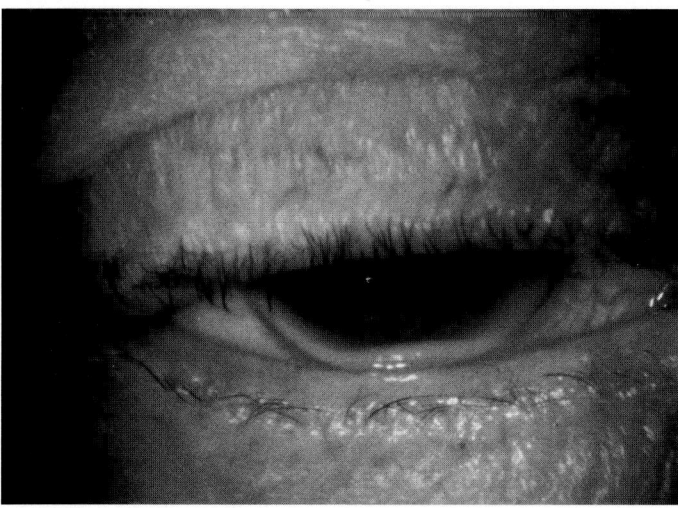

**FIGURE 14–16.** Culture-proven Staphylococcus epidermidis *endophthalmitis following uncomplicated cataract extraction in a diabetic man. Note the lack of lid edema and conjunctival hyperemia, which is usually, but not always, observed with endophthalmitis.*

ication to alleviate their symptoms. Pain may not be present in endophthalmitis caused by organisms of low virulence.

### Visual Acuity

The visual acuity generally will be reduced with infectious endophthalmitis. The possible exception is a smoldering *Propionibacterium acnes* endophthalmitis in which patients can have good vision.

### Ocular Motility

The ocular motility is generally not affected; however, with infectious endophthalmitis, the patient may have severe pain on movement of the globe.

### Pupil

The pupil is often markedly constricted and poorly reactive to light. There may be an afferent pupillary defect if irreversible retinal and/or optic nerve damage have already occurred.

### Retinoscopic Reflex

Due to the accumulation of cells in the anterior chamber and vitreous, the reflex is quite dim.

### Slit Lamp Examination

The conjunctiva, sclera, and episclera may be uniformly and markedly injected across the globe, although with some species the conjunctiva may be quiet. The cornea may be edematous. The anterior chamber is notable for marked cell and flare. A pupillary fibrotic membrane may be observed. In severe cases, a hypopyon sometimes may be observed in the anterior chamber. Capsular infiltrate may be observed.

### Intraocular Pressure

The IOP is classically elevated, although normal IOPs may be observed or hypotony may be observed due to rupture of the cataract incision and/or an infection resulting from a wound leak.

### Vitreous and Retinal Examination

Vitreous cells are observed and, in the more aggressive forms of endophthalmitis, clumps of cells may be noted in the anterior vitreous. Retinal findings may or may not include retinal hemorrhages and swelling of the optic nerve.

## Differential Diagnosis

The differential diagnosis of a patient who presents in the above fashion includes a sterile inflammatory process[48,49] (see discussion of uveitis in Chapter 15). In general, however, any patient who presents with ocular inflammation out of proportion to what would be expected in that time frame, should be suspected of having endophthalmitis. In these cases, a telephone consultation is mandatory. If it is determined that the patient with a significant postoperative iritis is probably not infected based on clinical findings, then the patient should be very closely observed. Such patients treated with a topical corticosteroid to suppress the inflammation should be reexamined within hours to see if there is any progression of the inflammation. It should, however, be noted that infectious endophthalmitis may temporarily improve with the use of topical steroids. Certainly any postsurgical inflammation that is noted to progress significantly within a few hours should be presumed infectious and immediately referred for consultation.

## Treatment, Follow-up, and Prognosis

Patients suspected of having endophthalmitis should be cultured by anterior chamber and/or vitreous tap (Table 14–6).

While waiting for the culture results, if clinical suspicion warrants, the patient is typically treated with intravitreal, subconjunctival, and topical antibiotics. Many surgeons will also perform a core vitrectomy to remove organisms and inflammatory debris as well as to enhance the therapeutic distribution and effectiveness of the antibiotics[40] (Figure 14–17). The benefit of using systemic antibiotics is controversial. A multicenter endophthalmitis vitrectomy study is now under way to evaluate the efficacy of performing a vitrectomy and the use of systemic antibiotics.[50]

Several factors influence the eventual outcome of patients developing endophthalmitis. Patients infected with *Staphylococcus epidermidis* have a better outcome than other infections. Driebe et al found that 78% of *Staphylococcus epidermidis* infections had a final visual acuity of 20/400 or better.[39] A study at Barnes Hospital found that the prognosis directly correlated with the presenting visual acuity. The sooner patients are treated, the better the outcome.[30]

Infectious endophthalmitis is a rare entity whose prognosis is directly dependent on the timeliness of the diagnosis. Clinicians should always suspect endophthalmitis when the inflammatory reaction is beyond what is expected. Prompt referrals are mandatory.

**TABLE 14–6. TREATMENT OPTIONS: ENDOPHTHALMITIS SUSPECTED**

Immediate referral for anterior chamber/vitreous tap
Possible vitrectomy
Topical, subconjunctival, and intravitreal antibiotics
Topical and oral steroids 24–48 h later

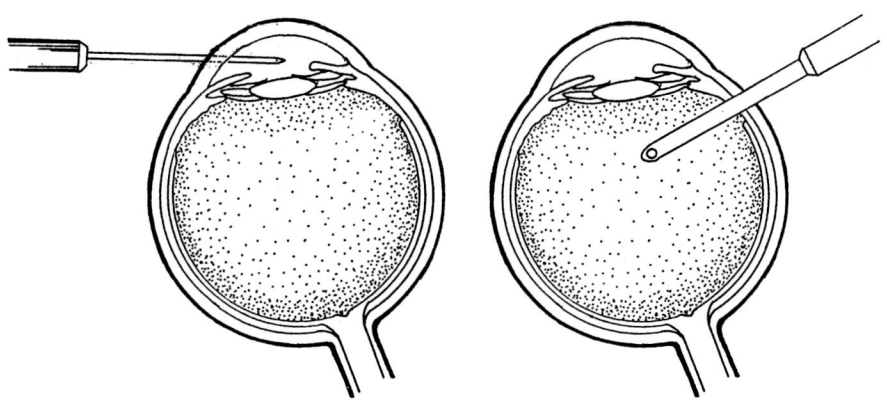

**FIGURE 14–17.** Patients suspected of having endophthalmitis should undergo an anterior chamber and vitreous tap to culture for the causative organisms.

## — IRIS PROLAPSE/VITREOUS TO THE WOUND —

As surgical techniques have improved, complications such as iris prolapse and vitreous to the wound are becoming exceedingly rare. However, they may be found in patients who had surgery some years ago, had intraoperative complications during modern cataract extraction, or have a history of ocular trauma.

### Background

The causes of iris prolapse are improper wound closure, postoperative trauma, and increased IOPs.[51] It is a rare, sight-threatening complication that requires immediate return to the surgeon for evaluation and treatment. Iris prolapse typically occurs early in the postoperative course. It may also occur later before wound healing is complete and may be associated with severe coughing or vomiting.

Vitreous to the wound is more common than iris prolapse. It generally occurs following intraoperative capsular rupture when the surgeon withdraws surgical instruments from the eye carrying vitreous with them. Due to the transparent nature of the vitreous, the surgeon may not note its presence during the surgery. It then becomes apparent at the first postoperative visit.

### Clinical Presentation and Assessment

A patient with iris prolapse often has noteworthy pain. The typical clinical presentation is a black or dark purple discoloration within a wound gape (Figure 14–18). In more severe cases, the iris may actually push through the wound in the shape of a fan (complete prolapse) causing a teardrop- or pear-shaped pupil with its apex pointing to the area of iris incarceration. There may also be intense conjunctival injection, possible wound leak with shallow or flat anterior chamber, and low IOP. It should be noted whether the conjunctiva covers the area of prolapse or whether the iris is exposed to the extraocular surface, as this may carry a higher risk of intraocular infection.

Iris prolapse may also occur later in the postoperative course and present in an incomplete fashion, with conjunctiva covering the area. The patient may be asymptomatic or may report a history of trauma, recurrent postoperative iritis, or an irregular pupil. There may be anterior chamber cells and flare or the chamber may be quiet. Inspection of the wound will show a black or purplish band in portions of the wound gape or just a few small blackish dots in the wound margin. A bleb formation is possible. There may also be a mildly distorted pupil, again, with its apex pointing to the prolapse.

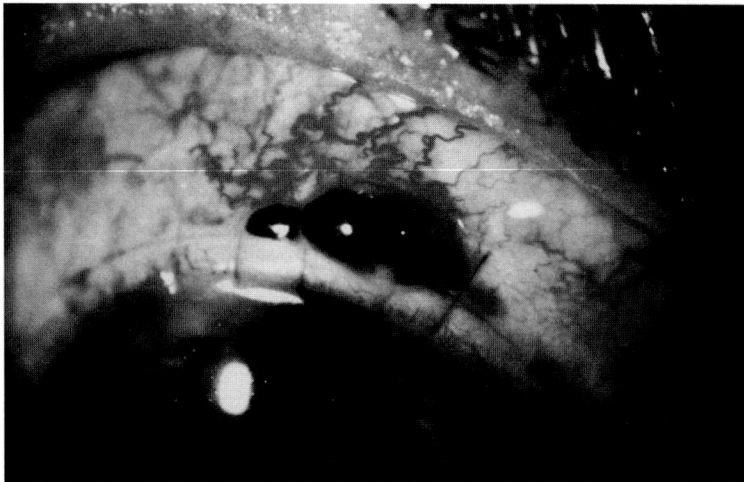

**FIGURE 14–18.** Iris incarceration to the wound.

A complicated surgery may result in vitreous to the wound. This occurs when there has been posterior capsular rupture and vitreous prolapses into the anterior chamber. The patient is generally asymptomatic but may note a peaked pupil. On slit lamp examination, the doctor may more easily appreciate vitreous in the anterior chamber if it has pigment adherent to its anterior face. Alternatively, there may be a small strand of vitreous through the pupillary area that is adherent to the wound margin ("vitreous wick syndrome"). This "wick" may distort the pupil as it stretches through the pupil to the wound (Figures 14–19 and 14–20). Careful detection by slit lamp inspection and gonioscopy are necessary, because vitreous to the wound carries a high incidence of cystoid macular edema[30] and vitreous loss increases the likelihood of retinal detachment.[52–54]

### Treatment, Follow-up, and Prognosis

Iris prolapse requires immediate attention, as it may result in improper wound healing, flat anterior chamber, and a chronically hypotensive eye (Table 14–7).

**FIGURE 14–19.** Peaked pupil secondary to vitreous to the wound.

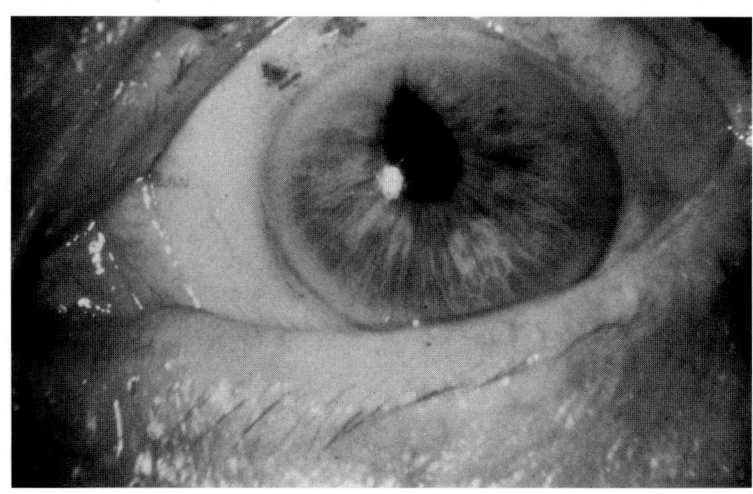

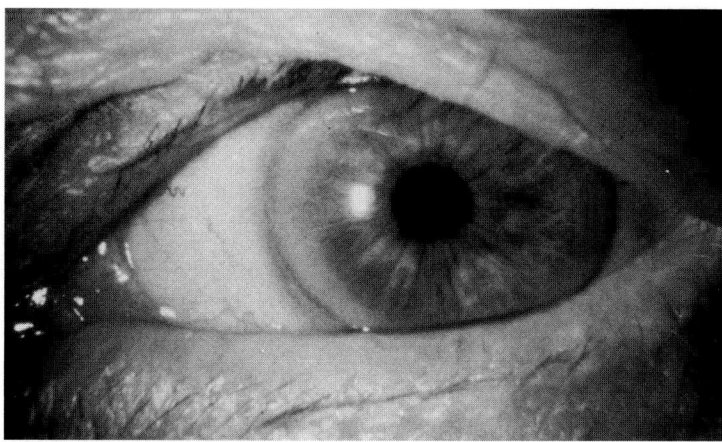

**FIGURE 14–20.** Round pupil following Nd:YAG laser vitreolysis of the vitreous to the wound in Figure 14–19.

It may also lead to chronic iridocyclitis with corneal decompensation, secondary glaucoma, or endophthalmitis (Figure 14–21). Surgical repair of iris prolapse is aimed at returning the iris to its preoperative position and restoring wound integrity (Figure 14–22). A surgical attempt may be made to open the wound gape further and push the iris into place. An iridectomy may also be employed to remove the portion of the iris in the wound gape. After the iris is removed from the wound area, resuturing to seal the wound firmly is completed. In cases where the iris is covered by conjunctiva, photocoagulation, cryotherapy, or chemical cauterization are alternative methods.[55]

In cases of iris prolapse and vitreous to the wound with a quiet asymptomatic eye, a review of the patient's records may be helpful in establishing when this occurred. A surgical consult should be offered to discuss risks and benefits of repair. In general, if the eye is quiet and there is conjunctiva over the wound, the surgeon may elect to do nothing but explain to the patient that he or she may be at higher risk for postoperative infection. If there is a history of recurrent intraocular inflammation or if the wound appears compromised due to the prolapse, the surgeon may elect surgical repair or other treatment. Follow-up would be determined by the procedures performed and surgeon preference.

Patients who have vitreous to the wound are at risk for cystoid macular edema (CME). Nd:YAG laser lysis of the vitreal strands has been shown to prevent this or alleviate chronic CME. There also is an increased risk of retinal detachment in patients with vitreous to the wound. Those with retinal breaks, lattice degeneration, and vitreoretinal traction are especially at risk. These patients need to be monitored carefully.

**TABLE 14–7. TREATMENT OPTIONS: IRIS PROLAPSE AND/OR VITREOUS TO THE WOUND**

Refer for surgical repair:
　Reposition and/or perform iridectomy
　Restore wound integrity
　Treat vitreous to the wound surgically or with laser

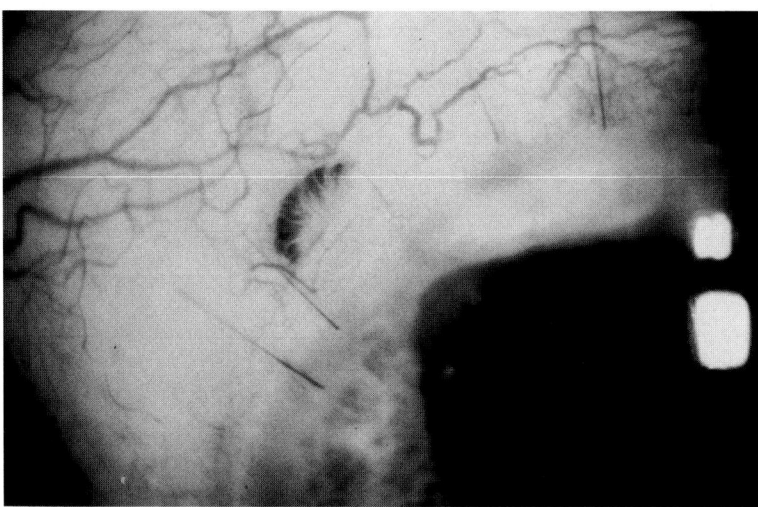

FIGURE 14–21. Iris incarceration to the wound with peaked pupil.

## INTRAOCULAR LENS DISLOCATIONS

We define IOL dislocation as a lens partially moved from its proper position but still attached to some tissue (subluxation) or one that is completely free of its tissue support (luxation). When the IOL moves suddenly to its new position, it is expelled. If the dislocation is slow, the IOL is extruded[56] (see Chapter 3). Intraocular lens dislocation must be differentiated from lens decentration and pupillary capture. Decentration occurs when the IOL is partially or totally off the visual axis but maintains most of its tissue support (Figure 14–23). Pupillary capture is present when the pupillary margin becomes located partially or completely anterior to an anterior chamber IOL or posterior to a posterior chamber IOL (Figures 14–24 and 14–25). IOL dislocations occur due to incorrect placement, incorrect size, or loss of structural support of the lens. Most dislocations today occur as a result of incorrect placement and/or loss of structural support.

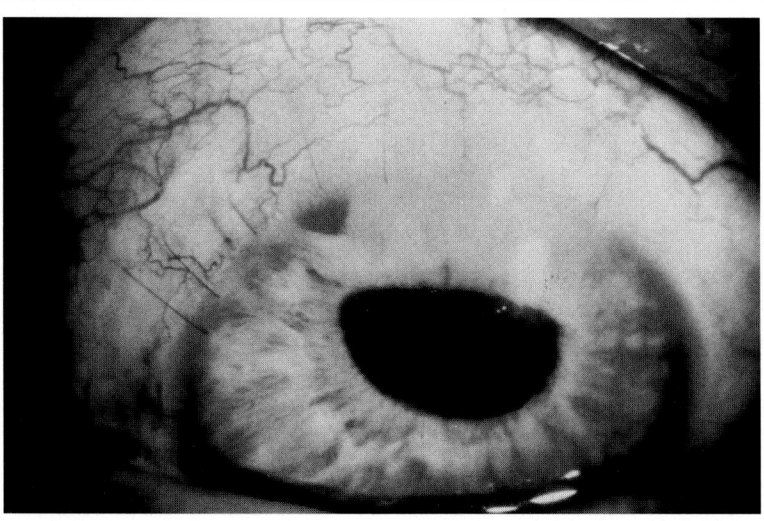

FIGURE 14–22. Repair of iris incarceration.

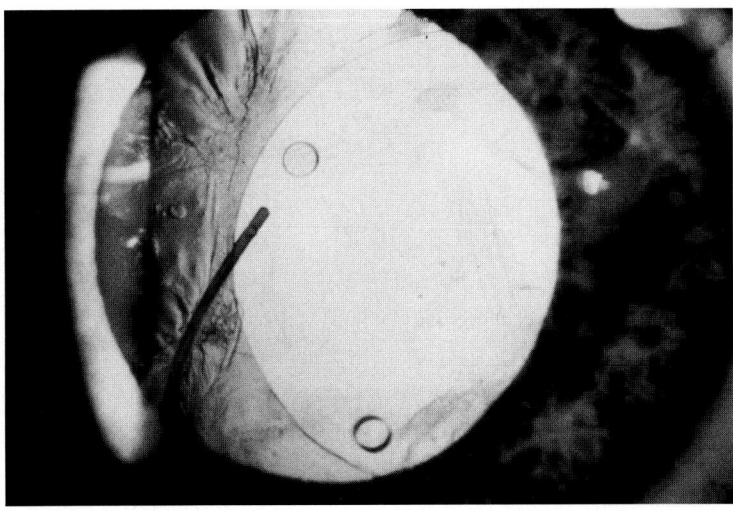

**FIGURE 14–23.** Decentration of a posterior chamber IOL.

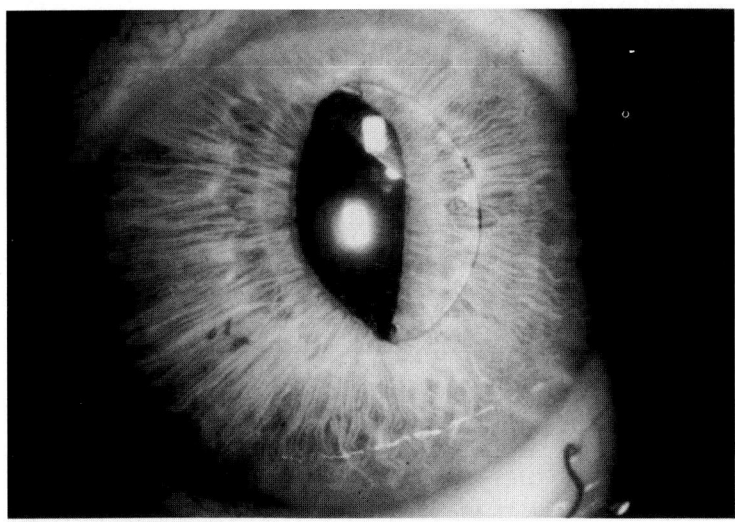

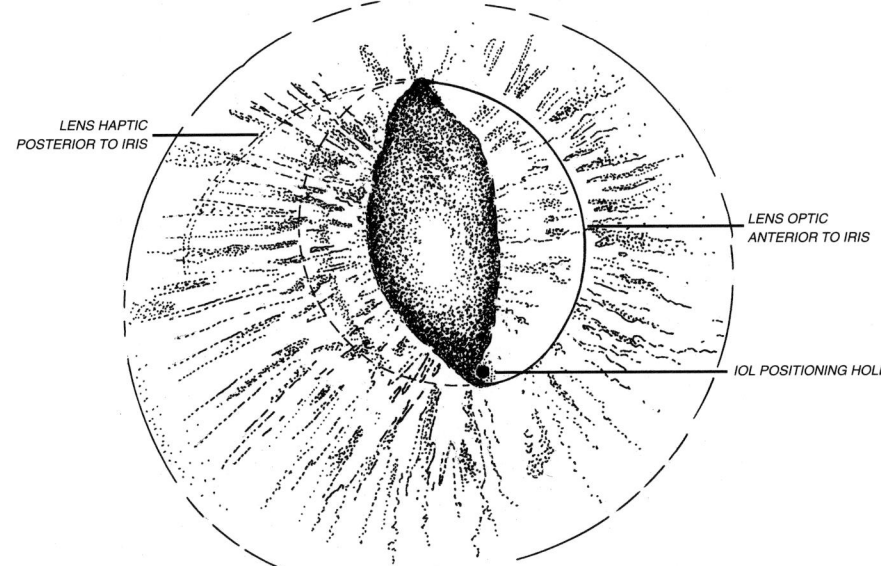

**FIGURES 14–24 AND 14–25.** Partial pupillary capture of a posterior chamber IOL.

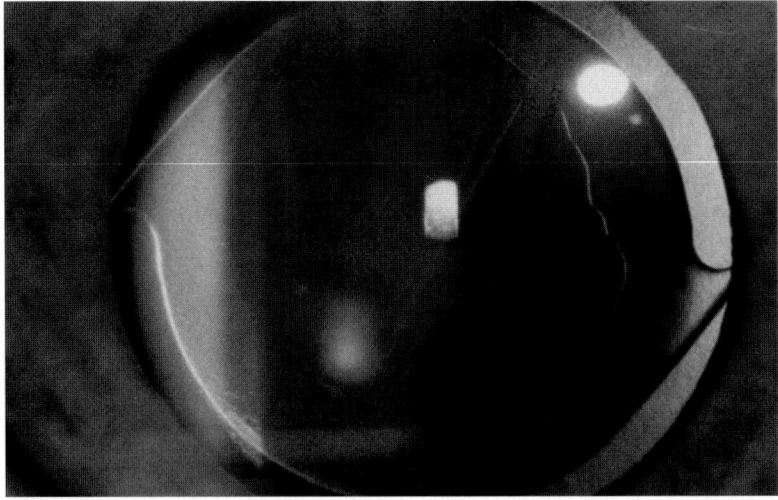

FIGURE 14–26. *A properly positioned posterior chamber IOL in the capsular bag.*

## Background

Posterior IOL dislocations and decentrations are best understood if capsular bag, zonular, and ciliary sulcus relationships to the lens implant are kept in mind. A surgery that is done by opening the capsule with capsulorhexis, placing the lens in the bag without side tearing of the capsule, and good attachment of the zonules offers an excellent chance of a well-centered, unmoving implant[57] (Figures 14–26 and 14–27) (see Chapter 3). "Can-opener" capsulotomy may lead to side rips in the bag that allow the lens haptics to escape the bag and result in "bag-sulcus fixation," where one of the haptics moves into the sulcus and thereby displaces the lens implant in that direction (Figure 14–21). Incorrect placement of the lens by the surgeon and creating a bag-sulcus placement will also cause this malposition.

The "sunset" syndrome may be observed with the loss of zonular support for the bag inferiorly (Figures 14–28 and 14–29). This results in a gradual drop of the lens out of the pupillary space. The sunrise syndrome may occur when the superior haptic of the intraocular lens is placed in the sulcus and the inferior haptic is fixated within the capsular bag. This will cause the lens to decenter superiorly and will take on the appearance of a rising sun. The "windshield-wiper" syndrome is excessive side-to-side movement of an anterior chamber IOL due to a small lens placed within the eye.

## Clinical Presentation and Assessment

A patient with a dislocated IOL generally reports subtle to marked blur or distortion and glare problems. They may or may not have symptoms of pain de-

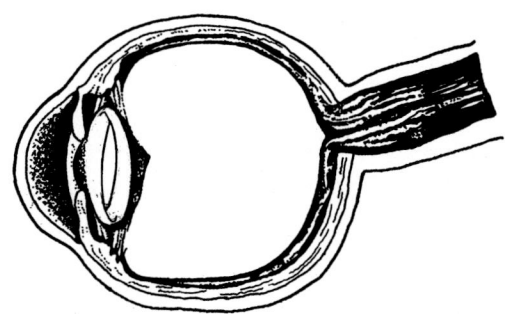

FIGURE 14–27. *Cross section of PC IOL in the capsular bag.*

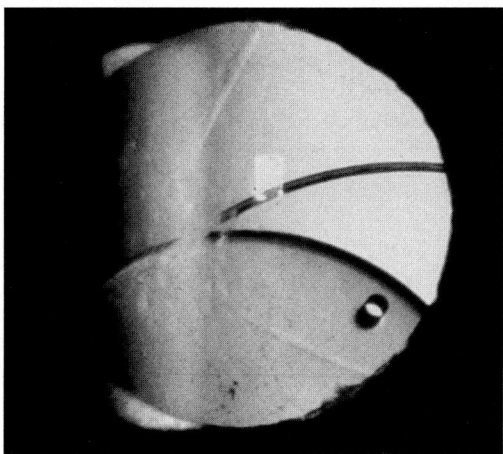

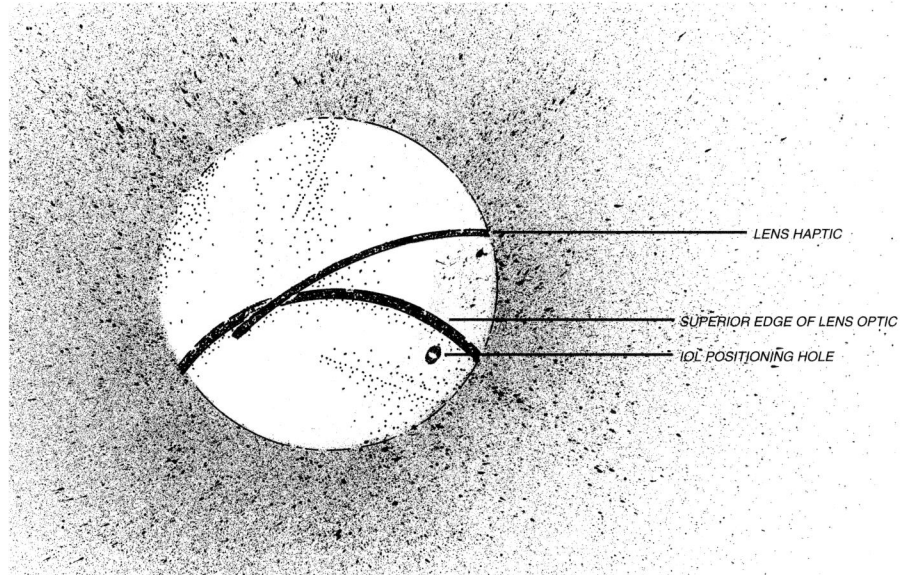

**FIGURES 14–28 AND 14–29.** Sunset syndrome observed following removal of a traumatic cataract due to disinsertion of zonules inferiorly.

pending on if the lens is dislocated in a position to cause irritation to vascular tissue. The patient should be examined at the slit lamp undilated to determine lens position under normal conditions and then after dilation to observe further the extent of dislocation.

## Differential Diagnosis

An IOL dislocation must be differentiated from a decentration and pupillary capture. The most frequent malposition of a posterior chamber lens is decentration. These are usually not of serious consequence as long as the optic axis of the patient is covered by the optic portion of IOL. Decentrations may be caused by misplacement of the IOL, such as in a bag-sulcus fixation, IOL haptic damage, or adhesions of the anterior capsule to the posterior capsule that move the IOL from its intended position. Decentrations may increase with time if capsular adhesions form around the haptics and move the IOL.

Pupillary capture is currently a rare occurrence with capsulorhexis and capsular fixation of an IOL. Pupillary capture occurs when the optic of the IOL enters the pupillary space and is entrapped by the iris as the pupil assumes its normal size following surgery (see Figures 14–24 and 14–25). The result of pupillary capture is a distorted pupil and possible chronic iritis.

## TABLE 14-8. TREATMENT OPTIONS: DISLOCATED IOLS

Refer to operating surgeon for consideration of repositioning or exchange
Advise patient to avoid strenous activities

## Treatment, Follow-up, and Prognosis

In the case of the sunset syndrome, an immediate return to the surgeon is necessary as surgical repair will likely be undertaken (Table 14–8). This repair is commonly aimed at securing the lens with the superior haptic sutured to the iris (Figures 14–28 to 14–30). If this fails, the surgeon may remove the lens implant and place an anterior chamber lens. If the lens is lost in the inferior sulcus or vitreous, an attempt may be made by the surgeon to retrieve the lens or the patient may be sent to a retinal specialist for an anterior vitrectomy and lens retrieval.

The sunrise syndrome may be treated by attempting to reduce the rotation of the lens by placing the lens haptics in the horizontal direction. This will be handled by return to the surgeon for repositioning or lens exchange.

Due to the potential for damage to the corneal endothelium, windshield-wiper syndrome also requires immediate return to the surgeon for either lens replacement or fixation by suturing the haptics to the iris.

In the case of pupillary capture, it should be reported to the surgeon, as the surgeon may want to reposition the IOL. In the presence of a posterior IOL and intact posterior capsular bag, an effort may be made in the office to reposition the IOL by dilating the pupil with an easily reversible mydriatic such as phenylephrine HCl 0.25% or tropicamide 1.0% (Mydriacyl). During mydriasis, the IOL should be inspected closely and any movement of the lens should be noted. Should the IOL reposition behind the iris plane following dilation, the pupil should be constricted with a strong miotic to trap the lens behind the iris. This has rarely worked in our experience, but should such an attempt be successful, the use of a miotic for a few weeks until adhesions hold the lens firmly behind the iris plane is suggested. Pupillary capture left untreated may result in chronic iritis. However, there are many cases of long-standing pupillary capture in which the patient is asymptomatic without any resulting chronic in-

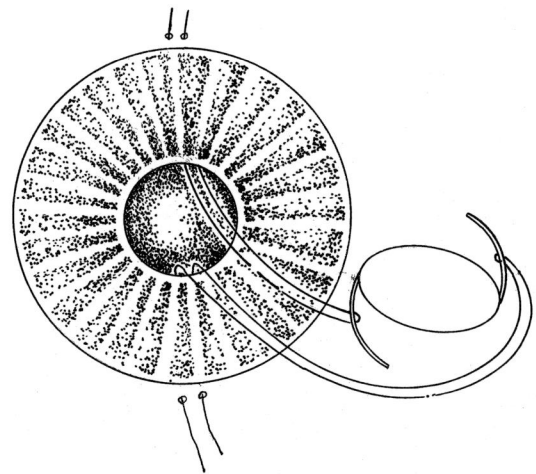

**FIGURE 14–30.** A posterior chamber IOL can be sutured to the iris if there is a lack of capsular support.

flammation. The prognosis of these cases is good, and intervention is usually not necessary.

Dislocations may gradually get worse over time. If symptoms and/or inflammation increase to significance, surgical intervention may be necessary.

## RETINAL BREAK/DETACHMENT

The possibility of retinal break or detachment following cataract surgery mandates periodic dilated fundus examination on all patients beginning during the early postoperative period and continuing at least annually. Appropriate patient counseling regarding potential symptoms is indicated, especially for patients at higher risk for developing rhegmatogenous retinal detachment, such as those with axial myopia, lattice degeneration, and/or a history of retinal detachment in the fellow eye.

### Background

A retinal tear is a break caused by vitreous traction, usually the result of strong vitreoretinal adhesion in an area of thin or weak retina (Figures 14–31 and 14–32). A flap (horseshoe) tear will appear as a strip of retina pulled anteriorly by the collapsing vitreous. The apex of a horseshoe tear usually points toward the posterior pole. In an operculated tear, a piece of retina that has torn completely free from the retinal surface will be observed floating in the vitreous in close proximity to the break. Hemorrhage, arising from the rupture of retinal vessels that cross retinal tears, may also be present.

Although the majority of breaks do not cause detachment, any retinal break may allow fluid from the vitreous to separate the sensory retina from the underlying pigment epithelium. Persisting traction with increasing liquefied vitreous in the subretinal space will eventually lead to retinal detachment (Figure 14–33). Such rhegmatogenous retinal detachments may involve anywhere from less than a quadrant of the retina to the entire retina including the macula.

The incidence of retinal detachment following extracapsular cataract extraction (ECCE) with nuclear expression or phacoemulsification has been determined to be low; averaging approximately 1%[58–60] (Table 14–9). Such incidence increases in eyes with vitreous loss and following intracapsular cataract extraction (ICCE), where disturbance of the vitreous is more likely[61–63] (Figure 14–34). Intraocular lens implants do not appear to influence the incidence of retinal detachment.

Most detachments occur within 6 months of surgery and thus may be a significant complication in the early postoperative course. Axial myopia, lattice degeneration of the retina, vitreoretinal tufts or tags, meridional folds, and a history of retinal detachment in the opposite eye are several of the predisposing factors for the development of rhegmatogenous retinal detachment in eyes following cataract extraction. The peripheral fundus must be examined carefully preoperatively for the presence of these factors, with consideration being given to the prophylactic treatment of any asymptomatic retinal breaks prior to cataract surgery.

### Clinical Presentation and Assessment

Patients experiencing a retinal tear or detachment following surgery may report the phenomena of floaters (entopsias) and flashing lights (photopsias).

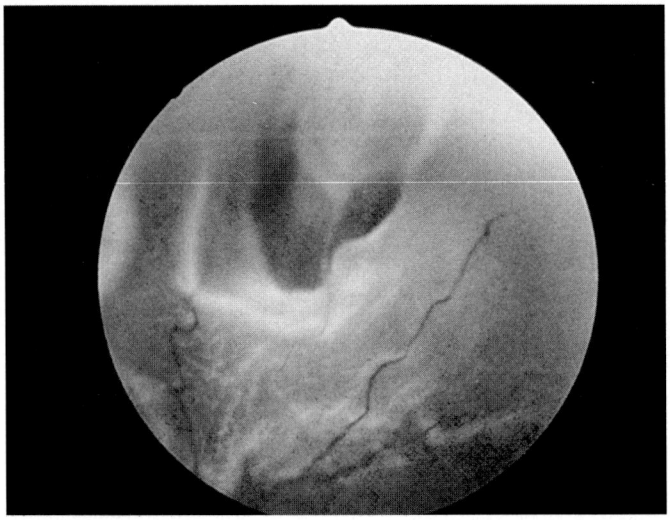

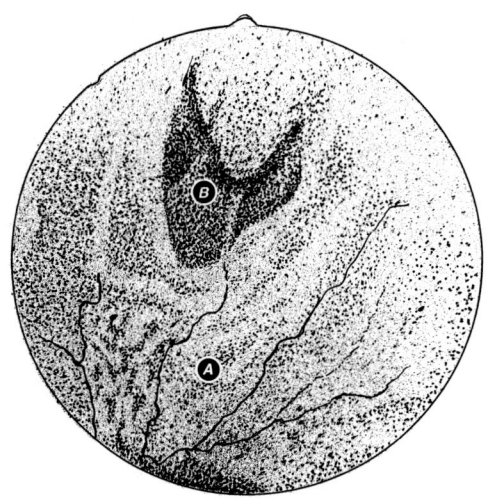

**FIGURES 14–31 AND 14–32.** A rhegmatogenous retinal detachment (A) with break (B).

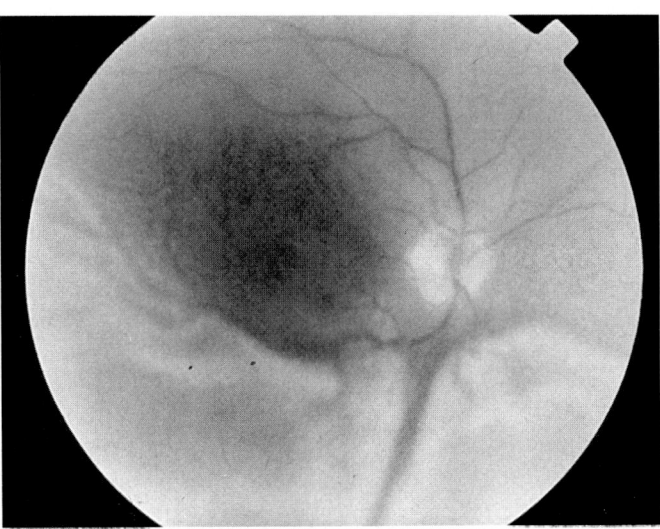

**FIGURE 14–33.** Retinal detachment.

**TABLE 14-9. INCIDENCE OF RETINAL DETACHMENT FOLLOWING CATARACT SURGERY**

| Type of Surgery | Incidence |
| --- | --- |
| Extracapsular cataract extraction | 0.8% to 0.9% |
| Intracapsular cataract extraction | 1.55% to 3.60% |

Furthermore, retinal detachment may elicit the symptoms of a peripheral shadow or dense curtain encroaching on central vision.

Such symptoms are reason for prompt dilation and thorough funduscopic examination (Table 14–10). Indirect ophthalmoscopy with scleral depression and/or slit lamp biomicroscopy, best performed with a contact lens, are required to make the definitive diagnosis and to rule out retinal breaks and detachment. During the early postoperative period in patients with sutureless incisions, scleral depression should be avoided unless absolutely necessary, particularly in the superior quadrants and over the incision site. In our clinic, patients needing a definitive peripheral retinal evaluation are first examined with a contact lens with a peripheral mirror. If any question still remains, they are then referred to a vitreoretinal surgeon for further examination.

Recent retinal detachments, that is, those manifesting during the first 2 weeks following surgery, will appear corrugated, semitransparent, and undulate with eye movements. The elevation will have convex edges and surfaces, and underlying choroidal detail will be obscured. Other clinical signs may include a lower IOP in the affected eye and the presence of pigmented cells in the vitreous or anterior segment. This "tobacco dust," also known as Shaffer's sign, is best observed through biomicroscopic examination of the anterior segment and anterior vitreous. Finally, any prolonged uveitis in an eye with a well-positioned IOL and the absence of an abnormal anterior uveovitreal relationship should prompt the doctor to dilate the patient's eye and determine if a retinal break or detachment is present.

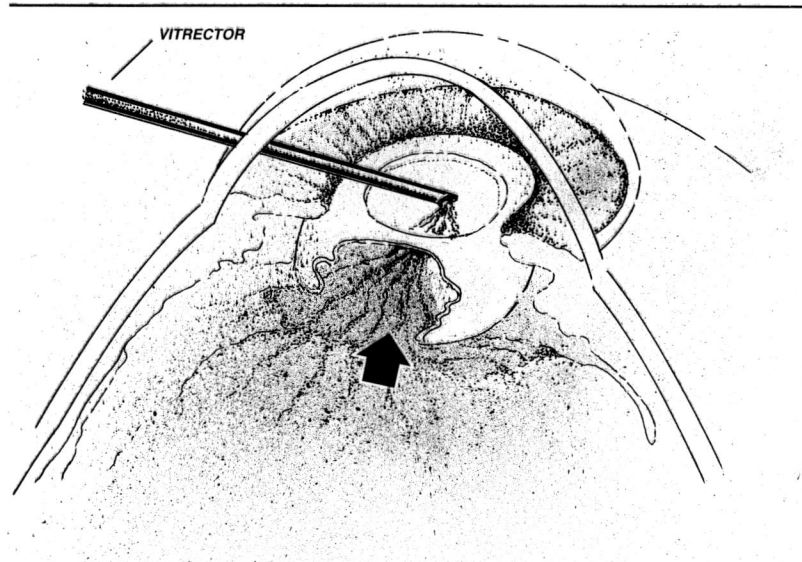

*FIGURE 14–34.* During cataract surgery, vitreous loss increases the risk of retinal detachment due to vitreoretinal traction.

**TABLE 14–10. CLINICAL SIGNS AND SYMPTOMS OF RETINAL DETACHMENT**

| Symptoms | Signs |
| --- | --- |
| Floaters, most notably numerous black "specs" | ± Decreased visual acuity |
| | ± Relative afferent pupillary defect |
| Flashing lights | ± Reduced IOP |
| Progressive "curtain" scotoma | Relative scotoma |
| | Anterior vitreous pigment cells, "Shaffer's sign" |
| | Retinal folds, subretinal fluid, retinal break |

## Differential Diagnosis

If a definite retinal break cannot be found in association with a retinal detachment, all other causes of retinal elevation must be considered and ruled out. These include exudative and tractional retinal detachment, retinoschisis, and choroidal detachment (see Chapter 15).

## Treatment, Follow-up, and Prognosis

Patients presenting with acute symptomatic tears or retinal detachment should be referred immediately to a vitreoretinal surgeon for treatment (Table 14–11). Patients should be advised to limit their activity and avoid ingesting liquid or solid foods in preparation for a promptly scheduled surgery with possible general anesthesia.

If a large vitreous hemorrhage is present, the surgeon may ask the patient to limit activity until the vitreous is clear enough to identify the break or breaks and provide a complete evaluation.

When a detachment is identified, surgery is scheduled as soon as possible. Most surgeries for rhegmatogenous retinal detachment require less than 2 hours and are performed under general and/or retrobulbar anesthesia. Techniques may include cryopexy, laser photocoagulation, scleral buckling, pneumatic retinopexy, or a combination thereof.

Surgical repair of a rhegmatogenous retinal detachment involves locating all of the retinal breaks and sealing them with diathermy, cryotherapy, or endolaser. Next, a scleral buckle or sponge is applied and, if needed, subretinal fluid must be drained. Pneumatic retinopexy is another technique used, especially for smaller superior breaks in which a bubble of expanding gas is injected into the vitreous to hold the detached retina in place and the breaks are then treated.

The prognosis for vision following retinal detachment is best in cases without macular detachment, although CME or macular pucker may still occur and

**TABLE 14–11. TREATMENT OPTIONS: RETINAL DETACHMENT**

Refer immediately to surgeon for repair
Counsel patient to limit activity
Avoid intake of food and liquids in anticipation of general anesthesia

affect final visual acuity. In the presence of macular detachment, degeneration of the photoreceptors results with subsequent poor postoperative visual acuity, with severity dependent on the duration of macular detachment.

Once stability of the retinal repair has been achieved, as determined by the retinologist through periodic postoperative follow-up visits, it is possible for the optometrist to comanage the ongoing eye care of the patient effectively. Care should include a thorough dilated fundus examination at least annually. Finally, the symptoms of retinal detachment must be reviewed with the patient and the patient must understand that immediate evaluation is necessary should these symptoms arise.

## REFERENCES

### Ocular Hypertension

1. Kooner KS, Dulaney DD, Zimmerman TJ: Intraocular pressure following extracapsular cataract extraction and posterior chamber intraocular lens implantation. *Ophthal Surg.* 1988;**19**:471–474.
2. Gross JG, Meyer DR, Robin AL, et al: Increased intraocular pressure in the immediate postoperative period after extracapsular cataract extraction. *Am J Ophthalmol.* 1988;**105**:466–469.
3. Naeser K, Thim K, Hansen T, et al: Intraocular pressure in the first days after implantation of posterior chamber lenses with the use of sodium hyaluronate. *Acta Ophthalmol.* 1986;**64**:330–337.
4. Rothkoff L, Biedner B, Blumenthal M: The effect of corneal section on early increased intraocular pressure after cataract extraction. *Am J Ophthalmol.* 1978;**85**:337–338.
5. Vu MT, Shields MB: The early postoperative pressure course in glaucoma patients following cataract surgery. *Ophthal Surg.* 1988;**19**:467–470.
6. Shields MB: *Textbook of Glaucoma.* 2nd ed. Baltimore: Williams & Wilkins; 1987:334–358.
7. Liesegang TJ: Viscoelastic substances in ophthalmology. *Surv Ophthalmol.* 1990;**34**:268–293.
8. Stamper RL, DiLoreto D, Schacknow P: Effect of intraocular aspiration of sodium hyaluronate on postoperative intraocular pressure. *Ophthal Surg.* 1990;**21**:486–491.
9. Tomey KF, Traverso CE: The glaucomas in aphakia and pseudophakia. *Surv Ophthalmol.* 1991;**36**:79–112.
10. Poleski SA, Willis WE: Angle-supported intraocular lenses: A goniophotographic study. *Ophthalmology.* 1984;**91**:838–840.
11. Evans RB: Peripheral anterior synechia overlying the haptics of posterior chamber lenses. *Ophthalmology.* 1990;**97**:415–423.
12. Vernon SA: Non-contact tonometry in the postoperative eye. *Br J Ophthalmol.* 1989;**73**:247–249.
13. Brencher HL, Kohl P, Reinke AR, Yolton RL: Clinical comparison of airpuff and Goldmann tonometers. *J Am Optom Assoc.* 1991;**62**:345–402.
14. Moseley MJ, Evans NM, Fielder AR: Comparison of a new non-contact tonometer with Goldmann applanation. *Eye.* 1989;**3**:332–337.
15. Patorgis C: Complications of cataract and implant surgery. *Optom Clin.* 1991:**1**(2):81–113.
16. Pollack IP, Brown RH, Crandall AS, et al: Prevention of the rise in intraocular pressure following neodymium-YAG posterior capsulotomy using topical 1% apraclonidine. *Arch Ophthalmol.* 1988;**106**:754–756.
17. Hill RA, Minckler DS, Lee M, et al: Apraclonidine prophylaxis for postcycloplegic intraocular pressure spikes. *Ophthalmology.* 1991;**98**:1083–1086.

18. Wiles SB, Mackenzie D, Ide CH: Control of intraocular pressure with apraclonidine hydrochloride after cataract extraction. *Am J Ophthalmol.* 1991;**111**:184–188.
19. Robin AL: Effect of topical apraclonidine on the frequency of intraocular pressure elevations after combined extracapsular cataract extraction and trabeculectomy. *Ophthalmology.* 1993;**100**:628–633.
20. Yaldo MK, Shin DH, Parrow KA, Lee SH, Lee SY: Additive effect of 1% apraclonidine hydrochloride to nonselective β-blockers. *Ophthalmology.* 1991;**98**:1075–1078.
21. Jaanus SD: Hyperosmotic agents. In Bartlett JD, Zimmerman TJ, Jaanus SD, et al (eds): *Ophthalmic Drug Facts*. St Louis: Facts and Comparisons; 1989:163–172.
22. Strelow SA, Sherwood MB, Broncato LJB, et al: The effect of diclofenac sodium ophthalmic solution on intraocular pressure following cataract extraction. *Ophthal Surg.* 1992;**23**:170–175.
23. Weinberger D, Lusky M, Debbi S, Ben-Sira I: Pseudophakic and aphakic pupillary block. *Ann Ophthalmol.* 1988;**20**:403–405.
24. Willis DA, Stewart RH, Kimbrough RL: Pupillary block associated with posterior chamber lenses. *Ophthal Surg.* 1985;**16**:108–109.
25. Samples JR, Bellows AR, Rosenquist RC, et al. Pupillary block with posterior chamber intraocular lenses. *Arch Ophthalmol.* 1987;**105**:335–337.
26. Shrader CE, Belcher CD, Thomas JV, Simmons RJ, Murphy EB: Pupillary and iridovitreal block in pseudophakic eyes. *Ophthalmology.* 1984;**91**:831–837.

## Wound Leak with Shallow Anterior Chamber

27. Jaffe NS, Jaffe MS, Jaffe GF: *Cataract Surgery and Its Complications,* 5th ed. St Louis: CV Mosby; 1990:361–364.
28. Weinstein GW: Cataract Surgery. In Tasman W (ed): *Duane's Clinical Ophthalmology,* Vol 5. Philadelphia: Harper & Row; 1991:7:38.

## Endophthalmitis

29. Smith RE, Nozik RA: *Uveitis.* 2nd ed. Baltimore: Williams & Wilkins; 1989:101–105.
30. Bohigian GM, Olk RJ: Factors associated with a poor visual result in endophthalmitis. *Am J Ophthalmol.* 1986;**101**:332–334.
31. Javitt JC, Vitale S, Canner JK, et al: National outcomes of cataract extraction/endophthalmitis following in-patient surgery. *Arch Ophthalmol.* 1991;**109**:1085–1089.
32. Pettit TH, Olson RJ, Foos RY, Martin WJ: Fungal endophthalmitis following intraocular lens implantation. *Arch Ophthalmol.* 1980;**98**:1025–1039.
33. Speaker MG, Milch FA, Shah MK, et al: Role of external bacterial flora in the pathogenesis of acute postoperative endophthalmitis. *Ophthalmology.* 1991;**98**:639–650.
34. Raskin EM, Speaker MG, McCormick SA, et al: Influence of haptic materials on the adherence of staphylococci to intraocular lenses. *Arch Ophthalmol.* 1993;**111**:250–253.
35. Alvarez O, Morales J, McCartney DL: Haemophilus aphrophilus endophthalmitis associated with a filtering bleb. Letter to ed. *Arch Ophthalmol.* 1991;**109**:618–620.
36. Wolner B, Liebmann JM, Sassani JW, et al: Late bleb-related endophthalmitis after trabeculectomy with adjunctive 5-fluorouracil. *Ophthalmology.* 1991;**98:**1053–1060.
37. Ormerod LD, Puklin JE, McHenry JG, McDermott ML: Scleral flap necrosis and infectious endophthalmitis after cataract surgery with a scleral tunnel incision. *Ophthalmology.* 1993;**100**:159–163.
38. Miller KM, Glasgow BJ: Bacterial endophthalmitis following sutureless cataract surgery. *Arch Ophthalmol.* 1993;**111**:377–379.
39. Driebe WT, Mandelbaum S, Forster RK, et al: Pseudophakic endophthalmitis. *Ophthalmology.* 1986;**93**:442–448.
40. Forster RK: Endophthalmitis. In Tasman W (ed): *Duane's Clinical Ophthalmology,* Vol. 4. Philadelphia: Harper & Row; 1989:1–21.

41. Mao LK, Flynn HW, Miller D, Pflugfelder SC: Endophthalmitis caused by streptococcal species. *Arch Ophthalmol.* 1992;**110**:798–801.
42. Maxwell DP, Baber WB: Acute postoperative endophthalmitis associated with dual strains of staphylococcus epidermidis. *Ophthal Surg.* 1992;**23**:222–224.
43. Ormerod LD, Ho DD, Becker LE, et al: Endophthalmitis caused by the coagulase-negative staphylococci. Disease spectrum and outcome. *Ophthalmology.* 1993;**100**:715–723.
44. Ormerod LD, Becker LE, Cruise RJ, et al: Endophthalmitis caused by the coagulase-negative staphylococci. Factors influencing presentation after cataract surgery. *Ophthalmology.* 1993;**100**:724–729.
45. Piest KL, Kincaid MC, Tetz MR, et al: Localized endophthalmitis: A newly described cause of the so-called toxic lens syndrome. *J Cataract Refract Surg.* 1987;**13**:498–510.
46. Ficker L, Meredith TA, Wilson LA, et al. Chronic bacterial endophthalmitis. *Am J Ophthalmol.* 1987;**103**:745–748.
47. Fox GM, Joondeph BC, Flynn HW, et al: Delayed-onset pseudophakic endophthalmitis. *Am J Ophthalmol.* 1991;**111**:163–173.
48. Apple DJ, Mamalis N, Steinmetz RL, et al: Phacoanaphylactic endophthalmitis associated with extracapsular cataract extraction and posterior chamber intraocular lens. *Arch Ophthalmol.* 1984;**102**:1528–1532.
49. Marak GE: Phacoanaphylactic endophthalmitis. *Surv Ophthalmol.* 1992;**36**:325–339.
50. Doft BH: Editorial. The endophthalmitis vitrectomy study. *Arch Ophthalmol.* 1991;**109**:487–488.

## Iris Prolapse/Vitreous to the Wound

51. Apple DJ, Mamalis N, Olson RJ, Kincaid MC: *Intraocular Lenses: Evolution, Designs, Complications, and Pathology.* Baltimore: Williams & Wilkins; 1989:312.
52. McDonnell PJ, Zenaida C, de la Cruz MS, Green WR: Vitreous incarceration complicating cataract surgery: A light and electron microscopic study. *Ophthalmology.* 1986;**93**:247–253.
53. Chambless WS. Incidence of anterior and posterior segment complications in over 3000 cases of extracapsular cataract extractions: Intact and open capsules. *J Am Intraocul Implant Soc.* 1985;**11**:31–32.
54. Coonan P, Fung WE, Webster RG, et al: The incidence of retinal detachment following extracapsular cataract extraction. *Ophthalmology.* 1985;**92**:1096–1099.
55. Jaffe NS, Jaffe MS, Jaffe GF: *Cataract Surgery and Its Complications,* 5th ed. St Louis: Mosby; 1990:581.

## Intraocular Lens Dislocations

56. Alpar J, Choyce P: Complications of anterior chamber lenses and management. In Percival P (ed): *Color Atlas of Lens Implantation.* St Louis: Mosby-Year Book; 1991:235.
57. Assia EI, Legler UFC, Merrill C, et al: Clinicopathologic study of the effect of radial tears and loop fixation on intraocular lens decentration. *Ophthalmology.* 1993;**100**:153–158.

## Retinal Break/Detachment

58. Javitt JC, Vitale S, Canner JK, et al: National outcomes of cataract extraction I. *Ophthalmology.* 1991;**98**:895–902.
59. Smith PW, Stark WJ, Maumenee AE, et al: Retinal detachment after cataract extraction with posterior chamber intraocular lens. *Ophthalmology.* 1987;**94**:495–504.

60. Laatikainen L, Tarkkanen A: Proliferative vitreoretinopathy after intraocular lens implantation. *Acta Ophthalmol.* 1985;**63**:380–382.
61. Sorensen KE, Baggesen K: Retinal detachment following intracapsular cataract extraction. *Acta Ophthalmol.* 1990;**68**:549–553.
62. Percival SPB, Anand V, Das SK: Prevalence of aphakic retinal detachment. *Br J Ophthalmol.* 1983;**67**:43–45.
63. Clayman HM, Jaffe NS, Light DS, et al: Intraocular lenses, axial length, and retinal detachment. *Am J Ophthalmol.* 1981;**92**:778–780.

# Early, 1- to 14-Day (Less Emergent) Complications

CHAPTER 15

## PTOSIS

Postoperative transient ptosis noted within 48 hours of the surgery is not uncommon. It is usually not a cause of concern unless it persists.

### Background

Although topical anesthesia is being used by some surgeons, most cataract surgeons standardly use retrobulbar or peribulbar anesthesia. The desired effect of the anesthesia is to achieve akinesia (paralysis of muscles) as well as anesthesia.[1] The muscles controlling lid elevation (levator palpebrae superioris and Müller's muscle) are all affected by peribulbar anesthesia and results in an inability to elevate the lid.[1-3] Although in most patients the anesthetic and akinetic effect has worn off by the 1-day postoperative visit, occasionally a more prolonged effect will result. Ptosis within a few days following surgery can also be a result of eyelid edema.

Other factors have been associated with postoperative ptosis that persists more than a few days (see discussion of late ptosis in Chapter 16).

### Clinical Presentation and Assessment

Patients may or may not report noticing the ptosis. They may also complain of temporary diplopia. Ptosis of variable degree and some extraocular muscle restriction may be observed on examination.

### Differential Diagnosis

Differential diagnosis of ptosis present within 24 to 72 hours of surgery is probably not necessary, because most cases improve with time. In the late postoperative period, one may consider whether the ptosis may be related to preoperative ptosis due to neurologic, muscular, or mechanical abnormalities (see discussion of ptosis in Chapter 16).

### Treatment, Follow-up, and Prognosis

Although most patients with early postoperative ptosis will improve quickly, some may persist. At the early postoperative visits, patients should be counseled that most cases of ptosis improve with time.

## DIPLOPIA

Prolonged akinesia (temporary paralysis of muscles) following cataract surgery occasionally persists for 24 hours or more. Assuming good visual potential in each eye, these patients will complain of diplopia.

### Background

Patients undergoing retrobulbar or peribulbar anesthesia develop akinesia of the extraocular muscles.[1] Most patients recover quickly from the anesthesia however, some may have a prolonged recovery of 24–48 hours resulting in diplopia.

### Clinical Presentation and Assessment

The patient describes diplopia. Ocular motility testing reveals a noncomitant strabismus with the vertical muscles most commonly affected.

### Differential Diagnosis

If the diplopia does not recover after 48 hours, other causes should be considered (see discussion of diplopia in Chapter 16).

### Treatment, Follow-up, and Prognosis

The patient should be reassured and followed.

## WOUND LEAK WITH WELL-FORMED ANTERIOR CHAMBER

When ocular hypotony is found during the first few postoperative weeks, a wound leak must be suspected (see Chapter 14). Even though a wound leak is present, there may be a well-formed anterior chamber and a normal-appearing posterior segment. This occurs when the flow of aqueous from the leak is low enough that aqueous production can still fill the anterior chamber. Jaffe suggests that this presentation may be more common than is generally thought in wounds tested 24 hours after surgery.[4]

### Clinical Presentation and Assessment

Although patients may have no symptoms, some report discomfort or blurred vision. Objectively, one finds low intraocular pressure (0–5 mm Hg) and normal corneal appearance or a waffled fluorescein pattern of the corneal surface after fluorescein instillation. Slit lamp examination of the anterior chamber

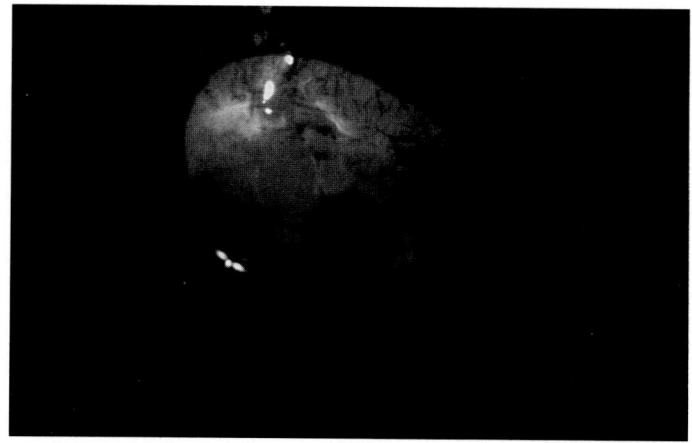

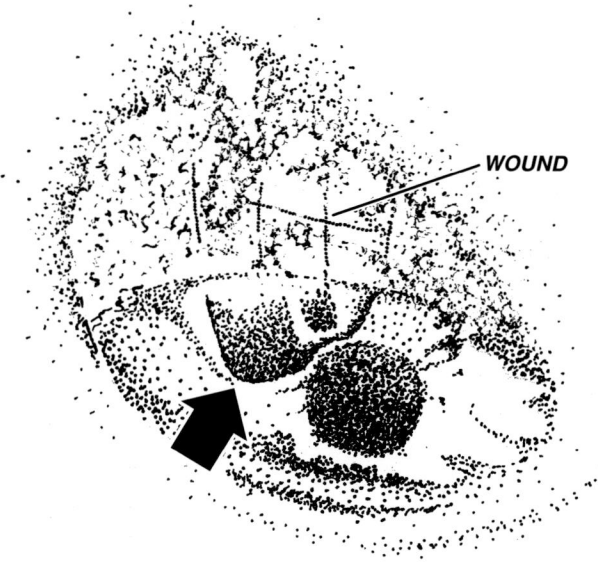

FIGURES 15–1 AND 15–2. Wound leak.

should include estimation of its depth and observation of inflammatory signs. The wound should be carefully inspected for vitreous or iris incarceration, poor apposition of the margins, or gaping. A Seidel test may be performed by placing sterile fluorescein sodium along the wound margin (Figures 15–1 and 15–2). If a leak is present, a clear stream of aqueous with a bright green border percolates from the wound and cascades down the cornea. (See the arrow in Figure 15–2.) To ensure against infection, any form of fluorescein instilled should be sterile. A single dose of 2% fluorescein sodium is excellent for this purpose, but a fluorescein strip wetted with a newly opened bottle of sterile saline may be used. Also, a newly opened fluorescein anesthetic preparation (Fluress) is appropriate. The eye should be dilated and choroidal and retinal detachment should be ruled out.

## Differential Diagnosis

The differential diagnosis for low intraocular pressure with formed anterior chamber is wound leak versus uveitis, ciliary body shutdown, choroidal detachment, and retinal detachment.

**TABLE 15–1. TREATMENT OPTIONS: WOUND LEAK WITH FORMED ANTERIOR CHAMBER**

| With Patch | Without Patch |
|---|---|
| Instill ciprofloxacin 0.3%, two drops in clinic | Begin ciprofloxacin 0.3%, one drop four times daily |
| Instill atropine 1.0%, one drop in clinic | Instill atropine 1.0%, one drop in clinic |
| Begin cephalexin, 250 mg by mouth four times daily | Begin prednisolone acetate 1.0%, one drop one to two times daily (tapered dosage) |
| Apply pressure patch | Begin cephalexin, 250 mg by mouth four times daily |
| Wear shield at night | Recheck in 24 h |
| Recheck in 24 h | |

## Treatment, Follow-up, and Prognosis

The management of a wound leak associated with well-formed anterior chamber is usually pressure patch application (Table 15–1). Some advocate the use of aqueous suppressants (carbonic anhydrase inhibitors), or beta-blockers, as they may slow the movement of aqueous through the leak by decreasing aqueous formation. However, there is no substantial clinical evidence to support this claim.

As a wound leak may lead to iris incarceration or shallowing of the anterior chamber, the patient needs to be monitored closely until the leak resolves. Patients are usually patched with a pressure patch, but in cases where the wound margins are irregular or there is wound gape, tissue adhesive with or without a soft lens may be used or the surgeon may elect to suture the area. In our clinic, patients are given additional prophylactic topical antibiotics. Fluoroquinolones such as ciprofloxacin 0.3% (Ciloxan) are used, and the patient is continued on oral antibiotics such as cephalexin (Keflex) until the leak resolves.

In most patients, the leak seals after a 12- to 24-hour pressure patch. If this fails, it is often attempted again. With multiple failures or shallowing of the anterior chamber, the patient is returned to surgery for further repair.

## ACUTE CORNEAL EDEMA

Corneal edema following cataract surgery is usually transient; however, it may be a serious complication resulting in permanently reduced vision. Postoperative corneal edema is clinically divided into acute cases and chronic cases (see discussion of chronic corneal edema in Chapter 16). (See Color Plate 15–1.)

### Background

Acute postoperative corneal edema usually occurs within the first or second postoperative day. Edema of this nature frequently resolves within 2 weeks of surgery, but rarely it may persist for 2–3 months. Acute postoperative corneal edema is thought to be the result of intraoperative hydration of the cornea, tran-

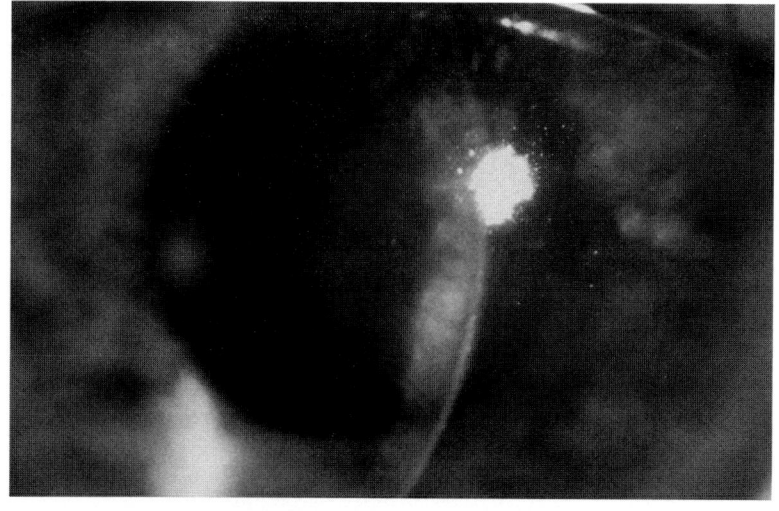
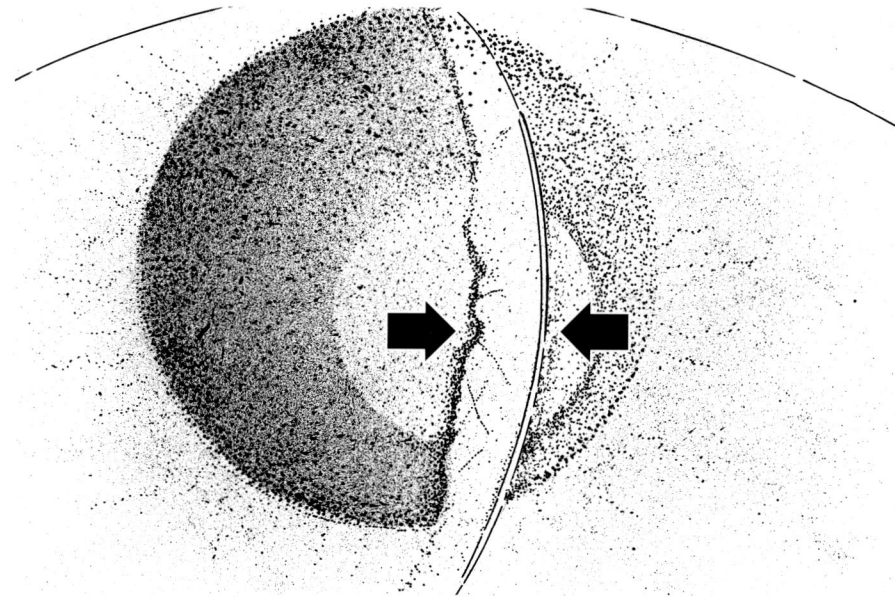

**FIGURES 15–3 AND 15–4.** Postoperative corneal edema; note the thickened stroma centrally.

sient loss of endothelial cell function resulting from surgical trauma/inflammation, and/or acute rise in intraocular pressure.

## Clinical Presentation and Assessment

The chief patient complaint with corneal edema is blurred vision. The patient may also complain of a foreign body sensation or pain. The patient may note worse vision in the mornings and then improvement later in the day. Objectively, one should closely observe all layers of the cornea with the biomicroscope. Examine for epithelial microcysts and/or bullae, stromal thickening, and folds (Figures 15–3 and 15–4). If the corneal edema is judged to be the result of intraoperative hydration of the cornea or endothelial "shutdown" from surgical trauma, the edema usually presents clinically as stromal folds (Figures 15–5 and 15–6). Further examine for anterior chamber inflammation and other sources of decreased vision: capsular clouding or abnormal retinal findings (especially cystoid macular edema and retinal detachment).

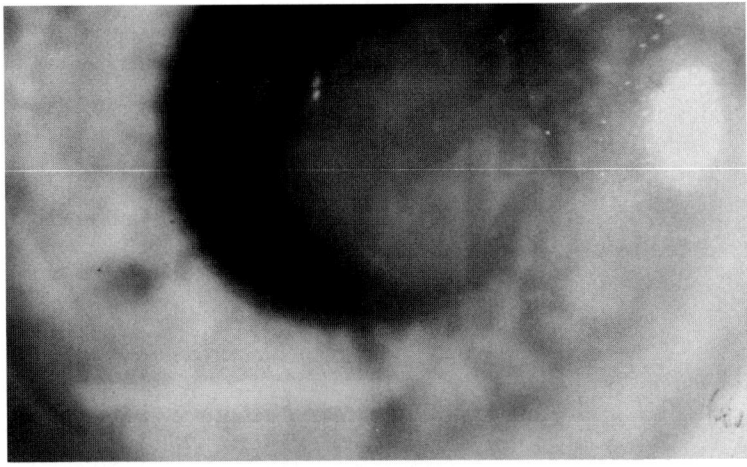

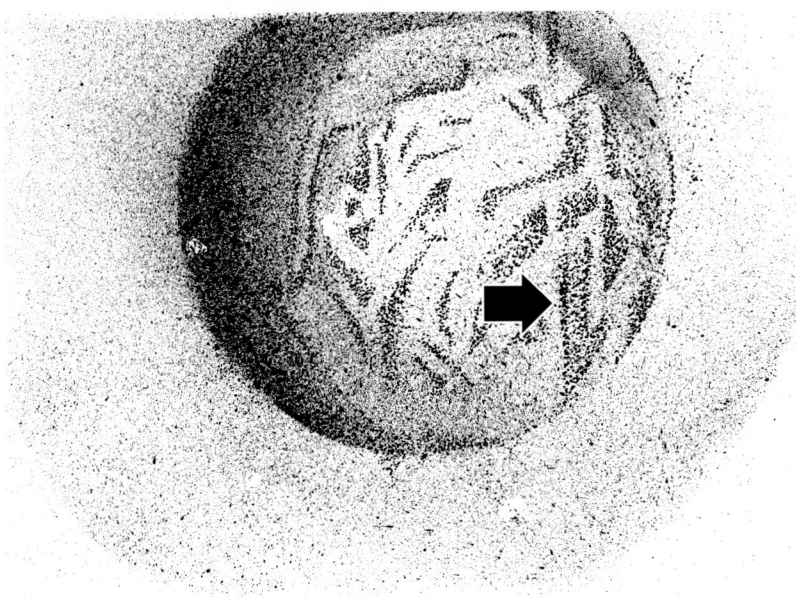

**FIGURES 15–5 AND 15–6.** Postoperative corneal edema with folds in Descemet's membrane.

### Differential Diagnosis

The symptoms of decreased vision necessitate ruling out retinal detachment. Once corneal edema is determined as the source of symptoms, differentially diagnose between that secondary to inflammation, hydration, and trauma versus that due to high intraocular pressure.

### Treatment, Follow-up, and Prognosis

Unless bullous keratopathy is present, patients with moderate corneal edema may be followed with normal postoperative treatment until the edema resolves, which usually occurs in 1–2 weeks (Table 15–2). If excessive inflammation is present, consider increasing the dosage of the postoperative steroid. If bullous keratopathy is present, then topical hyperosmotics may be used four to eight times a day to reduce the epithelial edema.

When the cause of the corneal edema is the result of intraocular pressure (IOP) rise, the treatment should be directed at lowering the IOP. Beta-blockers, if not contraindicated, are usually successful in lowering postopera-

### TABLE 15-2. TREATMENT OPTIONS: CORNEAL EDEMA

**Traumatic/Endothelial Loss**
  Maintain normal antibiotic/steroid solution
  Consider hyperosmotic ointment at night if bullae present
  IOPs > 21 mm Hg, consider adding beta-blocker, one drop twice daily
  Follow weekly
  Penetrating keratoplasty is indicated if no improvement after 3 mo follow-up

**Inflammatory**
  Maintain on antibiotic
  Prednisolone acetate 1.0%, one drop every 2–3 h
  Consider hyperosmotics drops or ointment if bullae present
  Consider beta-blocker if IOP > 21 mm Hg
  Follow weekly

**Ocular Hypertension**
  Maintain on antibiotic/steroid solution
  Lower IOP (see Table 14–1)

---

tive pressure rises that are less than 35 mm Hg. Intraocular pressures of 35–45 mm Hg usually require beta-blockers and carbonic anhydrase inhibitors (CAIs). Intraocular pressure greater than 45 mm Hg may require beta-blockers, CAIs, apraclonidine HCl (Iopidine), and oral hyperosmotic agents (see discussion of ocular hypertension in Chapter 14). Miotics are less often used in the early postoperative period due to their tendency to increase already present intraocular inflammation.

## HYPHEMA

Perhaps one of the most unnecessarily alarming surgical sequelae following cataract surgery is a postoperative hyphema. The doctor's insecurity in observing this condition is generally based on two factors. First of all, the patients often have a dramatic loss of vision and may present in a state of panic, and second, the seriousness of a surgical hyphema is erroneously thought to correspond to that of a traumatic hyphema. In reality, most surgical hyphemas are quite benign with rare exception. (See Color Plates 15–2 through 15–4.)

### Background

The incidence of hyphema following cataract extraction and implantation of an intraocular lens (IOL) varies from 1.5% to 5% and is dependent on many different factors.[5–8] These numbers are consistent with our experience of a 5% incidence of postoperative hyphema, which we have defined as any amount of red blood cells in the anterior chamber.[8]

Patients who have neovascularization of the iris, for whatever reason, are at increased risk, as are those individuals who have Fuchs' heterochromic iridocyclitis.[9] In this form of uveitis, abnormal trabecular vessels may be present increasing the risk of a hyphema at the time of cataract surgery. Also, if a patient has preexisting posterior synechiae that are broken at the time of surgery, or if there is manipulation of the iris tissue by the surgical instruments, then the risk is increased. Perhaps the greatest risk factor for developing a hyphema

### TABLE 15-3. HYPHEMA: PREDISPOSING FACTORS

Incision position
Amount of surgical cauterization
Fuchs' heterchromic iridocyclitis
Iris neovascularization
Manipulation of the iris
Intrinsic clotting defects
History of anticoagulant therapy

postsurgically occurs with patients who are taking anticoagulants. Gainy et al found a 12% incidence of hemorrhagic complication in patients who were treated with warfarin (Coumadin) compared with zero in a control group.[10]

The position of the incision is a major factor in postoperative hyphema. Patients with a posterior scleral incision are more likely to develop a hyphema than those whose incisions are in the nonvascularized cornea. In the case of clear corneal incisions, Roberts et al have shown that even patients taking anticoagulants have a low rate of hyphema.[11] The degree of cautery applied at the time of surgery will determine the susceptibility of bleeding. The surgeon must weigh the benefits of heavy cautery to reduce hemorrhaging versus the problem of increased scarring with excessive cauterization. Our cataract surgeons, utilizing the pocket incision, have claimed that due to the wound entry into the anterior chamber through clear cornea, the sealing corneal flap will prevent blood cells from entering the anterior chamber from the scleral and conjunctival wound. Whether or not this type of incision carries a lower incidence of hyphema has not been definitively proven. If performed, iridotomies increase the risk of hyphema due to severence of the iris vessels (Table 15–3).

## Prophylactic Measures

A number of prophylactic measures have been advocated in an effort to reduce the incidence of postoperative hyphemas. Prior to the use of posterior chamber IOLs, iridotomies were a routine procedure when performing cataract extraction. Today, however, with the current posterior chamber IOL that is properly angulated and placed in the bag, the risk of pseudophakic angle closure is minimal and most surgeons avoid the routine use of an iridectomy. This lowers the risk of postoperative hyphema. Thermal cautery applied to the wound area to blanch the conjunctival vessels also reduces the incidence of hyphema; however, its benefit must be weighed against the side effects from the cautery that include increased astigmatism and delayed healing.

Probably the biggest controversy revolves around the question as to whether anticoagulants such as warfarin (Coumadin) or aspirin should be discontinued prior to cataract extractions. In 1985, Stone et al[12] conducted a survey of members of the American Intraocular Implant Society. In this survey, they asked about the discontinuance of anticoagulants prior to cataract surgery, and the occurrence of postoperative complications. Of ophthalmologists responding, the group that did not discontinue the anticoagulants reported no long-term effects from hemorrhagic complications. Those doctors who did discontinue the anticoagulants prior to surgery reported that there were a number of serious systemic complications, which included thrombotic complications and cerebral vascular accidents.[12]

McMahan has also studied long-term effects of hemorrhagic complications in patients who are maintained on anticoagulants prior to cataract surgery.[13] He reviewed 2178 cataract surgery patients, 28 of whom were on anticoagulants in a prospective study. McMahan found that in the anticoagulated patients undergoing cataract surgery, there were no significant long-term sight-threatening complications resulting from being maintained on anticoagulant medications.[13] Gainy et al[10] also studied 50 patients receiving long-term warfarin sodium therapy. This study was divided into three groups: (1) those who were maintained on warfarin and had cataract extraction, (2) those who had warfarin discontinued prior to surgery, and (3) a control group who were not on anticoagulants. They found that the risk of hemorrhagic complications in the warfarin-treated groups (1 and 2) was 12% compared with 0% in the control group (3). Gainy et al[10] did not, however, find any significant difference in outcome between groups 1 and 2: that is, those patients who were maintained on warfarin and those patients who had their warfarin discontinued prior to surgery. Hall et al[14] found the incidence of postoperative hyphema to be approximately 6% in patients who were maintained on anticoagulants. In none of the patients was there any long-term visual effects from hemorrhage. Others have also agreed that maintaining patients on their anticoagulants does not pose a significant risk to the patient from hemorrhagic complications.[15]

From all of the above studies, it seems that maintaining the patients on anticoagulants prior to cataract surgery is supported from a risk-benefit viewpoint. Nevertheless, this subject is considered controversial and some surgeons discontinue anticoagulant therapy prior to cataract extraction.

## Clinical Presentation and Assessment

Patients with early hyphema usually present at their day 1 postoperative visit complaining of reduced vision. Sometimes, however, the hemorrhage may occur later, delaying symptoms from 2–14 days following surgery. Vision loss is due to the dispersal of red blood cells in the anterior chamber that absorb light and therefore significantly reduce the visual acuity. Patients usually describe hazy vision. If a clot hyphema is present, the symptoms may mimic those of a retinal detachment; that is, a shade or dark shadow to the edge of the vision. Symptoms may diminish quickly due to settling of the red blood cells. Often patients are understandably quite frantic due to their precipitous loss of vision. Usually no pain is described unless the intraocular pressure (IOP) also is elevated. The patient may also describe a difference in the color of the irides, as the red blood cells will make the iris on the affected side appear more reddish brown compared with the fellow eye.

The assessment of a hyphema involves taking the visual acuity, careful examination of the wound area, and evaluation of the anterior segment without excessive manipulation of the globe. The IOP should be checked by applanation tonometry as ocular hypertension may occur.

Hyphemas may be classified according to their presentation: layered, diffuse, clot, and eightball (Figures 15–7 to 15–9). The diffuse type, or microhyphema, is the most common. In this form, red blood cells are dispersed in the anterior chamber and are not sufficient enough to accumulate in the form of a clot or layer in the inferior aspect of the angle. In examining a patient with a diffuse hyphema, one may often find streaks of blood on the corneal endothelium, as well as tan to reddish brown colored cells circulating in the anterior chamber that resemble sand particles. Often iris details are obscured due to the dense accumulation of blood cells. Since the site of the hyphema is most often from the vessels in the cataract incision, it is common to see a clot of blood suspended from the wound superiorly. This often has a fibrinoid appearance and may be suspended in the anterior chamber or attached by strands to the iris and/or cornea. If there is a sufficient quantity of dispersed red blood

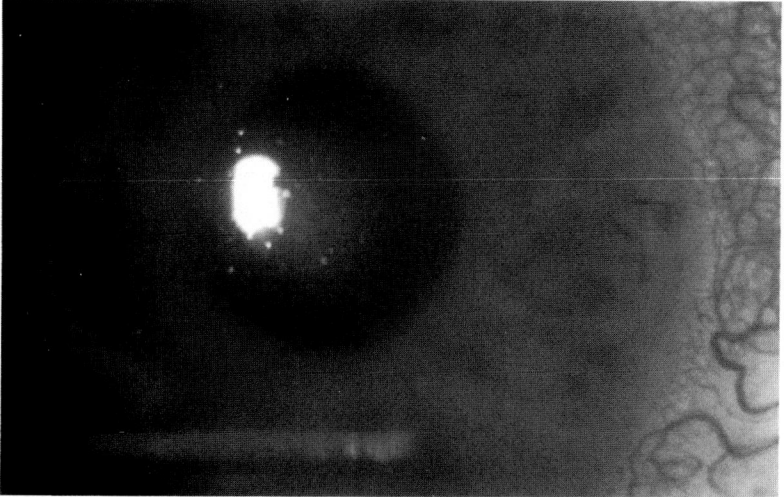

**FIGURE 15–7.** Diffuse hyphema following cataract surgery. The diffuse red blood cells block vision and create heterochromia.

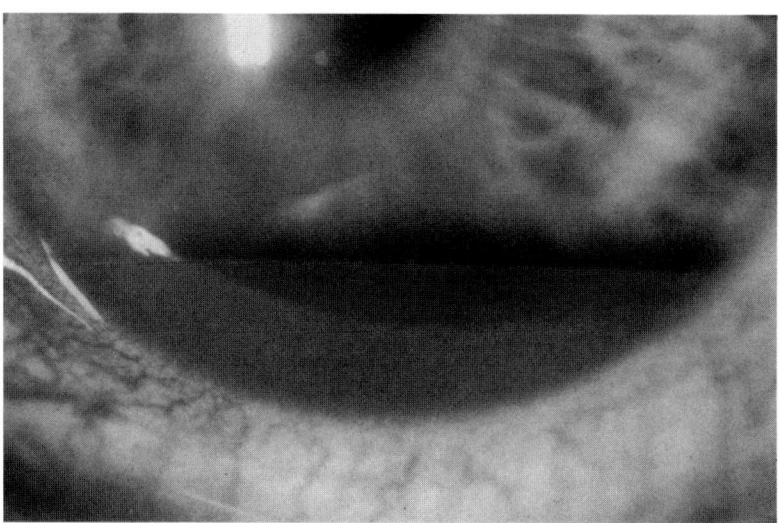

**FIGURE 15–8.** Layered hyphema.

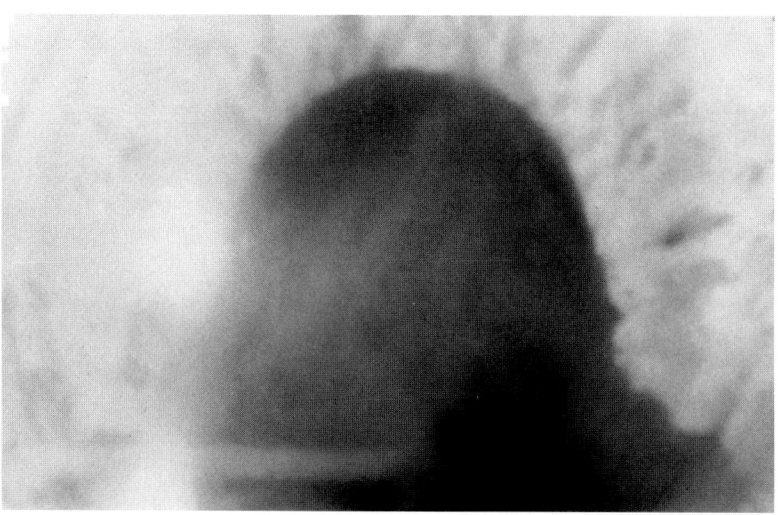

**FIGURE 15–9.** Fibrinoid clotted hyphema from an incisional vessel.

cells, then a layer of blood may form in the inferior portion of the anterior chamber angle. In rare cases, due to an excessive bleed, the entire anterior chamber may be observed to be filled with a mass of dark brown coagulated red blood cells. This has a very hard fibrinoid appearance and is termed an eightball hyphema (see Figure 4–23).

## Differential Diagnosis

Prior to assuming that the hyphema is from the surgical incision, one must be careful to rule out other causes. Patients with diabetes or other retinal ischemic disease should have their irides examined meticulously for the presence of rubeosis iridis. In addition, those with Fuchs' heterochromic iridocyclitis are more susceptible to developing hyphemas in the postsurgical period due to fine vessels that grow in the trabecular meshwork.

## Treatment, Follow-up, and Prognosis

In most cases, management is directed toward reassuring the patient and addressing his or her concerns.

We typically continue our routine antibiotic/steroid postoperative regimen when a hyphema is encountered (Table 15–4). Although there are no studies supporting the benefit of topical steroids in treating postsurgical hyphemas, it has been demonstrated that traumatic hyphemas resolve quicker with a lower incidence of rebleed when oral steroids are administered.[16] Presumably this is due to the ability of the steroid to decongest the inflamed vascular network. For this reason, in patients whose surgical hyphemas do not resolve as quickly as anticipated, it may be reasonable to increase the frequency of their topical steroids. Due to the side effects of systemic steroids, we do not advocate their use routinely for uncomplicated postsurgical hyphemas. The patient also is asked to limit their activities for several days and to keep the head elevated at night by using an extra pillow. An eye shield is sometimes given to the patient to wear at night for protection. We also advise our patients to avoid taking aspirin unless otherwise prescribed by their primary health care provider.

Occasionally, the IOP may be significantly elevated. According to Shields,[17] an elevated IOP of 40 to 50 mm Hg can be tolerated for 5–6 days provided that the optic nerve is healthy. In the presence of a compromised optic nerve, even IOPs below 30 mm Hg may result in loss of ganglion cells. Also, if the IOP is

### TABLE 15–4. TREATMENT OPTIONS: HYPHEMA

Continue antibiotic/steroid regimen
Limit activity
Avoid anticoagulants, unless already prescribed
Monitor IOP and consider the following treatment (mm Hg):
- 30–35  Beta-blocker, one to two drops (in office); follow-up in 2–3 days.
- 35–45  Add acetazolamide (Diamox) 250 mg by mouth, once. Recheck IOP within 24 h.
- 45–55  Add apraclonidine 1% (Iopidine) in office, two drops 20 min apart; check IOP in 1 h. Recheck IOP within 4 h.
- 55+    Add oral 50% glycerin (Osmoglyn) 2 oz over ice; if diabetic, use 45% w/v solution isosorbide (Ismotic). Keep patient until pressure is below 35 mm Hg. Recheck IOP within 4 h.

Recheck in 1–3 d

### TABLE 15-5. HYPHEMA: POTENTIAL COMPLICATIONS

| | |
|---|---|
| Psychologic distress | Endocapsular hematoma (rare) |
| Reduced visual acuity (temporary) | Vitreous hemorrhage (rare) |
| Ocular hypertension (temporary) | Ghost cell glaucoma (rare) |
| Corneal blood staining (rare) | |

elevated markedly for several days in association with a hyphema, blood cells may be pushed through the corneal endothelium into the stroma resulting in blood staining.

In a patient without previously diagnosed glaucoma and an IOP of 30 mm Hg or greater, antihypertensive therapy is temporarily administered in our clinics. If no contraindications exist, a single drop of a topical beta-blocker will usually suffice, with a follow-up IOP check within 24 hours. With more elevated intraocular pressures (>35 mm Hg), or in a glaucoma patient with previously diagnosed optic nerve damage, 250–500 mg of oral acetazolamide (Diamox) and/or a single drop of 1% apraclonidine HCl (Iopidine) are administered in addition to the beta-blocker. The IOP should then be rechecked later the same day. One should avoid drastic lowering of the IOP, as this may induce a rebleed. For this reason, depression of the auxiliary wound that releases aqueous as a means to reduce the IOP should be avoided.

### Hyphema Complications

The most common complication with a postoperative hyphema is psychologic distress in both the patient and doctor (Table 15–5). The patient should be reassured that in most cases the postoperative hyphema should clear and their vision has an excellent chance of being restored to normal. We reviewed the records of 25 patients with hyphema seen at Pacific Cataract and Laser Institute.[8] Of these patients, all were found to achieve the expected level of visual acuity at their 5-week postoperative visit without any significant visual compromise due to the hyphema (Table 15–6). We also found that the incidence of pressure elevation was less than 10% and transient in nature (Table 15–7). Only two patients experienced an IOP of greater than 35 mm Hg, and in all cases the postoperative IOP at 5 weeks was equal to or lower than the preoperative IOP. In counseling patients with hyphema, however, one should state that there is a small risk that pressure could be significantly elevated (>35 mm Hg).

Eightball hyphemas occur when there is excessive bleeding in the anterior chamber associated with a fibrin "pseudocapsule." These should be evacuated surgically within the first week if rapid resolution does not occur.

Vitreous hemorrhage may occur following cataract surgery from different mechanisms. A hyphema in the presence of a broken posterior capsule can re-

### TABLE 15-6. PACIFIC CATARACT & LASER INSTITUTE HYPHEMA STUDY

| Visual Acuity Outcome at 6 Weeks |
|---|
| 25 hyphemas in 500 eyes studied |
| 22 patients had 20/30 vision or better |
| 2 patients had vision of 20/30 to 20/50[a] |
| 1 patient had visual acuity of 20/200[a] |

[a] Visual acuity consistent with preexisting retinal disease.

### TABLE 15-7. PACIFIC CATARACT & LASER INSTITUTE HYPHEMA STUDY

| 1-Day IOP |
|---|
| 25 hyphemas in 500 eyes studied |
| 22 patients had normal IOP |
| 1 patient had IOP between 25 and 35 mm Hg |
| 2 patients had IOP > 35 mm Hg |
| All 25 patients had normal IOP at 5 weeks postoperatively |

sult in red blood cell accumulation in the vitreous humor. Also, it has been postulated that without hyphema and an intact capsule, vitreous hemorrhage may occur as a result of zonular traction.[18]

If there is hemorrhage into the vitreous, one should monitor the eye for ghost cell glaucoma, which may occur within the first month of surgery.[17] As opposed to red blood cells in the anterior chamber, cells in the vitreous clear slowly. With time, the normal red blood cells degenerate to become biconcave, tan colored, and more rigid. These rigid ghost cells do not pass readily through the pores of the trabecular meshwork; hence, the increased IOP.[17] Ghost cell glaucoma is generally transient, with resolution occurring after the degenerated cells have passed through the trabecular meshwork.

Another special consideration is the patient with hyphema who has previously documented retinal vascular disease. Patients with diabetic retinopathy and retinal vascular occlusions should be carefully followed if a postoperative hyphema occurs. As the blood is resorbed, the doctor should carefully evaluate the iris and angle for any signs of neovascularization. The pupil should then be dilated for a careful evaluation to rule out proliferative retinopathy. If a postoperative hyphema does not clear as expected, a consultation with a vitreoretinal surgeon and/or B-scan ultrasonogram is advised to rule out posterior segment disease.

A recently described complication of postoperative hyphema is endocapsular hematoma (Figures 15–10 and 15–11). This entity, described by Hagan and Gaasterland, occurs when red blood cells accumulate between the posterior capsule and the IOL.[19] Red blood cells in this position are sequestered and are not cleared as usual by the aqueous currents of the anterior chamber. This persistent hemorrhage will markedly decrease the visual acuity and has been shown to disperse very well with neodymium:yttrium-aluminum-garnet (Nd:YAG) capsulotomy.[19]

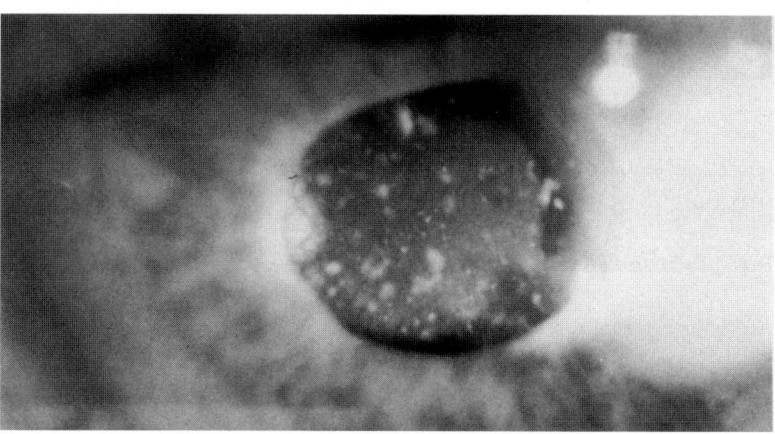

**FIGURE 15–10.** Endocapsular hematoma following cataract extraction and anterior vitrectomy; note the blood sequestered behind the intraocular lens.

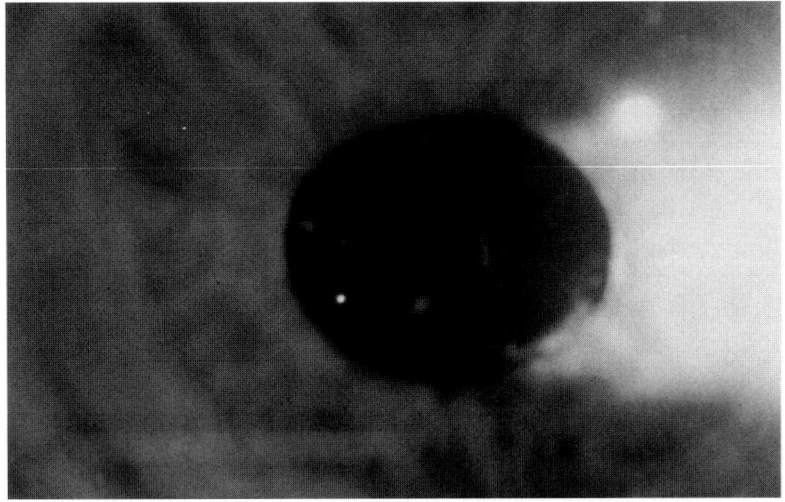

**FIGURE 15–11.** Following Nd:YAG capsulotomy, endocapsular hematoma shown in Figure 15–10 is dispersed with clearing of vision.

The prognosis of a patient who experiences a postsurgical hyphema is excellent. The most common disability is to the patient's psyche; therefore, it is of paramount importance to provide compassionate reassurance.

Although most postsurgical hyphemas carry an excellent prognosis, there are certainly exceptions. We have had one postoperative patient who developed a large eightball hyphema with a fibrin clot on the IOL that required surgical evacuation. Another patient with advanced glaucoma also required surgical evacuation due to elevated IOP from a large layered hyphema. In individuals with eightball hyphemas or markedly elevated IOPs with hyphema, early surgical intervention is probably warranted.

## UVEITIS

With the advent of modern surgical advancements, including capsular bag placement of the posterior chamber IOL, small sutureless wound incision, shortened surgical time, and ocular anti-inflammatory medication, the incidence of postoperative inflammatory complications experienced in the earlier days of cataract surgery has been drastically reduced. Nevertheless, as with any surgical technique, the body's immunologic response may induce unwanted side effects. In this section, we address those sequelae and complications associated with this response.

### Background

At the 1-day postoperative visit, the eye should be fairly comfortable with mild cells and flare, mild lens debris, and mild conjunctival injection. This mild uveitis is a normal sequela and usually resolves within 1–2 weeks with the use of postoperative topical steroid suspensions or solutions. Occasionally, the inflammatory reaction may be more severe in the early postoperative period due to surgical trauma, hypersensitivity to irrigating solutions or IOL polishing compounds, viscoelastics, prior history of iritis, physiologic lens anaphylaxis, infection, or mechanical irritation from the implant.[20]

Patients who have traumatic surgeries may experience a postoperative iritis that exceeds that which is expected. Most commonly this may be seen in patients with dense cataracts requiring extended phacoemulsification time, in those who dilate poorly resulting in iris trauma, and in those who have had intraoperative complications, such as a broken capsule with vitreous loss.

The "toxic lens syndrome" may occur due to an inflammatory reaction to residual substances from the sterilization process on the IOL surface.[21] In the earlier days of IOL manufacturing, this accounted for a significant number of severe inflammatory reactions, including cases of sterile endophthalmitis.[20,21] Now, however, due to improved sterilization techniques, it is quite rare.

Phacoanaphylactic endophthalmitis following an uncomplicated extracapsular cataract extraction (ECCE) with posterior chamber IOL has been described by Apple.[21] Histopathologic findings in a patient whose eye was enucleated due to severe iritis confirmed this diagnosis. Apple concluded that the patient developed a hypersensitivity reaction to her own lens protein that precipitated the inflammatory reaction.[21] Phacoanaphylactic endophthalmitis presents following trauma or cataract surgery when residual lens material is not tolerated. Clinically, a uveitis develops days to weeks following disruption of the lens with inflammatory cells present in the aqueous and vitreous. A granulomatous uveitis occurs with mutton-fat keratic precipitates and posterior synechia formation. An initial improvement may be noted with corticosteroids only to worsen as they are tapered. Often the uveitis will improve following the removal of the residual lens fragments. Although the above clinical findings should raise the suspicion of phacoanaphylactic endophthalmitis, its definitive diagnosis can only be made histologically.[22]

Fibrinoid inflammatory pupillary membranes may be associated with moderate to severe postoperative iritis (Figures 15–12 and 15–13). Walinder et al[23] have found that these membranes occur in about 15% of cataract surgery cases and are more frequent in patients with pseudoexfoliation. They suggest that this occurs due to a breakdown of the blood aqueous barrier. Nishi found approximately an 8% incidence and suggested that it may be a result of lens-induced iritis due to a proliferation of lens epithelial cells.[24] Quality assurance/improvement studies reveal a much lower incidence in our setting. Others have found an optically clear membrane surrounding a posterior chamber IOL on postmortem histopathologic examination and have hypothesized that this was due to intraoperative and postoperative bleeding.[25]

Retained viscoelastics may temporarily suspend red blood cells and inflammatory debris in the anterior chamber and mimic a plastic iritis. This retained material may increase anterior segment inflammation.[26,27]

The mechanical effects of the IOL can induce unwanted inflammatory reactions. Any implant that is in continuous contact with the vascularized tissues of the eye can be a potential problem. Inflammatory complications from iris-fixated as well as closed-loop and rigid anterior chamber IOLs are well documented.[28-31] Posterior chamber IOLs may also cause a greater than expected inflammatory reaction, particularly if they are placed in the ciliary sulcus or suture fixated to the iris.[32,33] Performing a continuous tear capsulotomy and implantation of the intraocular lens in the bag will help maintain the blood aqueous barrier and reduce postoperative inflammation.

Patients who have preexisting uveitis should be counseled preoperatively and informed of their risk of greater than usual postoperative inflammation. Since their blood-aqueous barrier is already compromised, it is not unusual for such patients to experience a more severe and prolonged inflammatory reaction. Surgery should be deferred until the eye has been quiet and stable for several months and more intensive steroid therapy may be required preoperatively, intraoperatively, and postoperatively. Careful patient selection and placement of an IOL in the bag may result in successful outcomes in patients with a history of uveitis[34,28] (Chapter 7).

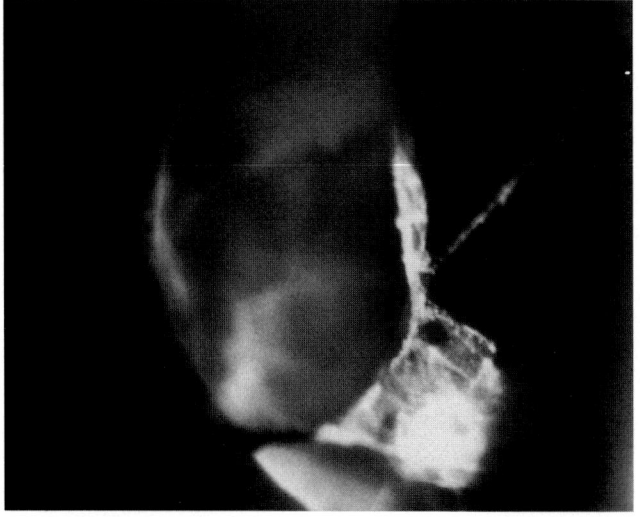

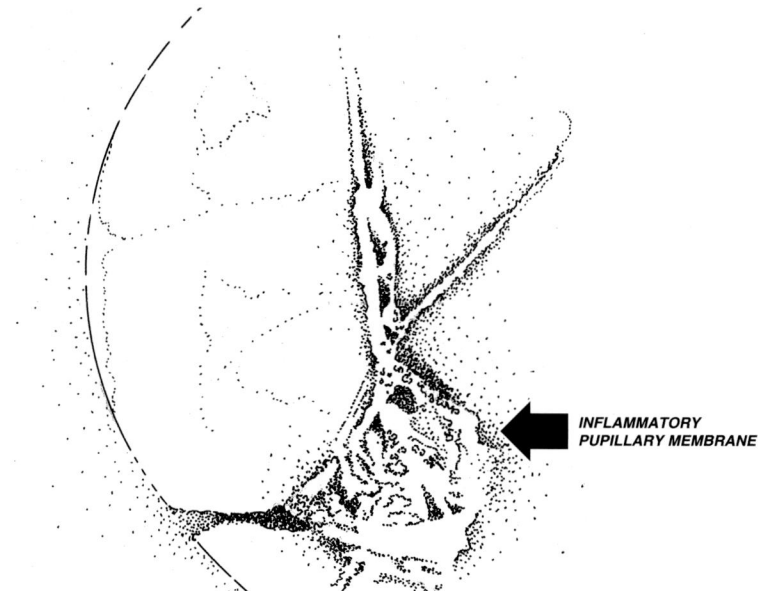

**FIGURES 15–12 AND 15–13.** Sterile fibrinoid uveitis following cataract extraction.

INFLAMMATORY PUPILLARY MEMBRANE

## Clinical Presentation and Assessment

The patient with uveitis typically complains of tenderness or pain, sensitivity to light, and blurry vision. Visual acuity may be reduced due to corneal edema, or less likely, macular edema. Pupillary examination will usually be remarkable for a miotic pupil on the affected side. The IOPs should be checked, and they may be reduced or elevated.

The slit lamp and external examination reveal a "hot" eye with conjunctival and episcleral injection. The cornea may be edematous due to cellular precipitation on the endothelium. The most notable findings are cells and flare in the anterior chamber that may be variable in degree and are not always directly proportional to the patient's symptoms. Some patients with mild cells and flare are in great discomfort, whereas others with a moderate reaction may be less symptomatic. The inferior aspect of the anterior chamber angle should be examined for layering of white blood cells (hypopyon), which indicates either a severe sterile iritis or possibly infectious endophthalmitis. The patient should

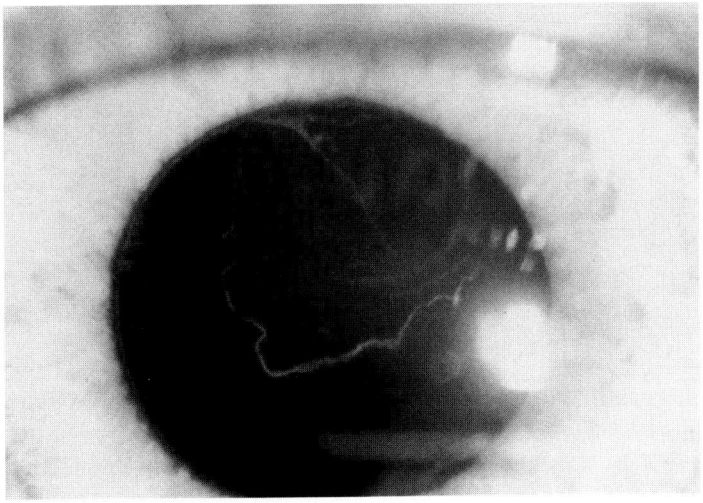
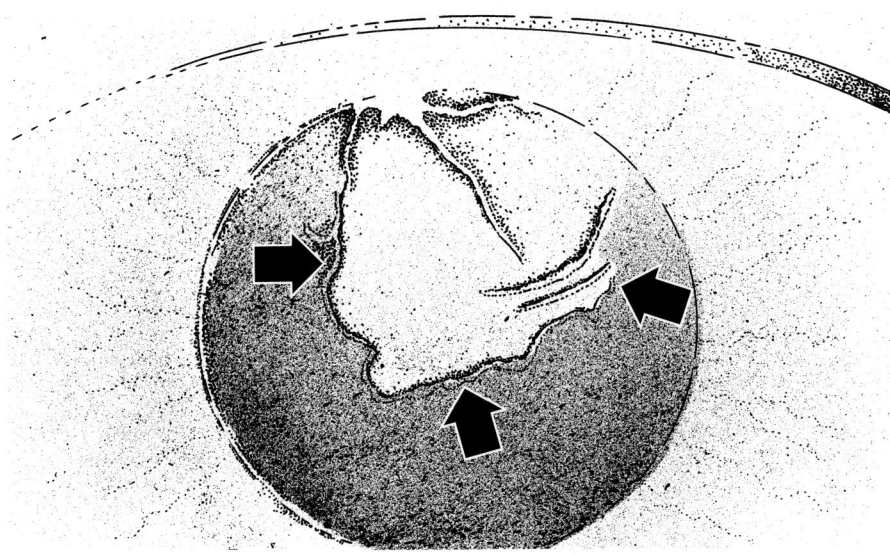

*FIGURES 15–14 AND 15–15.* Fibrin on the anterior surface of an IOL in a young patient following cataract extraction. This membrane cleared with topical steroid treatment.

be dilated/cyclopleged for diagnostic and therapeutic purposes. The pupillary space should be assessed for fibrin deposition on the IOL and small pieces of retained cortex that may be discovered along the edge of the pupil. Examination of the vitreous and fundus to rule out associated posterior segment disorders should be performed. A few cells may be seen in the anterior vitreous due to spillover from the anterior inflammation; however, dense cellular clumping should alert the clinician to the possibility of infectious endophthalmitis.

Fibrinoid membranes along the edge of the pupil or attached to the IOL may occasionally be observed, especially in young patients (Figures 15–14 and 15–15). These membranes occur within the first several weeks of surgery and show a complete resorption with administration of topical or subconjunctival steroids. They are associated with a moderate to severe anterior chamber reaction and resemble a cobweb. In severe cases, the membrane may completely occlude the pupil. When a fibrinoid membrane is observed, the clinician should carefully evaluate the eye for signs that may be suspicious of an infectious endophthalmitis. Clinical symptoms and signs that should arouse suspicion include severe pain, lid edema, hypopyon, and clumps of cells in the vitreous. If inflammatory signs are more than expected and there is suspicion of endophthalmitis, the operating surgeon should be consulted immediately.

## Differential Diagnosis

Any patient who presents during the postoperative course with greater than expected iritis should be suspected of having infectious endophthalmitis (see discussion of endophthalmitis, in Chapter 14). Although a hypopyon is often present, it may not always be observed in infectious endophthalmitis. In addition, the presence of cells in the anterior chamber and decreased vision necessitates thorough retinal evaluation to rule out cystoid macular edema (CME) and retinal detachment.

## Treatment, Follow-up, and Prognosis

In the absence of a history of surgical trauma, the clinician should suspect other causes of the inflammatory reaction (see Differential Diagnosis above). In some instances, patients or a caretaker may be instilling their drops incorrectly. If this is suspected, have the patient or responsible person demonstrate the technique of drop instillation in the office or inspect the bottle to ascertain if the correct medication is being used properly.

The goal in managing acute postoperative iritis is to reduce the inflammatory response to prevent unnecessary scarring, as well as corneal and macular edema. This is best achieved with topical corticosteroids, cycloplegics, and possibly topical nonsteroidal anti-inflammatory drugs (NSAIDs) (Table 15–8). In moderate to severe postoperative iritis, prednisolone acetate 1% every 2–4 hours will usually be adequate therapy. Rarely, hourly drop instillation and/or a steroid injection may be necessary. Topical cycloplegics/mydriatics are indicated in moderate to severe cases to increase comfort and to prevent posterior synechiae. After the anterior chamber reaction has subsided, the cycloplegic is discontinued, and the steroids may then be tapered and discontinued.

If the IOP is significantly elevated, topical antiglaucoma medications are used. Mild IOP elevations (<30 mm Hg) may be observed without treatment if there is no history of glaucoma or retinal vascular occlusive disease and if the optic nerve is healthy. In many cases, treating the inflammation with corticosteroids also reduces IOP due to clearing of inflammatory debris from the trabecular meshwork. IOPs of 30 or greater are generally treated first with a beta-blocker, assuming no contraindications, and if adequate IOP is not achieved,

### TABLE 15–8. TREATMENT OPTIONS: EARLY POSTOPERATIVE UVEITIS

| Moderate | Severe |
| --- | --- |
| Prednisolone acetate 1%, one drop every 3 h while awake | Rule out endophthalmitis |
| Continue steroids until < 1+ cell reaction, then taper | Topical scopolamine 0.25%, one drop twice a day |
| Topical cycloplegia is optional (Homatropine HBr 5%, one drop, two to three times per day) | Topical prednisolone acetate 1%, one drop every 1–2 h while awake |
| | Consider |
| |    Topical dexamethasone ointment every night |
| |    Referral for subconjunctival injection of steroid |
| |    Referral for oral prednisolone |
| | Continue steroids until < 1+ cell reaction, then taper |

then a carbonic anhydrase inhibitor (CAI) should be considered. One should avoid using miotics in ocular hypertension secondary to inflammation, as they increase capillary permeability, exacerbate inflammation, and increase the risk of posterior synechiae.

In patients with postoperative iritis, it is recommended to continue their topical steroids at full dose (every 2–4 hours) until the inflammatory signs have almost completely dissipated (less than 1+ cells). At this time, the steroid drops may be tapered. In most cases, patients with postoperative iritis respond well to topical treatment.

## INTRAOCULAR LENS DECENTRATION/PUPILLARY CAPTURE

Lens decentration or pupillary capture may or may not create problems for the patient and are managed accordingly. (See Color Plates 15–5 and 15–6.)

### Background

Lens decentration is one of the leading causes of explantation of posterior chamber IOLs and occurs when an IOL is partially or totally off the visual axis but still maintains most of its tissue support. Decentrations are dependent on lens loop fixation. That fixation is largely affected by radial tears of the capsular bag during surgery and lens loop style.[35] Lenses asymmetrically fixated with one loop in the capsular bag and the other loop in the ciliary sulcus are at greatest risk for decentration. As the bag collapses and fibroses around the lens haptics, the lens may be moved toward the haptic with the least support (Figures 15–16 and 15–17).

Pupillary capture occurs when the pupillary margin becomes partially or totally anterior to an anterior chamber lens and posterior to a posterior chamber lens. The incidence is reported at 0.3% to 3.1% of the time.[36,37] Pupillary capture may occur early in the postoperative period because of mechanical factors during or immediately following surgery. It also may occur late as a result of lens displacement in the case of anterior chamber lenses or iridocapsular synechiae that contract the iris behind a posterior chamber lens. Many current posterior chamber IOLs have anterior angulated haptics to help position the optic portion of the IOL more posteriorly. The more rigid polymethylmeth-

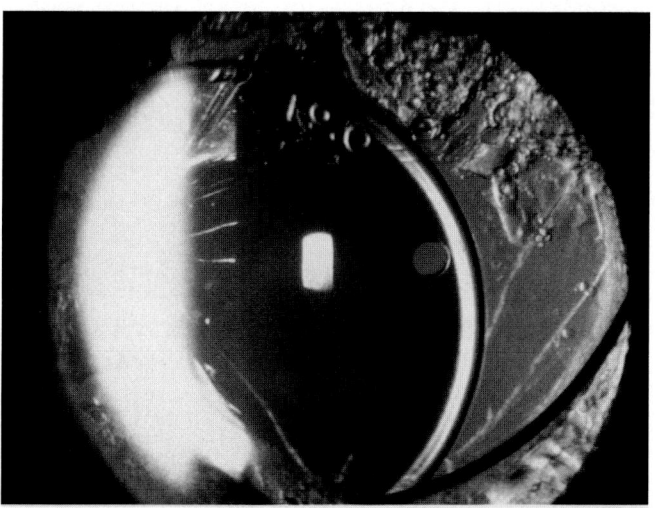

**FIGURE 15–16.** Decentration of posterior chamber IOL due to bag-sulcus fixation.

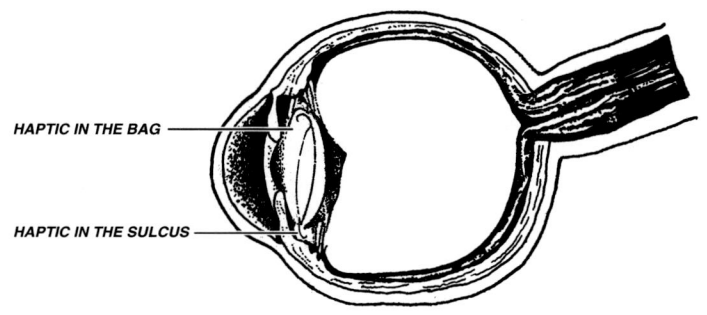

**FIGURE 15–17.** Cross section of PC IOL with bag-sulcus fixation.

acrylate (PMMA) lenses are thought to be less susceptible to pupillary capture. In addition, a lens placed in the capsular bag with a small anterior capsular opening helps to avoid this complication.

## Clinical Presentation and Assessment

Patients may be asymptomatic or complain of blur and distortion depending on the amount of lens decentration. Patients with pupillary capture may note an irregular pupil and visual disturbance. Pupillary capture may also precipitate chronic iritis and its symptoms secondary to iris irritation.

On examination, one may find induced astigmatism and/or increased myopia of 1.00 to 3.00 diopters if a posterior lens implant undergoes complete pupillary capture into the anterior chamber.[38] At the slit lamp, the doctor should observe the eye predilation and postdilation to determine evidence of the extent of decentration. In the case of pupillary capture without a capsular bag, the eye should not be dilated. The decentration or pupillary capture may be recorded and quantified by drawing or photography. One must assess the extent to which the decentration or capture contributes to patient symptoms.

## Differential Diagnosis

Symptoms from lens decentration must be differentiated from other refractive problems (ie, corneal astigmatism). Pupillary capture should be differentiated from pupillary block, which would occur acutely and present with high IOP and pain.

## Treatment, Follow-up, and Prognosis

The best scenario is avoidance of lens decentration and pupillary capture altogether via surgical technique that utilizes capsulorhexis with no capsular bag radial tears,[35] angulated rigid IOL haptics, or silicone lenses placed firmly posteriorly in the capsular bag.[38] Nevertheless, any patient who presents with these findings in the early postoperative period should have a consultation with the surgeon for consideration of IOL repositioning or exchange.

In the presence of decentration postoperatively, reassurance and patient education are the first form of management (Table 15–9). The decentration of the lens should be recorded and reported to the surgeon. As long as the patient remains asymptomatic, no further action beyond prudent follow-up need be taken. More serious decentrations may cause mild visual symptoms such as halos around lights or extra images from bright objects and are more common in patients with larger pupil sizes. If the patient is dissatisfied with his or her current visual status, a consultation with the surgeon is suggested. If the de-

**TABLE 15-9. TREATMENT OPTIONS: IOL DECENTRATION/ PUPILLARY CAPTURE**

Consult surgeon for consideration of lens repositioning or exchange.

---

centration moves positioning holes or the edge of the IOL near the optic axis, it may cause severe vision impairment, with the patient seeing through both an aphakic and pseudophakic optic axis in the latter case. These patients are best managed by repositioning or replacement of the IOL.

If a patient presents with pupillary capture and reports a long history of a misshapen pupil and/or there are signs of adhesions from the iris to the lens, then the lens may be left in place if there are no other signs of IOL inflammation. Records of the previous lens position and postoperative course may be sought. Any complaints of visual disturbance or signs of anterior segment inflammation should be recorded and surgeon consultation for repositioning or surgical repair may be undertaken.

## CHOROIDAL DETACHMENT

Choroidal detachment following cataract surgery occurs when serous fluid or blood accumulates in the suprachoroidal space causing the ciliary body and choroid to detach from the underlying sclera. A choroidal detachment is termed an exudative or a transudative detachment if it is caused by fluid accumulation in the suprachoroidal space and a hemorrhagic detachment if blood accumulates. Exudative choroidal detachments secondary to a wound leak are formed when low IOP allows a hydrostatic pressure drop in anterior uveal veins, so that fluid may pass into the suprachoroidal space. The proteins in plasma then add an osmotic force that draws more fluid into the space increasing the fluid detachment.[39]

The choroid is more firmly attached to the sclera and globe posteriorly as a result of adhesions around the optic nerve, posterior ciliary nerves, and vortex veins. Therefore, most choroidal detachments occur as ciliary body and anterior choroidal separations[39,40] (Color Plate 15–7 and Figure 15–18). Because the ciliary body is detached, it may decrease aqueous production, which then may produce or exacerbate hypotony of the globe.[41]

### Background

Jaffe has divided postcataract choroidal detachments into three groups: (1) those occurring immediately after surgery, (2) those occurring 7–21 days after surgery, and (3) those occurring months to years after surgery.[41] Although there is disagreement concerning the true etiology of early exudative choroidal detachments, they may be due to low IOP at the time of surgery when the eye is open and appear as small low-lying elevations that resolve spontaneously in most cases. Hoffman and associates reported a 37% incidence of limited choroidal hemorrhage in eyes undergoing intracapsular cataract extraction.[42] The choroidals that occur in the 7- to 21-day range are extensions of early choroidals or are associated with loss of wound integrity. With modern sutures and scleral tunnel incisions, these types of choroidal detachments have been vastly reduced. Late choroidal detachments are of unknown origin but may be associated with trauma.

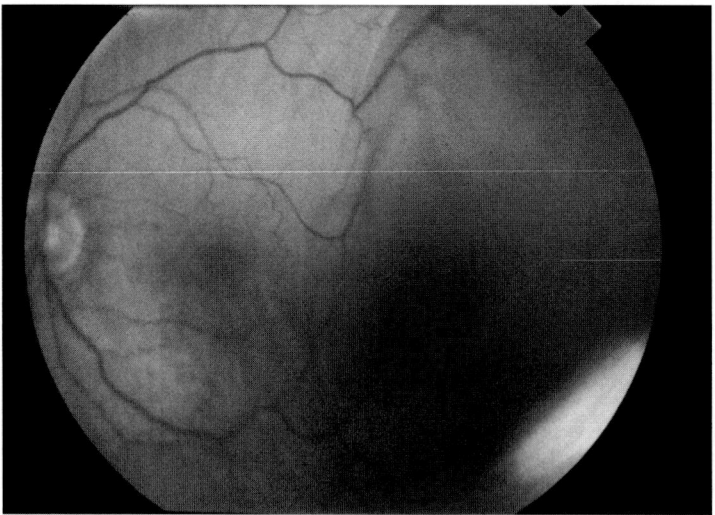

**FIGURE 15–18.** Choroidal detachment.

### Clinical Presentation and Assessment

A patient with choroidal detachment following cataract surgery may be asymptomatic or may subjectively report poor vision and ocular discomfort. Objectively, the typical patient would present with low IOP, positive Seidel sign (wound leak), and shallow anterior chamber (see Chapter 14). In rare cases, a wound leak may not be observable and the anterior chamber may be well-formed. The fundus examination would show large dark mounds that involve the anterior fundus and, if large enough, will be separated only by vortex veins. The choroidal elevations will not wave with normal ocular movement as in retinal detachment. Hemorrhagic detachments appear more reddish, whereas exudative ones have a more brown appearance.[43] When large enough and involving the visual axis, choroidals will cause decreased vision. If the edges of separate mounds are in contact with each other, this is termed a "kissing choroidal."

### Differential Diagnosis

The differential diagnosis of choroidal detachment is retinal detachment and, depending on appearance and presentation, choroidal melanoma.

### Treatment, Follow-up, and Prognosis

Small, asymptomatic choroidal detachments may be monitored and normal postoperative medications continued. When an exudative choroidal detachment with shallow anterior chamber and wound leak is found, consultation with the surgeon is necessary. Timely evaluation and management is important, as choroidal detachment may, with continued shallow anterior chamber, form permanent anterior synechia and lead to persistent glaucoma. Kissing choroidals are an emergency due to the risk of retinal detachment (Table 15–10).

The treatment of a postoperative choroidal detachment is divided into medical and surgical. First-line medical treatment consists of aggressive cycloplegia with agents such as scopolamine 0.25% or atropine 1%. Some advocate the use of oral steroids to reduce inflammation and encourage choroidal reattachment.

**TABLE 15–10. TREATMENT OPTIONS: CHOROIDAL DETACHMENTS**

Rule out wound leak. If present, treat[a]
Consult with surgeon

**With formed anterior chamber:**

Treat with topical prednisolone acetate 1%, one drop every 2–4 h and atropine sulfate 1%, one drop two to four times per day

**With shallow anterior chamber:**

Treat maximally with above recommendations
Consider adding oral steroids

[a] See Chapter 14, Wound Leak with Shallow Anterior Chamber Angle, and Chapter 15, Wound Leak with Well-formed Anterior Chamber Angle.

Aqueous hyposecretion agents (carbonic anhydrase inhibitors) such as acetazolamide (Diamox) have also been advocated in an attempt to percolate less aqueous through the wound area, which enhances wound healing. Slowing the flow of aqueous posteriorly may also contribute to reduction of choroidal detachment. The use of these hypotensives is certainly controversial, and the rationale for its use is not well documented.

If medical management of choroidal detachment in the presence of wound leak fails and the eye remains hypotonic for a period of a week, the surgeon may attempt a surgical procedure to repair the wound and decrease the choroidal detachment. The surgeon will direct this repair at trying to establish wound integrity by reforming the anterior chamber with either air or fluid. A suprachoroidal tap and drainage of the detachments may be performed to restore attachment of the choroid to the underlying sclera. If the surgery is successful, the choroidal detachment often disappears over a period of a few weeks and long-term sequelae are negligible.

## ANTERIOR ISCHEMIC OPTIC NEUROPATHY

Anterior ischemic optic neuropathy (AION) has been reported to be associated with cataract surgery.[44] Because it may leave the patient with poor vision, early recognition and differential diagnosis is essential.

### Background

Anterior ischemic optic neuropathy may occur in one of two forms, arteritic or nonarteritic, and is due to an infarct of the anterior aspect of the optic nerve (Table 15–11). Although the exact mechanism is unknown, many investigators believe the infarct is due to a compromised peripapillary, choroidal, and posterior ciliary arterial supply. It is highly associated with systemic vascular disorders such as arteriosclerosis and hypertension. The vast majority of presentations involve the prelaminar portion of the optic nerve. However, there are reported cases where retrobulbar infarct has occurred.[45]

It is controversial as to whether or not modern cataract surgery can precipitate AION. An extensive study of the complications of cataract surgery shows a very low incidence of 0.07%.[46] Large studies of the general nonsurgical population concerning the occurrence of AION in the second eye following its pres-

**TABLE 15-11. CLINICAL PRESENTATION OF ANTERIOR ISCHEMIC OPTIC NEUROPATHY**

| Arteritic vs Nonarteritic AION | |
|---|---|
| **Nonarteritic** | **Arteritic** |
| Associated symptoms: Vision loss, headache, occasional loss of color vision | Associated symptoms: Vision loss, possible temporal artery and scalp tenderness, headache, jaw claudication, general malaise, and weight loss |
| Visual acuity: Generally in the 20/50 to 20/100 range | Visual acuity: Generally 20/100 or worse |
| Positive afferent pupillary defect | Positive afferent pupillary defect |
| Optic disc appearance: Edematous may be sectoral; possible nerve fiber layer, hemorrhage and narrowed arterioles | Optic disc appearance: Pale and edematous with less swelling due to greater ischemia |
| Visual field loss: Arcuate or altitudinal, mild to severe | Visual field loss: Severe altitudinal; usually involves both hemifields |

ence in the first eye report an approximate 30% to 40% bilaterally in patients without cardiovascular disease. This rises to an approximately 40% to 60% chance of second eye involvement in patients with systemic hypertension, diabetes mellitus, or both.[47] Nonarteritic AION has been associated with cataract extraction and may occur during the early postoperative course or months to years after the surgery.[48] Carroll reported that patients undergoing uncomplicated cataract extraction who developed AION in the first eye had an approximately 50% chance of suffering it in the second eye within a year of surgery.[44] In his study, only eyes undergoing cataract surgery developed anterior ischemic optic neuropathy.

It has been suggested that anterior ischemic optic neuropathy in the immediate postoperative period may be precipitated by a sudden change in IOP or compromise of the systemic vascular system during complicated surgery.[49] Hayreh described this as postcataract extraction AION that was associated with high IOP following surgery and showed disc edema and/or splinter hemorrhages in the early postoperative course.[50] He concluded that when the perfusion pressure (blood pressure minus the IOP) was compromised in these patients, the stage was set for collapse of the optic nerve vascular system and the initiation of ischemia. Modern methods of ECCE with less manipulation of the eye pressure may reduce the risk of anterior ischemic optic neuropathy.

Patients who have had AION in one eye, whether or not associated with cataract extraction, should be counseled preoperatively that there is some evidence that undergoing intraocular surgery, such as cataract extraction, may increase the likelihood of the occurrence of this event in the second eye. Patients also should be advised that they carry a high risk, approximately 50%, of AION occurring in the second eye regardless of whether they undergo surgery or not.

## Clinical Presentation and Assessment

Patients with AION typically present with sudden, painless loss of vision, usually involving fixation. When examining the patient, the goal is to determine the etiology of the vision loss as well as differentiating between arteritic and nonarteritic AION (Tables 15-11 and 15-12).

## TABLE 15–12. CLINICAL ASSESSMENT OF ANTERIOR ISCHEMIC OPTIC NEUROPATHY

| Ocular | General |
|---|---|
| Visual acuity | Question patient concerning history of jaw ache, headache, scalp tenderness, general malaise |
| Visual field | |
| Pupillary testing | Laboratory blood work: |
| IOP measurement |    Erythrocyte sedimentation rate (ESR) |
| |    Complete blood count (CBC) with differential and platelet count |
| |    Antinuclear antibody (ANA) |

A history should be obtained to rule out associated symptoms of temporal arteritis such as scalp tenderness, jaw ache, or headache. Visual acuity is reduced to the 20/50 to 20/100 level, and an afferent pupillary defect is almost always present. The anterior segment and vitreous appear normal. The classic finding is that of optic disc inflammation with sectoral or complete nerve head swelling (Figures 15–19 and 15–20). There are often accompanying nerve fiber layer hemorrhages and edema, and the arteries are typically narrowed. Arteritic AION usually presents with a pale, swollen disc. Visual field testing shows altitudinal field loss, which may involve fixation (Figure 15–21). The field loss in the arteritic form is generally more severe.

The arteritic form of AION is associated with cranial arteritis and/or polymyalgia rheumatica and may result in bilateral blindness and death. Therefore, an erythrocyte sedimentation rate (ESR) is mandatory and needs to be done immediately. The most common test done is a Westergen erythrocyte sedimentation rate and values over 20 should be considered for temporal artery biopsy. Additional laboratory tests should include a complete blood count (CBC) with differential and a platelet count. An antinuclear antibody (ANA) is also obtained because of the association of the arteritic form of AION with polyarteritis nodosa and other inflammatory diseases.

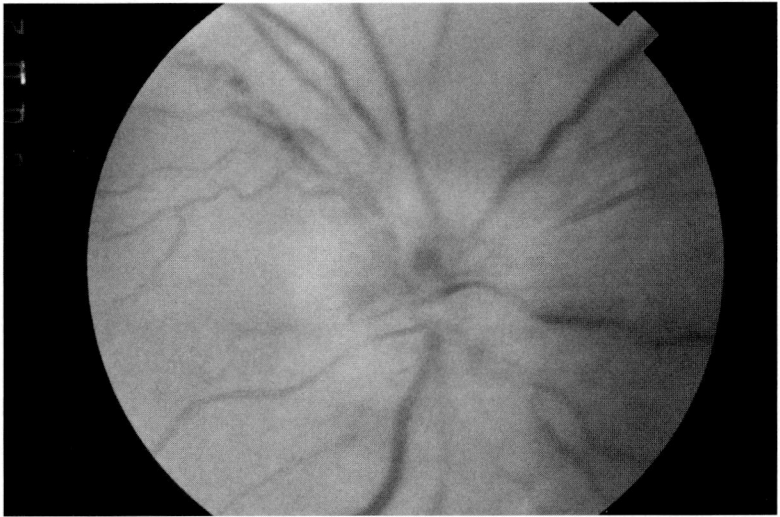

**FIGURE 15–19.** Ischemic optic neuropathy (nonarteritic).

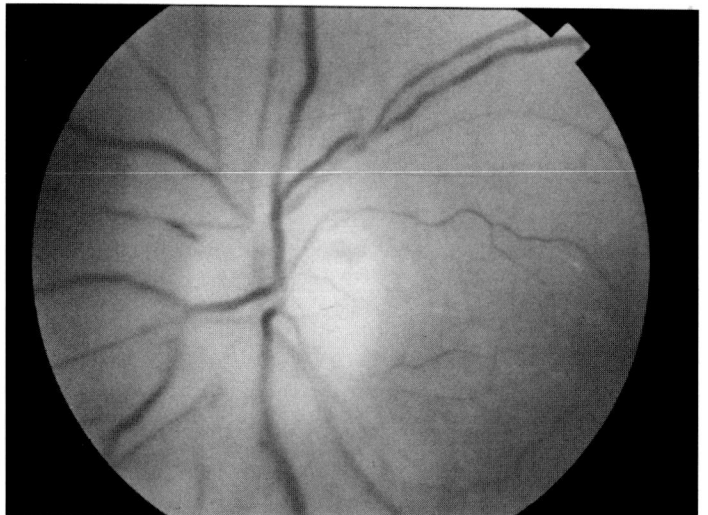

**FIGURE 15–20.** Ischemic optic neuropathy (arteritic).

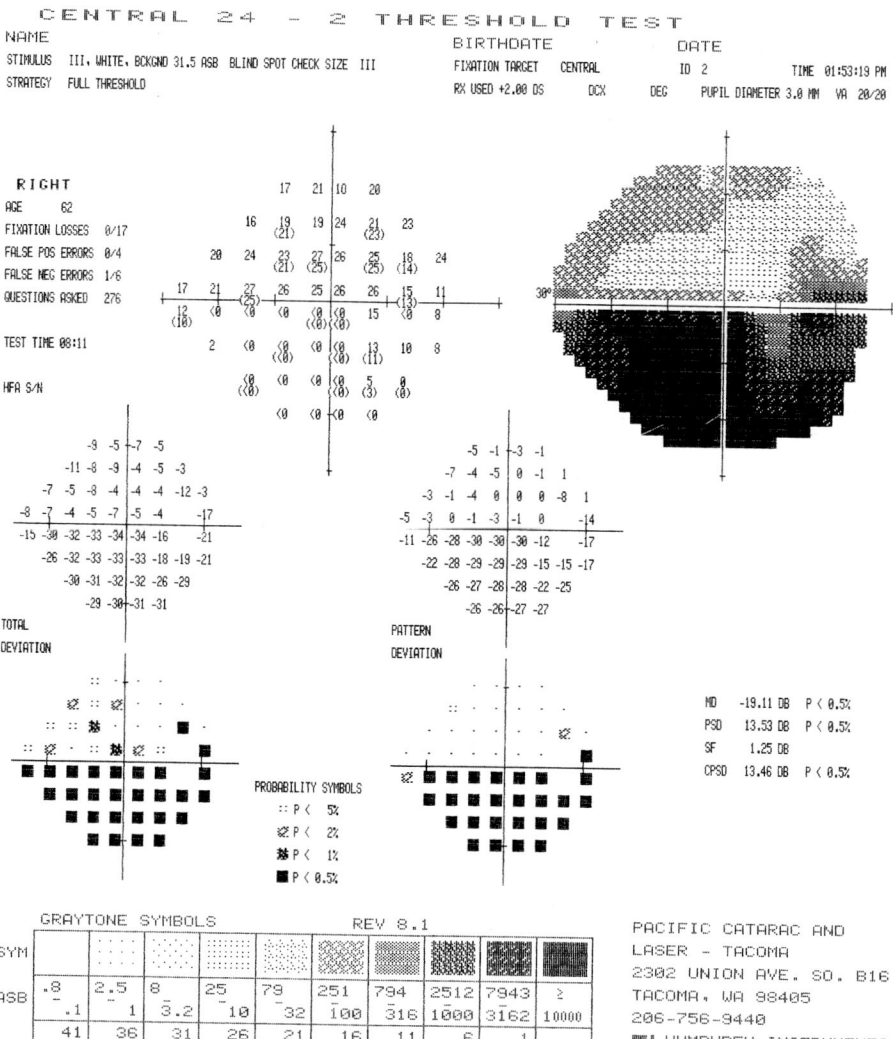

**FIGURE 15–21.** Altitudinal field loss due to ischemic optic neuropathy.

**TABLE 15–13. TREATMENT OF NONARTERITIC ANTERIOR ISCHEMIC OPTIC NEUROPATHY**

Treat underlying systemic hypertension or vascular disease

In cases of progressive visual loss over 1–4 wk, optic nerve decompression may be considered

Use of oral steroids is controversial

## Differential Diagnosis

This painless loss of vision in a postoperative patient must first be differentiated from hyphema and retinal detachment. If AION is diagnosed, prompt differentiation between the nonarteritic and the arteritic forms, as already described, is required.

## Treatment, Follow-up, and Prognosis

The first step in treating AION is to order the appropriate laboratory tests to differentiate the nonarteritic from the arteritic form, and to lower IOP if elevated.

No treatment has been shown to be effective in the nonarteritic form of AION (Table 15–13). The patient should be evaluated by their family physician for associated cardiovascular and inflammatory systemic diseases.

In the case of arteritic AION, treatment is immediate administration of systemic steroids (Table 15–14). The patients should be counseled that the steroids are not immediately effective and, even with treatment, there is risk of further vision loss. In addition, if this is the first eye to be affected, they should be advised of the risk of loss in their other eye before the steroids become fully effective.

Patients usually regain some portion of their visual function. However, there are reports of progressive loss of visual field and acuity over a 6-week period.[51] The disc edema slowly resolves over a period of a few weeks and the patient is eventually left with some degree of optic atrophy. Visual acuity is usually affected. Approximately 42% of patients receive partial visual recovery regardless of the cause of AION.

Sergott and associates have advocated optic nerve decompression in cases of progressive AION.[52] They suggest optic nerve sheath decompression in patients with documented progressive loss of vision over a 4-week period. Decompression surgery improved vision in 12 of 14 patients in their study. Sadun has reviewed optic nerve sheath decompression for AION and reports that other

**TABLE 15–14. TREATMENT OF ARTERITIC ANTERIOR ISCHEMIC OPTIC NEUROPATHY**

Temporal artery biopsy. It is the only way to confirm disease

60–80 mg prednisone by mouth each day

If vision loss continues, intravenous methyl prednisolone, 1000 mg every 12 h for 5 days may be considered

When sedimentation rate drops and symptoms decrease, taper steroid

investigators have not shown such impressive results.[53] The Ischemic Optic Neuropathy Decompression Trial has been founded and should help determine the usefulness of this treatment for patients with progressive AION visual loss.

## REFERENCES

### Ptosis and Diplopia

1. Bruce RA, McGoldrick KE, Oppenheimer P: *Anesthesia for Ophthalmology.* Birmingham, AL: Aesculapius; 1982:34–47.
2. Warwick R, Williams PL: *Gray's Anatomy,* 35th ed. Philadelphia: W.B. Saunders; 1973:1122–1124.
3. Wang HS: Peribulbar anesthesia for ophthalmic procedures. *J Cataract Refract Surg.* 1988;**14**:441–443.

### Wound Leak with Well-Formed Anterior Chamber

4. Jaffe NS, Jaffe MS, Jaffe GF: *Cataract Surgery and Its Complications,* 5th ed. St Louis: CV Mosby; 1990:360–361.

### Hyphema

5. Grabow HB: Early results of 500 cases of no-stitch cataract surgery. *J Cataract Refract Surg.* 1991;**17**(suppl):726–730.
6. Francois J, Verbraeken H: Complications in 1,000 consecutive intracapsular cataract extractions. *Ophthalmologica.* 1980;**180**:121–128.
7. Cohen JS, Osher RH, Weber P, et al: Complications of extracapsular cataract surgery. *Ophthalmology.* 1984;**91**:826–830.
8. Maki MJ, Stanfield DL: *Primary Care of the Cataract Patient.* Presented at the American Academy of Optometry, Anaheim, CA, December 1991.
9. Mills DB, Rosen ES: Intraocular lens implantation following cataract extraction in Fuchs' heterochromic uveitis. *Ophthal Surg.* 1982;**13**:467–469.
10. Gainy SP, Robertson DM, Fay W, Ilstrup D: Ocular surgery on patients receiving long-term Warfarin therapy. *Am J Ophthalmol.* 1989;**108**:142–146.
11. Roberts CW, Woods SM, Turner LS: Cataract surgery in anticoagulated patients. *J Cataract Refract Surg.* 1991;**17**(suppl):309–312.
12. Stone LS, Kline OR, Sklar C: Intraocular lenses and anticoagulation and antiplatelet therapy. *Am Intraocular Implant Soc J.* 1985;**11**:165.
13. McMahan LB: Anticoagulants and cataract surgery. *J Cataract Refract Surg.* 1988;**14**:569–571.
14. Hall DL, Steen WH, Drummond JW, Byrd WA: Anticoagulants and cataract surgery. *Ophthal Surg.* 1988;**19**:221–222.
15. Shuler JD, Paschal JF, Holland GN: Antiplatelet therapy and cataract surgery. *J Cataract Refract Surg.* 1992;**18**:567–571.
16. Farber MD, Fiscella R, Goldberg MF: Aminocaproic acid versus prednisone for the treatment of traumatic hyphema. *Ophthalmology.* 1991;**98**:279–286.
17. Shields MB: *Textbook of Glaucoma.* Baltimore: Williams & Wilkins; 1982:318–325.
18. Littlewood KR, Constable IJ: Vitreous haemorrhage after cataract extraction. *Br J Ophthalmol.* 1985;**69**:911–914.
19. Hagan JC, Gaasterland DE: Endocapsular hematoma. *Arch Ophthalmol.* 1991;**109**:514–518.

## Uveitis

20. Apple DJ, Mamalis N, Loftfield K, et al: Complications of intraocular lenses: A historical and histopathologic review. *Surv Ophthalmol.* 1984;**29**:1–54.
21. Apple DJ, Mamalis N, Steinmetz RL, et al: Phacoanaphylactic endophthalmitis associated with extracapsular cataract extraction and posterior chamber intraocular lens. *Arch Ophthalmol.* 1984;**102**:1528–1532.
22. Marak GE: Phacoanaphylactic endophthalmitis. *Surv Ophthalmol.* 1992;**36**:325–339.
23. Walinder PK, Olivius EO, Nordell SI, Thorburn WE: Fibrinoid reaction after extracapsular cataract extraction and relationship to exfoliation syndrome. *J Cataract Refract Surg.* 1989;**15**:526–530.
24. Nishi O: Fibrinous membrane formation on the posterior chamber lens during the early postoperative period. *J Cataract Refract Surg.* 1988;**14**:73–77.
25. Wolter JR, Kleberger E: Surface reaction on a posterior chamber lens seven days after implantation. *Am Intraocular Implant Soc J.* 1985;**11**:599–602.
26. Liesegang TJ: Viscoelastic substances in ophthalmology. *Surv Ophthalmol.* 1990;**34**:268–293.
27. Lane SS, Lindstrom RL: Viscoelastic agents: Formulation, clinical applications, and complications. *Semin Ophthalmol.* 1992;**7**:253–260.
28. Chung YM, Yeh T: Intraocular lens implantation following extracapsular cataract extraction in uveitis. *Ophthal Surg.* 1990;**21**:272–276.
29. Gelender H: Corneal endothelial cell loss, cystoid macular edema, and iris-supported intraocular lenses. *Ophthalmology.* 1984;**91**:841–846.
30. Lim ES, Apple DJ, Tsai JC, et al: An analysis of flexible anterior chamber lenses with special reference to the normalized rate of lens explantation. *Ophthalmology.* 1991;**98**:243–246.
31. Moses L: Complications of rigid anterior chamber implants. *Ophthalmology.* 1984;**91**:819–825.
32. Apple DJ, Kincaid MC, Mamalis N, Olson RJ: *Intraocular Lenses.* Baltimore: Williams & Wilkins; 1989:225–254.
33. Busin M, Brauweiler P, Boker T, Spitznas M: Complications of sulcus-supported intraocular lenses with iris sutures, implanted during penetrating keratoplasty after intracapsular cataract extraction. *Ophthalmology.* 1990;**97**:401–406.
34. Hooper PL, RAO NA, Smith RE: Cataract extraction in uveitis patients. *Surv Ophthalmol.* 1990;**35**:120–144.

## Intraocular Lens Decentration/Pupillary Capture

35. Assia EI, Legler UFC, Merrill C, et al: Clinicopathologic study of the effect of radial tears and loop fixation on intraocular lens decentration. *Ophthalmology.* 1993;**100**:153–158.
36. Lindstrom RL, Herman WK: Pupil capture: Prevention and management. *Am Intraocular Implant Soc J.* 1983;**9**:201–204.
37. Laren M, Jagger J: Pathogenesis of pupillary capture after posterior chamber intraocular lens implantation. *Br J Ophthalmol.* 1986;**70**:886–889.
38. Bucci FA, Lindstom RL: Total pupillary capture with a foldable silicone intraocular lens. *Ophthamic Surg.* 1991;**22**:414–415.

## Choroidal Detachment

39. Jaffe NS, Jaffe MS, Jaffe GF: *Cataract Surgery and Its Complications,* 5th ed. St Louis: CV Mosby; 1990:376–380.
40. Brubaker RF, Pederson JE: Ciliochoroidal detachment. *Surv Ophthalmol.* 1983;**27**:281–289.

41. Chandler PA, Maumenee AE: A major cause of hypotony. *Am J Ophthalmol.* 1961;**52**:609–618.
42. Hoffman P, Oliver M: Limited choroidal hemorrhage associated with intracapsular cataract extraction. *Arch Ophthalmol.* 1984;**102**:1761–1765.
43. Smith SG, Lindstrom RL: *Intraocular Lens Complications and Their Management.* Thorofare, NJ: Slack; 1988:50.

## Anterior Ischemic Optic Neuropathy

44. Carroll FD: Optic nerve complications of cataract extraction. *Trans Am Acad Ophthalmol Otolaryngol.* 1973;**77**:623.
45. Quigley HA, Miller NR, Green WR: The pattern of optic nerve fiber loss in anterior ischemic optic neuropathy. *Am J Ophthalmol.* 1985;**100**:769–776.
46. Kline OR, Yang HK: A review of 1400 intraocular lens implant cases. *Cataract Intraocular Lens Med J.* 1981;**7**:262–278.
47. Beri M, Klugman MR, Koher JA, et al: Anterior ischemic optic neuropathy VII. Incidence of bilaterality and various influencing factors. *Ophthalmology.* 1987;**94**:1020.
48. Serramo LA, Beherns MM, Carroll FD: Postcataract extraction ischemic optic neuropathy (letter). *Arch Ophthalmol.* 1982;**100**:1177–1178.
49. Jaffe NS, Jaffe MS, Jaffe GF: *Cataract Surgery and Its Complications,* 5th ed. St Louis: CV Mosby; 1990:453.
50. Hayreh SS: Anterior ischemic optic neuropathy IV. Occurrence after cataract extraction. *Arch Ophthalmol.* 1982;**100**:1177.
51. Kline LB: Progression of visual defects in ischemic optic neuropathy. *Am J Ophthalmol.* 1988;**106**:199–203.
52. Sergott RC, Cohen MS, Bosley TM, Savino PJ: Optic nerve decompression may improve the progressive form of nonarteritic ischemic optic neuropathy. *Arch Ophthalmol.* 1989;**107**:1743–1754.
53. Sadun AA: The efficacy of optic nerve sheath decompression for anterior ischemic optic neuropathy and other optic neuropathies. *Am J Ophthalmol.* 1993;**115**:384–389.

# Intermediate to Late Complications

CHAPTER 16

## PTOSIS

Ptosis following cataract surgery is usually defined as a 2-mm drop of the eyelid from the superior limbus.[1] Postoperative ptosis is generally minor in severity but may rarely be visually or cosmetically significant.

### Background

The incidence of ptosis following cataract surgery has been reported to be as high as 13%.[2,3] Feibel et al have recently reported an incidence of 5.8% of patients following peribulbar anesthesia and 5.5% with a retrobulbar block.[4] We estimate that 1 per 1000–2000 of our patients require treatment for ptosis that persists beyond 120 days postsurgically. Although the exact mechanism is unknown, there are probably a variety of factors responsible. Suggested causes include trauma to the superior rectus muscle complex, levator aponeurosis disinsertion, eyelid edema, lid speculum trauma, prolonged patching, and direct myotoxicity from peribulbar anesthetics.[5–9] Kaplan and Jaffe believe that trauma to the superior rectus muscle complex is the most important factor.[7] In their prospective study, they found less ptosis in patients with cataract who had an episcleral bridle suture with a facial nerve block (retroauricular) than those with superior rectus bridle sutures with a lid block. The superior rectus bridle suture is passed around or through the muscle belly to stabilize the globe during surgery. Kaplan and Jaffe theorize that this compresses the muscular arteries resulting in vascular congestion and stasis that may affect the muscular attachments from the superior rectus to the levator and cause ptosis.[7] Rainin and Carlson have hypothesized that some cases of postoperative diplopia and ptosis can be a result of direct muscle toxicity from the local anesthetic.[8] This concept is supported by animal and human studies that have demonstrated by histologic examination damage to muscle fibers following anesthetic injection.[9,10]

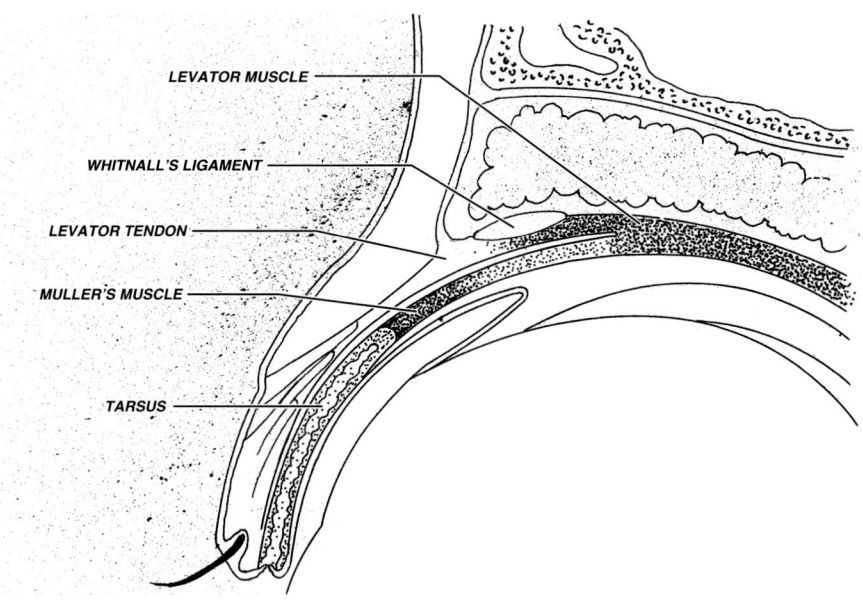

FIGURE 16–1. Anatomy of upper lid.

The damaged muscle fibers, however, were shown to regenerate.[10] This theory of muscle damage followed by regeneration correlates with the clinical observation of a transient postsurgical ptosis.

Linberg et al[11] have reported ptosis in seven patients following radial keratotomy performed under topical anesthesia using a rigid speculum to retract the lids. Because no bridle suture and no anesthetic injection were administered, Linberg et al theorize that the rigid lid speculum may have caused a dehiscence of the levator aponeurosis.[11] Cataract surgery also involves the use of a lid speculum; therefore, it seems reasonable to assume that a dehiscence of the levator aponeurosis plays a role in causing postoperative ptosis (Figure 16–1).

Postsurgical ptosis may possibly be minimized by using flexible lid retractors and avoiding bridle sutures.

## Clinical Presentation and Assessment

Following cataract surgery, the patient will usually complain of a lid droop or a "smaller eye" compared with the nonoperated eye. Ocular examination shows a ptosis variable in severity but usually mild. Good levator function is usually present (Figure 16–2).

## Differential Diagnosis

The various causes of acquired ptosis including neurogenic (Horner's syndrome) (Table 16–1), traumatic, myogenic, and mechanical ptosis should be ruled out.[12] History and preoperative examination records are most valuable in determining if the ptosis is surgically related. The onset of postsurgical ptosis will obviously correspond to the surgical event. If there is any doubt as to whether or not the ptosis was present preoperatively (if surgery was done elsewhere), examination of old photographs may be helpful. If there is continued doubt as to whether or not the ptosis is surgically related, neurologic work-up may be indicated.

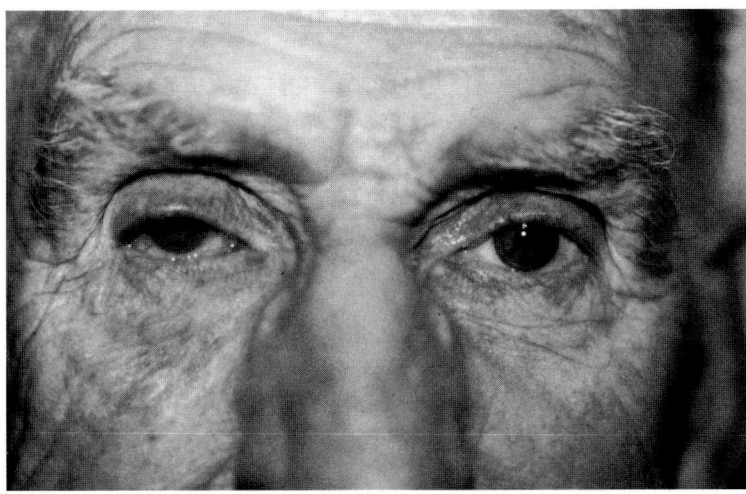

**FIGURE 16–2.** Postoperative ptosis.

## Treatment, Follow-up, and Prognosis

Postoperative ptosis may be transient or permanent. Kaplan et al found that in 44% of patients who developed ptosis postoperatively, an improvement was noted with time compared with 12% who worsened with time.[7] Similarly, dramatic improvement with time has been noted with even total traumatic ptosis.[13]

If the ptosis is secondary to anesthetic myotoxicity, a prolonged recovery would be expected. Although little information is available on the rates of regeneration of ocular muscle fibers, they may be extrapolated from laboratory studies.[8–10] Using these data, it is estimated that following anesthetic muscle tox-

**TABLE 16–1. NEUROGENIC PTOSIS: DIFFERENTIAL DIAGNOSIS**

|  | Compressive Third Nerve Palsy | Ischemic Third Nerve Palsy | Sympathetic Lesion |
|---|---|---|---|
| **Pupil** | 90% are mydriatic, nonresponsive | 90% are spared | Miotic, reactive to light and accommodation |
| **Extraocular Muscles** | SR, MR, IR, and IO paralysis | SR MR, IR, and IO paralysis | LR may be affected |
| **Eyelid Muscles** | Levator—complete ptosis | Levator—complete ptosis | Müller's muscle–partial ptosis |
| **Laboratory Tests** | CT/MRI scan CSF tap Cerebral angiography | Blood glucose Blood pressure Sedimentation rate CT/MRI | Cocaine Hydroxyamphetamine CT/MRI scan |
| **Common Causes** | Aneurysm Tumor Trauma | Diabetes Hypertension Giant cell arteritis Atherosclerosis | Trauma Tumor/infarction Vascular headache |
| **Other Signs** | Neurologic | Neurologic pain | Facial anhydrosis |
| **Management** | Neurologic evaluation | <40 years old: Full neurologic work-up >40 years old: Evaluate for DM/HBP; monitor | Neurologic evaluation |

SR, superior rectus muscle; MR, medial rectus muscle; LR, lateral rectus muscle; IR, inferior rectus muscle; IO, inferior oblique muscle; CSF, cerebrospinal fluid; DM, diabetes mellitis; HBP, high blood pressure; CT/MRI, computed tomography/magnetic resonance imaging.

**TABLE 16–2. PTOSIS: TREATMENT OPTIONS**

Rule out preexisting condition
Observation and reassurance
Consider surgical repair if ptosis persists for more than 6 months

icity, a minimum of 5–6 weeks would be required for complete muscle regeneration.[8]

Because most ptosis following surgery is mild and often improves with time, the best approach is to reassure the patient and observe. At least 6 months should elapse before deciding to refer the patient for surgical repair[7] (Table 16–2).

## DIPLOPIA

Certainly a very frustrating event arises when the postsurgical patient achieves excellent visual and anatomic results postoperatively but is unable to maintain single binocular fusion. The various causes and management of this rare complication are addressed.

### Background

Postoperative diplopia can be classified into monocular and binocular causes. Monocular diplopia in the operated eye may be a result of macular disease, media opacities, decentration of the intraocular lens (IOL), optical aberrations of the IOL, or uncorrected refractive error. Bifocal IOLs even when centered have been found to result in monocular diplopia.[14]

Binocular diplopia is due to a strabismus without sensory suppression. Postcataract surgery strabismus has been found to account for 8% of all surgically corrected strabismus in patients over 60 years of age.[15] Various causes of binocular diplopia following cataract surgery as described by Hamed[16] are:

1. Preexisting conditions such as disease that became symptomatic after removal of the cataract (muscle palsy, thyroid eye disease)
2. Disorders precipitated by prolonged occlusion by the cataract
3. Muscle and soft tissue damage by the surgery
4. Optical conditions resulting from pseudophakia and aphakia

Patients who have thyroid orbitopathy may show a marked inflammatory reaction following muscle surgery.[17] This has also been suggested as a possible cause of cataract postoperative diplopia by Hamed and Lingua.[18] These investigators reviewed 58 patients presenting with strabismus following cataract surgery. Of these, eight patients were found to have previously unsuspected thyroid orbitopathy based on clinical and radiologic examination. They suggested that the following factors could contribute to the development of diplopia postsurgically in a patient who preoperatively has asymptomatic thyroid orbitopathy[18]:

1. The orbital inflammation is exacerbated
2. An occluding cataract is removed clearing the image so that diplopia results
3. Coincidental occurrence

Therefore, it is suggested that any patient presenting with postoperative diplopia be evaluated to rule out a preexisting condition such as thyroid orbitopathy.

Other preexisting conditions can manifest in diplopia following cataract surgery. A patient with a diabetic sixth nerve palsy, for example, may be asymptomatic if a moderate cataract obstructs the vision. Following cataract surgery, however, the patient may report a "sudden diplopia" due to the improved retinal image. In a similar fashion, any preexisting condition that causes a strabismus may result in a sudden diplopia after the occluding cataract is removed.[16]

Horror fusionis is a rare complication following the removal of a dense cataract in an eye with previous amblyopia and strabismus.[19–21] This condition occurs when a strabismic patient is not able to fuse or suppress and thereafter has permanent intractable diplopia. It has been reported to occur in both children and adults following cataract surgery.[20] It is generally thought that a long-standing dense cataract may somehow break the suppression of a strabismic, amblyopic eye, and then following its removal, result in horror fusionalis.[19–21]

Direct injury or damage to the muscles or orbital soft tissues may also result in postoperative strabismus.[16,22–27] It is most commonly thought that the use of a bridle suture during cataract surgery is the primary cause.[22] Surgeons used bridle sutures in the past and some still do to fixate and stabilize the globe while performing cataract surgery. These sutures were placed by passing a suture needle underneath or through the belly of one of the recti muscles. The surgeon could then stabilize or manipulate the globe during surgery (Figure 16–3). This technique of globe fixation has been postulated to cause muscle damage by direct mechanical insult or by hypoxia from suture compression of the arteries of the muscle.[22] Fortunately, bridle sutures are used less frequently now than in the past for routine cataract surgery, which of course results in less frequent postoperative diplopia.

Direct damage to the muscle can also occur as a result of injury from the needle used during peribulbar or retrobulbar anesthesia[16] (Figure 16–4). It has been proposed that the needle may lacerate anterior ciliary vessels resulting in

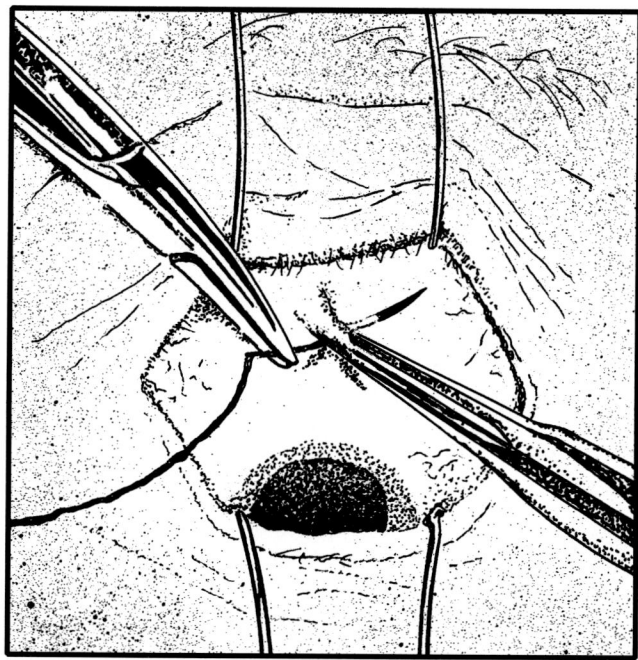

**FIGURE 16–3.** Bridle suture used to stabilize globe for cataract surgery.

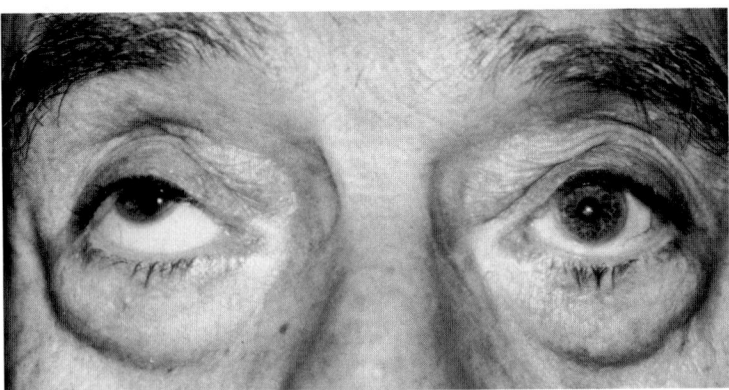

**FIGURE 16–4.** Muscle trauma due to retrobulbar anesthesia.

an intramuscular hematoma and edema.[16] The inferior muscles are at greatest risk, because they are the most common site of injection. An acquired Brown's syndrome has also been reported following a peribulbar injection in the superior nasal quadrant.[27]

Myotoxicity from the anesthetic has also been suggested as a cause of strabismus.[24–26] Rainin and Carlson have hypothesized that diplopia may be caused by muscle degeneration from exposure to the anesthetic and that recovery occurs as a result of muscle regeneration.[26]

Postoperative diplopia is most commonly due to optical factors. Patients who are rendered anisometropic and those with high astigmatism are particularly at risk. (See discussion of optical considerations below.)

## Clinical Presentation and Assessment

Subjectively, the patient with diplopia will report double vision. The first step is to determine if the diplopia is monocular or binocular by alternately occluding each eye. If monocular diplopia exists, the clinician should then concentrate on evaluating the uniformity of the media (cornea, lens, posterior capsule, and IOL). If the diplopia resolves with pinhole testing, this helps to confirm that the cause is either refractive error or media irregularity. Uncorrected astigmatism may result in monocular diplopia; therefore a refraction is mandatory. Careful slit lamp examination of the IOL through the nondilated and dilated pupil can uncover mild to moderate decentrations. If the edge of the implant or one of the fixation holes is observed through the nondilated pupil, then one is more suspicious of the IOL inducing the diplopia. If there is an iridotomy/iridectomy not covered by the lid, diplopia also may result. A posterior capsular opacity may also diffract light creating additional retinal images. Finally, once the media has been ruled out, the examiner should carefully assess the macula for disease.[23]

If the patient is experiencing binocular diplopia, the angle of strabismus should be measured in all fields of gaze. If the diplopia has persisted for more than a week, clinical and possibly laboratory tests should be performed to rule out thyroid orbitopathy. In this disease, the inferior muscles are usually first involved resulting in vertical strabismus. A forced duction test should therefore be performed if a strabismus persists following surgery. If eye movement is restricted with this test, then thyroid orbitopathy should be highly suspected. If the patient has not previously been diagnosed, physical examination and laboratory studies should be ordered. In some cases, neuroimaging of the orbits to rule out enlarged muscles will be necessary.

Additionally, other clinical signs that could indicate a preexisting condition should be investigated. Lid position, pupillary reactions, globe protrusion, cranial nerve deficits, and ocular movements may all be helpful in ruling out a preexisting condition.

## Differential Diagnosis

Diplopia following cataract surgery may be a direct result of the surgery; however, preexisting conditions should be ruled out. Thyroid orbitopathy may be exacerbated following surgery and manifest as a sudden diplopia.[17] Likewise, myasthenia gravis and muscle palsies may become symptomatic following the removal of an occluding cataract.[16] Review of preoperative data and old photographs as well as clinical and laboratory investigation may be warranted.

## Treatment, Follow-up, and Prognosis

Monocular diplopia due to refractive error is obviously best corrected by spectacle or contact lens prescriptions. If IOL decentration is the cause, there are two options for treatment. If no contraindications exist, the patient may be placed on a weak miotic agent (pilocarpine 0.5% to 1.0%) two or three times a day. If the miosis eliminates the patient's symptoms, then the patient may be given the option of continued miotic therapy or IOL repositioning or exchange.

After evaluating, ruling out, or treating other preexisting conditions, persistent binocular diplopia in which the patient is able to attain fusion may be treated with either prism spectacles or surgery. Because the strabismus may improve with time, prism correction is recommended for the first 6 months or until stability is reached.[23] During this period, either Fresnel prism lenses or ground-in prism may be used. We have had excellent success with Fresnel prisms, even in patients with large-angle strabismus. Low cost and ease of replacement make these prism lenses a very useful tool. They do, however, blur vision, are cosmetically apparent, and may discolor with time. After 6 months, the patient may be presented with the option of continuing with ground-in prism spectacles or undergoing surgery (Table 16–3).

## — OCULAR HYPERTENSION/GLAUCOMA —

Although transient spikes of the intraocular pressure (IOP) are common, long-term elevations following cataract surgery are much less frequent. The effect of cataract surgery on IOP has been extensively studied in glaucomatous as well as nonglaucomatous eyes. In 373 consecutive eyes undergoing cataract extraction, Radius et al found that those undergoing intracapsular cataract extraction averaged an 0.8 mm Hg rise in IOP, whereas those cataracts removed by extracapsular technique averaged an 0.8 mm Hg lowering of the intraocular pressure.[28] In 24 eyes with the preoperative diagnosis of glaucoma or ocu-

### TABLE 16–3. TREATMENT OF DIPLOPIA

Prismatic spectacle correction—Apply press-on Fresnel prisms for up to 3 months; when stable, formal spectacle correction with prism
Consider surgical realignment for large deviations
Consider vision therapy for small deviations

**TABLE 16-4. LATE OCULAR HYPERTENSION ETIOLOGY**

Steroid response
IOL effect (uveitis, glaucoma, hyphema syndrome)
Epithelial downgrowth (rare)
Pseudophakic angle closure

lar hypertension, the results were similar.[28] Others have found that in many cases patients who have glaucoma and undergo extracapsular cataract surgery with implantation of a posterior chamber IOL will have little or no long-term pressure elevation. Some may even show a lowering of the IOP from the preoperative level.[29,30] Nevertheless, after cataract extraction, patients may develop ocular hypertension/glaucoma in the late postoperative period due to a variety of mechanisms as described above (Table 16–4). Patients who are undergoing secondary implantation of an IOL are at a greater risk.[31]

## Open-Angle Glaucoma (see Table 16–4)

Preexisting glaucoma may be missed during the preoperative examination if the cataract obscures the view of the optic nerve. Patients with dense cataracts deserve a thorough examination of the optic nerve postoperatively, regardless of the intraocular pressure, as significant numbers of patients with cataract will have "normotensive glaucoma."

### *Steroid Induced*

#### *Background*

Because topical corticosteroids are routinely used following cataract surgery, susceptible individuals are at risk of developing steroid-induced ocular hypertension. Individuals who either have glaucoma or a family history of glaucoma are at greatest risk. The amount of elevation is dependent on the medication, concentration, and frequency of instillation. Of the commonly used topical steroid preparations, prednisolone acetate 1.0%, prednisolone phosphate 1.0%, and dexamethasone 0.1% are associated with a significantly higher risk of IOP response than is fluorometholone acetate[32] (Table 16–5).

Although the exact mechanism of increased IOP with steroids is uncertain, it is generally agreed that the steroid alters the normal aqueous outflow induced by the medication.

#### *Clinical Presentation and Assessment*

The patient has a history of topical steroid usage and may have a prior history of open-angle glaucoma, steroid response, or a family history of glaucoma. The

**TABLE 16-5. RISK OF INCREASING INTRAOCULAR PRESSURE WITH TOPICAL STEROIDS**

| Steroids with higher risk | Steroids with lower risk |
|---|---|
| Prednisolone preparations | Fluorometholone preparations |
| Dexamethasone | Medrysone |

IOP is found to be elevated in a quiet eye with an open angle usually weeks after instituting topical steroid use, although an IOP response can occur within days.[33]

### Differential Diagnosis

Steroid-induced ocular hypertension must be differentiated from primary open-angle glaucoma. This is done through knowledge of the patient using a corticosteroid preparation that correlates with a rise in the IOP.

### Treatment, Follow-Up, and Prognosis

The management of steroid-induced ocular hypertension is twofold: discontinue the steroid when possible and treat the IOP if necessary. If the anterior chamber is quiet, the steroid may be rapidly tapered or stopped. If the anterior chamber still shows an inflammatory reaction, the steroid may need to be slowly tapered over a week or so. An alternative would be to substitute a preparation with a lower steroid response potential; that is, fluoromethalone 0.1% for a more "potent" steroidal agent, such as prednisolone acetate 1%. A second alternative would be to substitute a nonsteroidal anti-inflammatory agent such as flurbiprofen, which has been shown to be effective in controlling postoperative inflammation and is probably less likely to affect the IOP.[34]

If there is significant iritis, the steroid is continued and the intraocular pressure should be controlled medically (Table 16–6). Prescription of an antiglaucoma medication is dictated by common sense. If the IOP is only moderately elevated (30 mm Hg or less), there is no preexisting glaucoma, and the anterior chamber is quiet, the steroid can be quickly tapered or stopped without adding an antiglaucoma medicine. If, however, the patient needs to be maintained on a steroid due to inflammation, if the IOP is very high, or if the patient has glaucomatous nerve damage, then a topical antiglaucoma medication is indicated. As a first choice, we prescribe a topical beta-blocker provided there are no systemic contraindications.

### TABLE 16–6. STEROID-INDUCED OCULAR HYPERTENSION: TREATMENT OPTIONS

**No Associated Intraocular Inflammation**

Discontinue or rapidly taper steroid

If optic nerve is healthy, follow without adding antiglaucoma medications, unless markedly elevated IOP (≥ 40 mm Hg) or other risk factors present

IOP should return to baseline in 1–4 wk

Permanent intraocular elevation requiring medical, laser, or surgery is rare

**Associated Intraocular Inflammation**

Depending on degree of inflammation, continue steroid, slowly taper, or switch to fluorometholone acetate 0.1% or 0.25%. Another alternative would be to substitute a topical nonsteroidal anti-inflammatory drug

Monitor IOP (mm Hg):

| | |
|---|---|
| 30–35 | Beta-blocker, one to two drops (in office); follow-up in 2–3 days. |
| 35–45 | Add acetazolamide (Diamox) 250 mg by mouth, once. Recheck IOP within 24 h. |
| 45–55 | Add apraclonidine 1% (Iopidine) in office, two drops 20 min apart; check IOP in 1 h. Recheck IOP within 4 h. |
| 55+ | Add oral 50% glycerin (Osmoglyn) 2 oz over ice; if diabetic, use 45% w/v solution isosorbide (Ismotic). Keep patient until pressure is below 35 mm Hg. Recheck IOP within 4 h. |

As inflammation subsides, taper and discontinue steroid

As IOP lowers, discontinue glaucoma medications

Following discontinuation of the steroid, the IOP is usually lowered within days to weeks. In rare cases, the IOP may remain elevated and require long-term medical therapy.

## Ocular Hypertension Secondary to IOL Irritation

Chronic inflammation may decrease trabecular filtration resulting in increased IOP.[35] A higher incidence of inflammatory complications have been found with rigid anterior chamber and iris-fixated IOLs compared with posterior chamber IOLs due to their direct contact with vascularized tissues.[36,37] Posterior chamber IOLs that are placed in the bag are at less risk than those that are sulcus fixated. The most classic example of this is the uveitis, glaucoma, hyphema (UGH) syndrome.

### Background

The UGH syndrome may be found with any IOL that touches vascularized tissues, but most notably with the iris-fixated and rigid anterior chamber IOLs (see Chapter 8). These implants are in direct contact with the iris and/or trabecular meshwork. With time, they chafe the tissues causing inflammation and/or dispersion of pigment or red blood cells.

Milder variants of the UGH syndrome may occur. Some patients may develop uveitis and/or glaucoma without hyphema. We have seen this occur in patients who have anterior chamber and iris-fixated IOLs as well as sulcus-fixated posterior chamber IOLs. In the latter, the haptics of the IOL may abrade the pigment epithelium of the iris resulting in dramatic iris transillumination defects and a clinical picture that resembles pigment dispersion syndrome (iris transillumination, endothelial pigment, and a trabecular pigment band)[38] (Figure 16–5).

### Clinical Presentation and Assessment

Classically, the patient with the UGH syndrome presents with elevated IOP, a layered hyphema, and iritis. Milder variants may occur in which the patient presents with a history of transient episodes of vision loss due to the occurrence of a microhyphema. In such cases, the doctor may need to evaluate the eye carefully for subtle signs such as hemorrhage on the capsule, red blood cells in the aqueous, or a small pool of red blood cells in the inferior angle, which

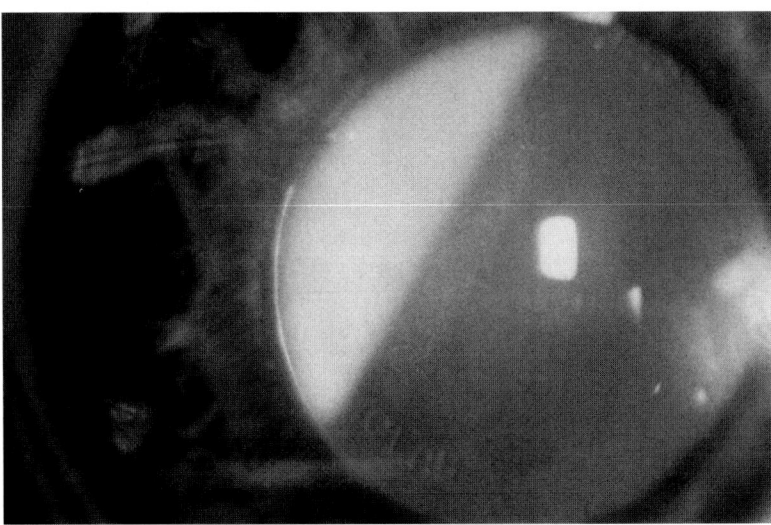

**FIGURE 16–5.** Iris transillumination secondary to posterior chamber IOL.

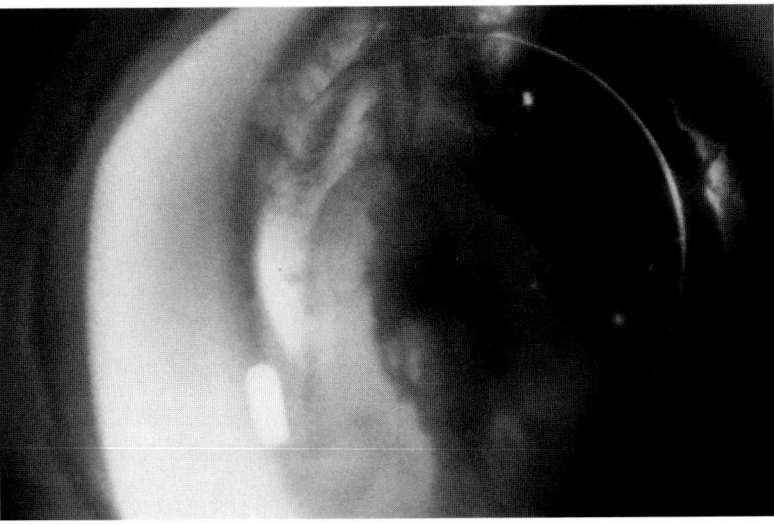

FIGURE 16–6. Uveitis glaucoma hyphema (UGH) syndrome with large central clot hyphema.

may only be observed by gonioscopy. The iris will typically show signs of trauma as evidenced by transillumination defects that correspond to points of IOL contact. The elevated IOP is due to obstruction of the trabecular meshwork from inflammatory debris, red blood cells, and pigment (Figures 16–6 and 16–7).

### Treatment, Follow-up, and Prognosis

The goal in managing patients with the UGH syndrome and its variants is to stabilize the condition medically and then consider explantation of the IOL with possible IOL exchange (Table 16–7). The goals of medical therapy are to reduce inflammation, lower the IOP, and reduce the risk of hyphema. Initially, topical steroids should be administered aggressively (prednisolone acetate 1.0% every 2–3 hours) and then tapered once the inflammatory reaction subsides. Assuming no systemic contraindications, the IOP is best lowered with a beta-blocker or carbonic anhydrase inhibitor (CAI). If the patient is taking anticoagulants, one should consult with the patient's family doctor to see if they may be discontinued. Limiting the activity of the patient may also inhibit traumatic contact of the IOL to the iris reducing the risk of a recurrent hyphema. Fol-

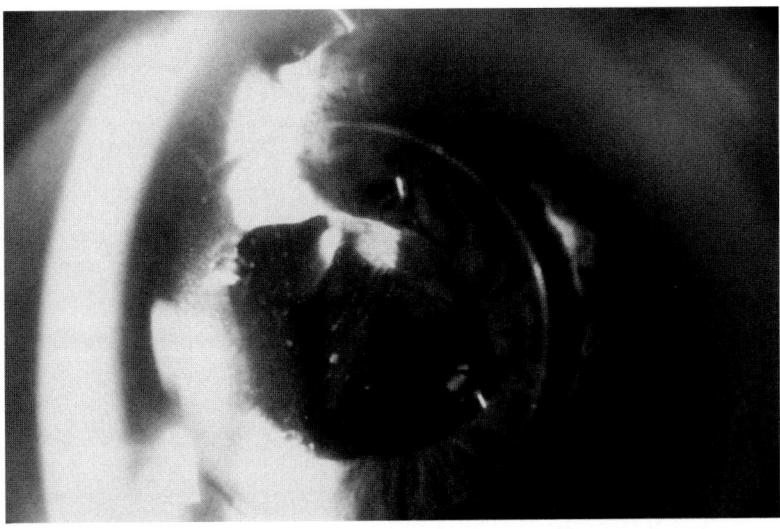

FIGURE 16–7. Same patient as in Figure 16–6 with resolution of the hyphema 1 day later.

**TABLE 16-7. INFLAMMATORY OCULAR HYPERTENSION SECONDARY TO IOL IRRITATION: TREATMENT OPTIONS**

Prednisolone acetate or phosphate 1%, one drop every 2–4 h, depending on severity of inflammation

Topical cycloplegics if no contraindications (such as iris-supported IOLs)

For control of IOP (mm Hg):

| | |
|---|---|
| 30–35 | Beta-blocker, one to two drops (in office); follow-up in 2–3 days. |
| 35–45 | Add acetazolamide (Diamox) 250 mg by mouth, once. Recheck IOP within 24 h. |
| 45–55 | Add apraclonidine 1% (Iopidine) in office, two drops 20 min apart; check IOP in 1 h. Recheck IOP within 4 h. |
| 55+ | Add oral 50% glycerin (Osmoglyn) 2 oz over ice; if diabetic, use 45% w/v solution isosorbide (Ismotic). Keep patient until pressure is below 35 mm Hg. Recheck IOP within 4 h. |

Treat underlying cause; eg, if uveitis, glaucoma, hyphema syndrome occurs, intraocular lens explant or exchange may be needed

---

lowing the reduction of the inflammatory reaction, one may consider administering a miotic to keep the pupil fixed. To prevent pseudophakic pupillary block, a patent iridectomy should be present before adding the miotic.

Explantation of the IOL is generally indicated after the condition is stabilized. The surgeon must decide whether to leave the eye aphakic or replace the explanted lens with a modern flexible anterior chamber IOL or posterior chamber IOL sutured into the ciliary sulcus (see Chapter 11).

## Closed-Angle Glaucoma

An acute form of pseudophakic pupillary block may occur in either the early or late postoperative periods (Table 16–8). When late postoperative pseudophakic angle closure is encountered, it is usually due to an anterior chamber IOL rotating to occlude the iridectomy. The clinical features and management of this condition have already been covered (see discussion of closed-angle with pupillary block in Chapter 14).

### Synechial Angle Closure

#### Background

Progressive synechial closure of the angle has been found to occur with angle-supported IOLs.[39,40] A high incidence of angle and iris abnormalities have especially been found with the rigid anterior chamber IOLs.[36] Modern flexible anterior chamber lenses with point fixation are at less risk of causing progressive synechial closure, because a smaller area is in contact with the trabecular meshwork. Posterior chamber IOLs also have been associated with progressive peripheral anterior synechiae.[41,42] This more commonly occurs in those patients

---

**TABLE 16-8. PSEUDOPHAKIC ANGLE CLOSURE ETIOLOGIES**

| | |
|---|---|
| Pseudophakic pupillary block | Iris incarceration to the wound |
| Progressive synechial closure | Epithelial downgrowth |

with sulcus-fixated IOLs and in those with IOLs who have anterior vaulted haptics.[39]

PAS may also occur as a direct surgical complication leading to chronic ocular hypertension/glaucoma.[41] If the anterior chamber collapsed following surgery due to choroidal detachments, hypotony, or pseudophakic angle closure, the prolonged contact of the iris to angle in the presence of inflammation may cause permanent adhesions. For this reason, any postoperative collapse of the anterior chamber should be treated as expeditiously as possible.

### Clinical Presentation and Assessment
The diagnosis of synechial angle closure is ascertained by careful gonioscopy. Peripheral anterior synechiae (PAS) are seen that initially "bury" the haptics and later may progress to involve larger areas of the angle.

### Treatment, Follow-Up, and Prognosis
The management of synechial angle closure is most successful with medications that decrease secretion of aqueous (beta-blockers and CAIs). Miotics may also be tried, but they may not be effective if large areas of the angle have been covered by the synechiae and are contraindicated if active inflammation is present. The mechanism of action of the miotic, which is to open the pores of the trabecular meshwork to increase outflow, is obviously ineffective if there is no trabecular meshwork available for filtration. In severe cases, the IOL may need to be explanted. When closed-loop IOLs are explanted, the haptics may need to be cut, and removed in pieces[36] (see discussion of explantation in Chapter 11).

## Epithelial Downgrowth

### Background
Epithelial downgrowth, also called epithelial ingrowth, is a rare condition that has been reported to occur in approximately 0.1% of eyes following cataract surgery.[41] These numbers were compiled before most modern surgical techniques and are therefore considerably higher than what one would expect with today's methods. This complication occurs following cataract surgery with poor wound apposition. An epithelial membrane grows through the wound and progressively covers the corneal endothelium, iris, and anterior chamber angle. This results in corneal edema and a severe form of glaucoma.[39]

### Clinical Presentation and Assessment
Visual acuity is markedly reduced and the IOP is elevated. A translucent membrane can be observed on the corneal endothelium and surface of the iris. An endothelial line is observed corresponding to the leading edge of the invading epithelial cells. A wound gape is often observed.

### Differential Diagnosis
Iris incarceration in the wound may also result in ocular hypertension (see discussion of iris prolapse in Chapter 14). The ocular hypertension that occurs is best treated with beta-blockers, CAIs, or filtering surgery.

Other forms of closed-angle glaucoma without pupillary block include fibrinous ingrowth, retrocorneal membranes, and neovascular glaucoma. Fibrinous ingrowth results when there is a break in Descemet's membrane and endothelium allowing a fibrovascular membrane to grow in the anterior chamber. Retrocorneal membranes are thought to be due to repeated corneal trauma that causes the proliferation of metaplastic endothelial cells. In neovascular glaucoma associated with pseudophakia, the mechanism is thought to be chronic inflammation. This precipitates a fibrovascular membrane that occludes the angle. Both of these forms are quite serious and typically require aggressive surgical procedures to preserve sight.

### Treatment, Follow-up, and Prognosis

Aggressive surgical procedures are necessary in order to remove the progressive epithelial membrane and most eyes do very poorly. The goal of therapy is to preserve the structure of the globe and possibly retain some usable vision.

## CHRONIC CORNEAL EDEMA/CORNEAL DECOMPENSATION

Chronic corneal edema following cataract surgery (also referred to as pseudophakic bullous keratopathy [PBK] when epithelial bullae are present) is the most common visually disabling complication of cataract surgery. Pseudophakic bullous keratopathy, if untreated, may lead to corneal decompensation. In the United States, pseudophakic bullous keratopathy is the most frequent cause of penetrating keratoplasty.[43,44]

## Background

The pathogenesis of PBK is secondary to direct or indirect damage to the corneal endothelium.[45] With sufficient damage and cell loss, the endothelium loses its ability to keep the cornea detergesced and clear. This allows aqueous to enter the corneal stroma causing swelling and translucence. If the epithelium becomes edematous, the cells eventually collapse allowing fluid accumulation between the epithelium and Bowman's membrane and leading to the formation of bullae. This entire process of endothelial cell loss, stromal edema, epithelial edema, and bullae formation is termed corneal decompensation.

Direct endothelial damage may occur both intraoperatively and postoperatively (Table 16–9). Intraoperative damage occurs when surgical instruments, the IOL, or crystalline lens material make contact with the corneal endothelium.[46] Endothelial cell damage may also occur intraoperatively as the result of changes in the pH and chemical composition of the aqueous due to irrigating solutions[47,48] and from hydraulic forces associated with irrigating the anterior chamber.

Although endothelial cell damage cannot be reversed once it occurs, the surgeon may attempt to limit the amount of intraoperative endothelial cell damage through surgical technique. The use of viscoelastic agents in complicated cases and for corneas with preexisting corneal endothelial disease can limit surgical endothelial trauma.[49,50] Endocapsular phacoemulsification (versus phacoemulsification in the anterior chamber) also limits endothelial cell damage by reducing contact of crystalline lens material to the corneal endothelium and by reducing aqueous turbidity[51] (see Chapter 10).

### TABLE 16–9. CAUSES OF CHRONIC CORNEAL EDEMA

| Intraoperative | Postoperative |
| --- | --- |
| Corneal contact by surgical instruments, IOL, physiologic lens material | IOL contact with endothelium |
| pH or chemical endothelial toxicity | Chronic inflammation |
| Hydraulic endothelial loss | IOP elevation |

Direct endothelial cell damage may occur postoperatively from constant or intermittent contact of the IOL with the corneal endothelium. This occurs most commonly with dislocated iris-fixated IOLs, less commonly with angle-supported anterior chamber IOLs, and rarely with posterior chamber IOLs.[52-54]

Indirect corneal endothelial damage may occur postoperatively as the result of chronic intraocular inflammation or from acute intraocular pressure rise. The release of inflammatory mediators in chronic intraocular inflammation has a toxic effect on the corneal endothelium resulting in endothelial cell damage. Chronic intraocular inflammation results when the IOL is in contact with vascular tissue. This type of contact is obviously most common with anterior chamber IOLs but may also occur with sulcus-fixated posterior chamber IOLs. Posterior chamber IOLs that are positioned within the capsular bag are less likely to produce chronic intraocular inflammation, since they are isolated from contact with vascular tissue.

Chronically elevated IOP may produce corneal endothelial cell damage as well as optic nerve damage. Intraocular pressure of 40 mm Hg or greater has the potential of producing corneal edema and endothelial cell damage. Causes of such pressure rises are discussed elsewhere (see discussion of ocular hypertension in Chapter 14).

## Clinical Presentation and Assessment

The patient may present with gradually decreasing vision associated with a range of other symptoms from intermittent foreign body sensation to acute pain. Objectively, one should perform a complete ocular examination to rule out all sources of decreased vision. Specifically, at the biomicroscope, one may observe signs of chronic inflammation (ciliary flush, mild cells and flare in the anterior chamber), corneal epithelial microcysts or bullae, corneal stromal folds and thickening, and/or endothelial disease such as Fuchs' dystrophy. Observe the type and position of the IOL, any signs of corneal touch, IOL instability, or vitreous in the anterior chamber. If vitreous is present, specifically note contact with cornea. Intraocular pressure is an important finding, as high IOP may be associated with the corneal decompensation.

Clinically, a patient who has IOL touch to the corneal endothelium may present with frank pseudophakic bullous keratopathy or may present with subtle signs of intermittent IOL touch, and endothelial cell counts, if taken, may be lowered. Clinical signs of intermittent IOL touch include ciliary flush, anterior uveitis, local corneal changes, and cystoid macular edema (CME).

## Differential Diagnosis

The differential diagnosis of chronic corneal edema and decompensation are similar to that of acute corneal edema (see discussion of acute corneal edema in Chapter 15). One must rule out other sources of decreased vision and pain in order to determine if the cornea is the source of the symptoms.

Keratitis secondary to sensitivity to postoperative topical medications (medicamentosa) may also present after a few weeks and has been confused with early corneal decompensation. These patients will have decreased vision and possible foreign body sensation with a coarse epithelial keratitis and staining. This reaction can be found with any postoperative topical drug, but beta-blockers and aminoglycosides are common offenders.

Medicamentosa patients do well by stopping all topicals and using nonpreserved lubricants until the cornea clears, which may take a few weeks. Oral hypotensives and antibiotics may be substituted for topical therapy if needed.

**TABLE 16–10. CHRONIC CORNEAL EDEMA: TREATMENT OPTIONS**

Lower elevated IOP: topical beta-blocker, one drop twice daily, or acetazolamide, 250 mg by mouth, twice daily
Topical hyperosmotics: 2% or 5% saline, one drop every 2–4 h and/or ointment at bedtime
Suppress anterior chamber and ciliary body inflammation: prednisolone acetate 1%, one drop every 2–4 h
Bandage lens for pain due to epithelial bullae if present
Surgical IOL repositioning, exchange, or explantation

---

After the cornea clears, topical hypotensives can be reintroduced in glaucomatous patients with close follow-up for possible reoccurrence.

### Treatment, Follow-up, and Prognosis

Patients presenting with postoperative intraocular inflammation should be promptly placed on appropriate medical therapy to avoid endothelial cell damage (Table 16–10). Patients with chronic uncontrollable postoperative intraocular inflammation may need referral to a surgeon for consideration of IOL removal, repositioning, or exchange (see discussion of uveitis in Chapter 15).

The initial treatment for chronic corneal edema is to control the intraocular inflammation and IOP medically. The inflammation may be treated aggressively with topical steroids (one drop every 2–4 hours), whereas the IOP should be lowered with antiglaucoma medications. To control discomfort, corneal microcysts and bullae should be treated with topical hyperosmotic drops applied every 1–4 hours and/or hyperosmotic ointment at bedtime. If vision and comfort are acceptable to the patient with these treatment regimens, the patient may be maintained at a low dosage for as long as needed with regular follow-up visits to evaluate stability.

If symptoms are not controlled and/or progress, a corneal consultation or return to the cataract surgeon is necessary. Pseudophakic bullous keratopathy, if untreated, may result in corneal decompensation. Sequelae of corneal decompensation include severe vascularization, scarring, ulceration, corneal melting and perforation, and endophthalmitis.

In the early course of corneal decompensation, IOL exchange may prevent progression to PBK. Coli and associates[55] have shown that patients with anterior chamber and iris-fixated IOLs showing early signs of corneal decompensation and endothelial cell loss are good candidates for IOL exchange. These investigators exchanged posterior chamber, iris sutured, scleral sutured, or sulcus-fixated IOLs as replacements and performed anterior vitrectomy when the posterior capsule was broken. Seventy-one percent of their patients had the same or improved vision after surgery. Of the ones who failed, 75% had beginning endothelial cell counts of 500/mm or less.

The final treatment for PBK and corneal decompensation is penetrating keratoplasty. The prognosis for success of corneal grafts for pseudophakic bullous keratopathy is quite good. Recent studies have shown 90% clear grafts with good vision approximately 75% of the time.[56]

There is also a close association of CME with PBK. This may limit the visual success of penetrating keratoplasty depending on the severity and duration of the CME.[56,57] It is therefore prudent when pursuing penetrating keratoplasty after making the diagnosis of PBK to educate patients that long-standing associated CME may permanently limit visual potential.

## LATE HYPHEMA

### Microhyphema (White-out Syndrome)

Microhyphemas (see discussion of hyphema in Chapter 15) have been reported by Johnson et al in patients who have had cataract extraction with a posterior chamber implant placed in the ciliary sulcus.[58] In these patients, iris transillumination defects have been observed immediately overlying the haptics of the implant indicating an abrasive effect on the pigment epithelium of the iris (see Figure 16–8). Patients usually present with the complaint of a sudden loss of vision described as a "white-out," which may clear rapidly within hours. On examination, in addition to the transillumination defects, there are red blood cells observed circulating in the anterior chamber and the visual acuity may be moderately to markedly reduced. In other patients, however, by the time of clinical presentation, many of the red blood cells have been resorbed and minimal anterior chamber findings are observed. (See Color Plates 16–1 through 16–3.)

Miotics and mydriatics have been used to prevent iris chafing, and on occasion, the IOL may need to be removed and/or exchanged. We have observed a patient with a sulcus-fixated three-piece posterior chamber IOL who developed a microhyphema syndrome. By exchanging the IOL with a single-piece polymethylmethacrylate (PMMA) angulated IOL, also fixated in the sulcus, the microhyphemas subsided. It was thought that the point of haptic fixation to the optic was a major source of abrasion in this patient.

By using a single-piece polymethylmethacrylate IOL and properly placing it into the capsular bag, the problem of microhyphema can be minimized.

### Uveitis-Glaucoma-Hyphema Syndrome

(See discussion of uveitis in Chapter 15, and of ocular hypertension/glaucoma and chronic iritis in this chapter).

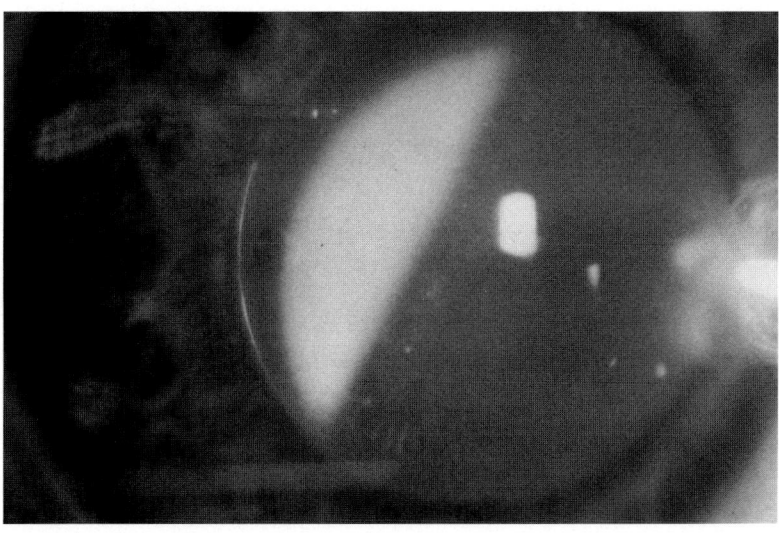

**FIGURE 16–8.** Iris transillumination defects in IOL white-out syndrome.

## — CHRONIC IRITIS

A patient is said to have chronic iritis when the inflammation persists longer than several months despite treatment (see discussion of endophthalmitis in Chapter 14 and of uveitis in Chapter 15).

### Background (Table 16–11)

Patients who have a history of preexisting uveitis should be counseled preoperatively and prepared for prolonged postoperative inflammation and the increased risk of a poor visual result (Table 16–11). Complications encountered following cataract surgery are dependent on the uveitis syndrome and occur more frequently in actively inflamed eyes. Some of the more common postoperative problems include cystoid macular edema, glaucoma, and ocular hypotony.[59] Patients with uveitis, however, can have successful outcomes by appropriate selection and preoperative management of their condition[59] (see discussion of history of iritis in Chapter 7).

The type and position of the IOL are strongly correlated with the susceptibility to develop chronic iritis. It is well known that IOLs whose fixation involves contact with vascularized tissues are at highest risk.[60-63] At greatest risk, therefore, are patients with iris-fixated and rigid anterior chamber IOLs, then modern flexible anterior chamber IOLs, and then sulcus-fixated posterior chamber IOLs. With capsular bag placement of a modern posterior chamber IOL, the incidence of chronic iritis has been significantly reduced.

The UGH syndrome is a well-known entity caused by IOL irritation.[62] It may occur weeks to years after cataract surgery. The lenses most often associated with this syndrome are the iris-fixated and rigid anterior chamber IOLs, which have now been abandoned by US surgeons due to their many complications. The UGH syndrome occurs due to the abrasive effect of the IOL on the uveal tissues and, in its classic form, presents with a layered hyphema, iritis, and ocular hypertension. Milder sequelae of tissue chaffing include the "white-out" and "pigment-dispersion" syndrome[64-66] (see Figures 16–5 to 16–8). In the white-out syndrome, recurrent microhyphemas result in an episodic loss of vision usually in a patient with an iris-fixated IOL. When these patients present to their doctor, clinical signs may be subtle or absent. Careful evaluation may reveal hemorrhage in the inferior angle observed only with the goniolens or on the IOL or anterior vitreous face. Sometimes circulating red or white blood cells may be observed in the anterior chamber.[65,66] A pigment dispersion–like syndrome also has been described associated with posterior chamber IOLs as well as iris- and angle-fixated lenses.[67] These patients typically show iris transillumination defects at points of IOL contact, sometimes have a mild low-grade uveitis, and may have glaucoma.

Retained lens material may induce a chronic inflammatory reaction and should be suspected if an iritis persists. Lens cortex will hydrate and appear

**TABLE 16–11. CHRONIC IRITIS: ETIOLOGIES**

| |
|---|
| IOL lens irritation to vascularized tissues |
| Retained lens fragments |
| Indolent endophthalmitis |
| Miotics |
| Retinal tears/detachment |
| Preexisting uveitis exacerbated by surgery |

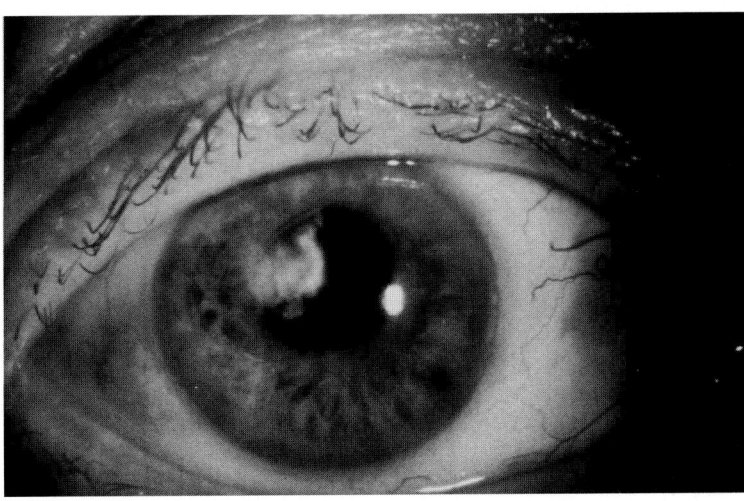

FIGURE 16–9. Retained cortex.

like fluffy white cotton candy in the anterior chamber or may be observed along the pupillary margin between the iris and IOL (Figure 16–9 and Color Plate 16–4.) Retained nucleus appears more solid and waxy in nature and is often yellow-brown in color with a layered appearance (Figure 16–10). Although iritis is present in both retained lens material and retained nucleus, it is more severe with the latter. In addition to iritis, patients with retained nuclear fragments have a high incidence of postoperative complications, including corneal decompensation, chronic glaucoma, and retinal detachment.[68] For this reason, the prompt removal of retained nuclear material in the early postoperative period is imperative.

Miotics have long been associated with an increase in vascular permeability. These antiglaucoma medications should be avoided if a significant iritis is present, because they will exacerbate the inflammatory reaction. The exception is a patient with glaucoma who must be maintained on miotic medications postoperatively. These patients may have a prolonged inflammatory reaction following surgery and should be treated accordingly.

Although most forms of endophthalmitis will present within 72 hours of the surgery, endophthalmitis may present as a moderate, smoldering iritis if the

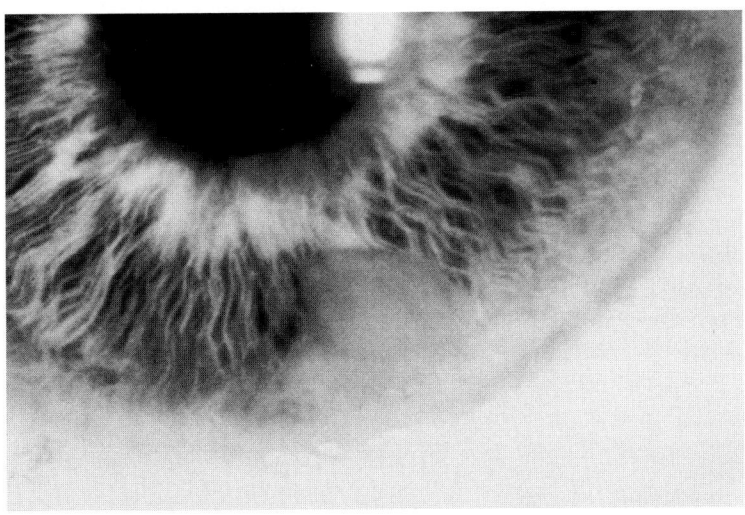

FIGURE 16–10. Retained nucleus at 5:00 in the anterior chamber.

organisms are localized within the capsular bag. An Nd:YAG (neodymium:yttrium-aluminum-garnet) capsulotomy may inadvertently disperse the bacteria resulting in a severe inflammatory reaction. *Propionibacterium acnes* is a well-known cause of localized delayed endophthalmitis.[69]

Endophthalmitis due to organisms of low virulence such as the coagulase-negative staphylococci also can present as a chronic uveitis[70] (see discussion of endophthalmitis in Chapter 14.)

## Clinical Presentation and Assessment

The clinical signs and symptoms of chronic iritis are much the same as with acute postoperative uveitis but are sometimes less severe. The patient may complain of photophobia, mild to moderate pain, and mildly decreased vision. Conjunctival injection and anterior chamber cells and flare may be present. In some cases, no cells/flare will be observed; however, other signs may be observed such as keratic precipitates (KPs) and/or lens precipitates that appear as dry pigmented "smudges" on the anterior IOL surface. The capillaries of the iris may become markedly dilated and tortuous resembling rubeosis iridis. If the iritis is recurrent, examine carefully for iris transillumination and red blood cells in the anterior chamber on the IOL or vitreous face. Measurement of IOP is critical to identify the UGH syndrome or related syndromes. Gonioscopy may be necessary to identify subtle hyphema, retained lens material, or other angle anomalies. Anterior chamber lenses may develop peripheral anterior synechiae around the haptics creating a "cocoon." If the patient has a posterior chamber IOL, gonioscopy should be used to rule out a malpositioned loop protruding through the iris into the angle as a cause of chronic iritis.[71] Cystoid macular edema (CME) should be ruled out if the visual acuity is reduced.

All patients with chronic iritis following surgery should have a dilated vitreoretinal examination to rule out a retinal detachment. Uveitis can be a late sign of a chronic rhegmatogenous retinal detachment (see discussion of retinal detachment on page 222).

## Differential Diagnosis

If the patient reports decreased vision, all potential sources of this symptom should be ruled out. Retinal detachment must be ruled out by dilated fundus examination. Once iritis is diagnosed, the doctor must attempt to determine the etiology. In addition to retinal detachment, other possible causes of chronic postoperative iritis include retained lens material, use of miotics, irritation due to IOL contact with vascularized tissues, infectious endophthalmitis, and exacerbation of preexisting uveitis.

## Treatment, Follow-up, and Prognosis

The goal in managing chronic iritis following cataract surgery is to (1) identify the cause, (2) eliminate the cause if possible, and (3) suppress the inflammation with topical/subconjunctival steroids (Table 16–12). If recurrent iritis existed preoperatively, aggressive preoperative, intraoperative, and postoperative control of inflammation with corticosteroids is advocated.

Patients with chronic iritis secondary to an IOL are candidates for IOL explantation with or without exchange. The decision to explant an IOL is made by the operating surgeon on an individual basis and is dependent on several factors (see Chapters 7 and 11):

## TABLE 16–12. CHRONIC IRITIS: TREATMENT OPTIONS

**Irritative**

Prednisolone acetate 1%, one drop, two to four times daily, then taper when anterior chamber has < grade 1+ cells

May need to maintain on low-potency steroids; ie, fluoromethalone acetate 0.1%, one drop one to two times daily indefinitely

If vision/comfort cannot be achieved, may need to refer for explantation or intraocular lens exchange

**Retained Lens Fragment**

Nucleus
  Refer back to operating surgeon to consider removal

Cortex
  Topical steroid: prednisolone acetate 1%, one drop every 2–4 h, then taper when remnant is resorbed and anterior chamber has < grade 1+ cells
  May need to maintain on low-potency steroids for 1–2 mo until inflammation resolves
  If cortical remnant is 3–4 mm in size, refer back for aspiration

---

1. Type of intraocular lens: rigid anterior chamber and iris-fixated lenses carry a poorer prognosis if left in the eye and the associated inflammation may not be controlled by medications alone.
2. Length of inflammation.
3. Associated conditions such as CME, glaucoma, and corneal edema.
4. Motivation of the patient.

Patients with the UGH syndrome may be treated over the short-term with beta-blockers, CAIs, and topical steroids to control their high IOP and inflammation. However, once stabilized, they would be candidates for lens explantation and exchange.

Retained nucleus is almost always surgically removed. Even small pieces may induce a severe inflammatory reaction with corneal decompensation, glaucoma, and retinal detachment.[68] Small pieces of retained cortex may be monitored while maintaining the patient on topical corticosteroids to suppress the associated inflammation. Large pieces of cortex may need to be removed by aspiration.

Chronic postoperative iritis is best treated initially with prednisolone acetate 1% four times a day for mild cases and every 2–3 hours for moderate to severe cases. Cycloplegics are also indicated for moderate to severe anterior chamber reactions. In some cases, patients may need to be gradually tapered from a more potent corticosteroid to one that is milder such as fluorometholone. Long-term low-dose topical steroids may need to be prescribed for a chronic uveitis secondary to IOL irritation. A mild topical corticosteroid may need to be maintained indefinitely to prevent vision loss and discomfort. We have successfully prescribed a maintenance dose of fluoromethalone 0.1%, used once daily, to several patients with rigid anterior chamber IOL-induced chronic iritis. These patients are also counseled about the increased risk of infection and increased IOP due to long-term topical steroid use.

A vitreous tap should be considered if an infection is suspected. Consideration of an infectious etiology should be entertained in nonresponsive chronic iritis of undetermined etiology or if a significant iritis occurs following Nd:YAG capsulotomy.

One possible complication of chronic iritis includes keratic and IOL precipitates. An Nd:YAG precipitotomy may effectively remove IOL precipitates

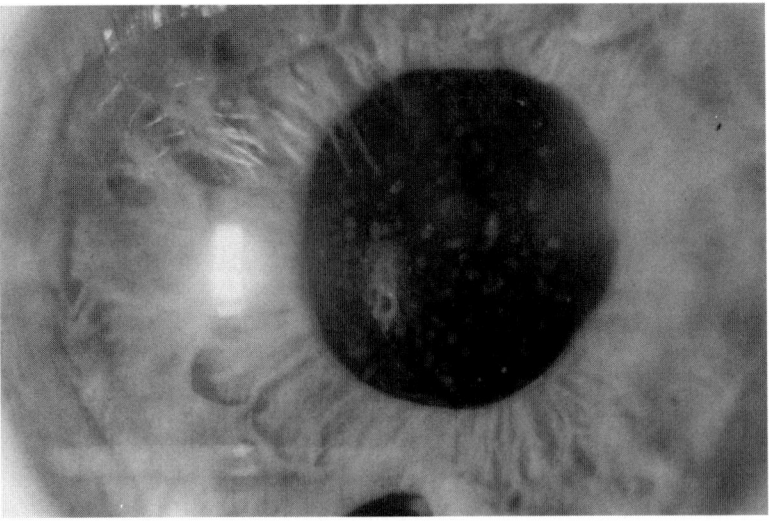

FIGURE 16–11. IOL precipitates.

and improve vision, although the precipitates often recur (Figures 16–11 and 16–12).

## POSTERIOR CAPSULAR OPACITIES/ ND:YAG CAPSULOTOMY

A posterior capsular opacity (PCO) is a clouding or thickening of the posterior lenticular capsule following phacoemulsification and other forms of extracapsular cataract extraction (ECCE). Sometimes this is called a secondary cataract, aftercataract, capsular fibrosis, or epithelial pearls. (See Color Plate 16–5.)

### Background

A PCO may occur as soon as a few days to weeks after surgery. With ECCE, up to 50% of eyes develop a PCO within 5 years of surgery.[72,73] In general, the younger the patient, the greater the risk. Opacification is caused by proliferation and migration of lens epithelial cells and their derivatives following ECCE.

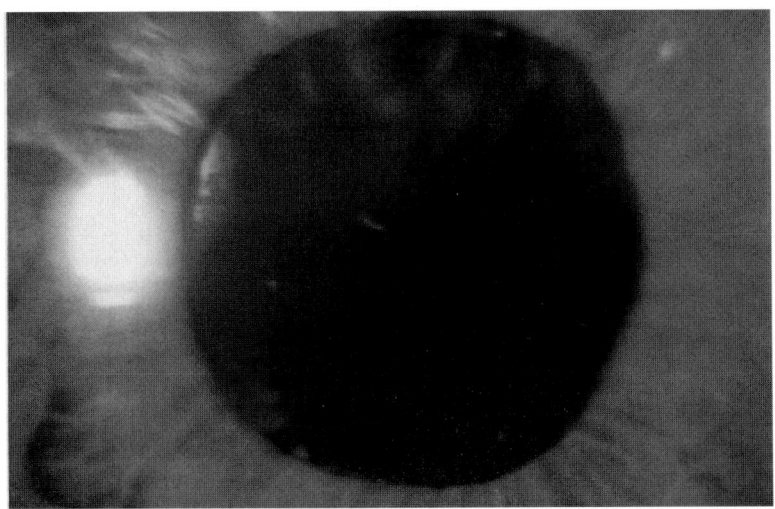

FIGURE 16–12. Dispersal of IOL precipitates in Figure 16–11 following Nd:YAG precipitotomy.

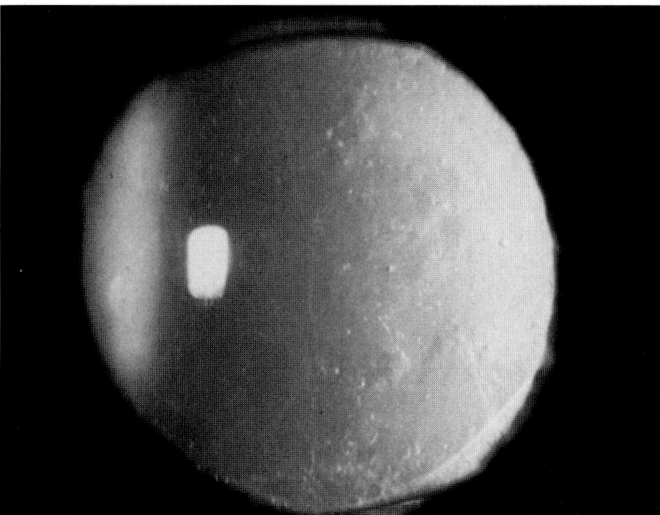

**FIGURE 16–13.** Mild posterior capsular opacification.

Fibrous or pseudofibrous metaplasia of lens epithelial cells into myofibroblasts results in fibrosis, which can lead to capsular clouding, contraction, and folds.[72,74,75] Early fibrous opacities tend to be white and wispy, but they may become dense, white opacities as they mature (Figures 16–13 and 16–14).

This proliferation of epithelial cells often forms a uniform, clear thickening of the capsule (fibrous membrane), which may be difficult to observe with the biomicroscope. As the thickening progresses, it tends to become uneven with a Swiss cheese–like appearance forming a reticular (netlike) capsular thickening. In severe cases, globular opacities, called pearls, may form (Figures 16–15 and 16–16).

In addition, problems secondary to lens epithelial cell remnants, such as IOL decentration due to stress on the capsular bag or excessive distortion of IOL loops, phacotoxic or phacoanaphylactic inflammatory reaction, poor view of the peripheral fundus, and soft IOL surface distortion, may occur. Finally, with possible widespread use of bifocal or multifocal IOLs in the future, the

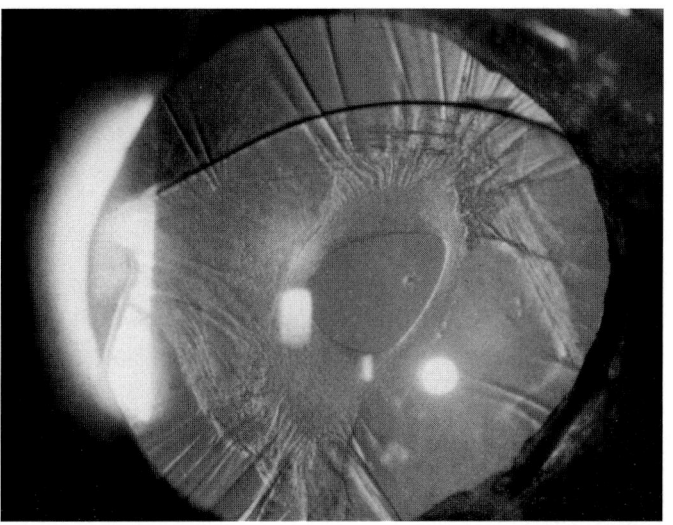

**FIGURE 16–14.** Anterior capsular contraction.

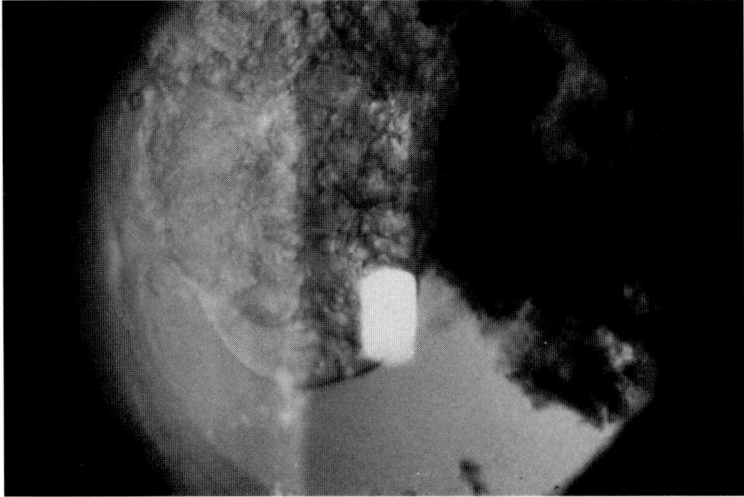

**FIGURE 16–15.** Severe posterior capsular opacification (on left) with adjacent retained cortex (on right).

near-perfect centration needed for these lenses may be hindered by remnants of lens epithelial cells distorting the capsular bag following ECCE.[72]

In addition to epithelial cell proliferation, there are other causes of capsular opacification.[72,75] Postsurgical inflammation may result in protein accumulation resembling KPs or spicules. White blood cells may form a dustlike layer on the capsule. Residual lens cortex from incomplete aspiration may become trapped between the posterior chamber IOL and the posterior capsule (Figure 16–17). Trapped cortical remnants usually swell with absorbed water to take on a white, fluffy appearance. Unlike cortical material in the anterior chamber, posteriorly entrapped cortical material may not resorb readily. Red blood cells and blood stains from a hyphema may also be entrapped between the posterior chamber IOL and posterior capsule (see Figures 15–10 and 15–11). Pigment cells liberated from the iris or ciliary body during surgery may cling to the posterior capsule and cause clouding. Some slow-growing low-virulence bacteria, such as *Propionibacterium acnes,* may become sequestered in the posterior capsule and form a smooth bacterial colony that mimics a true PCO. This may be accompanied by chronic anterior uveitis. If this capsular opacity

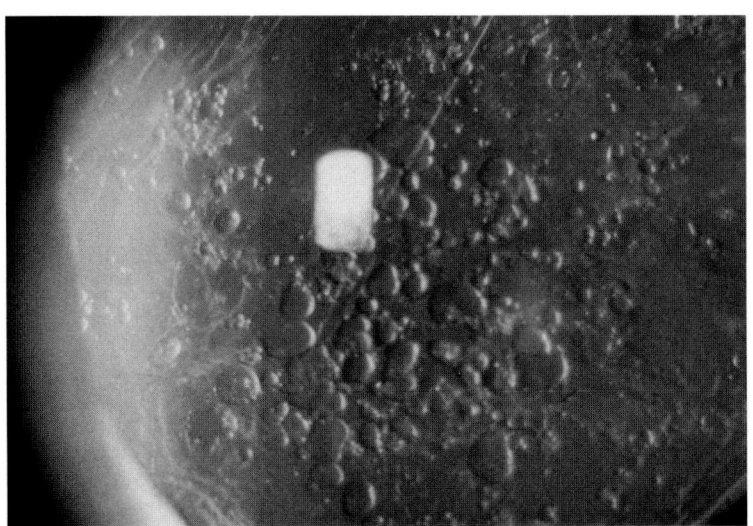

**FIGURE 16–16.** Elschnig pearls.

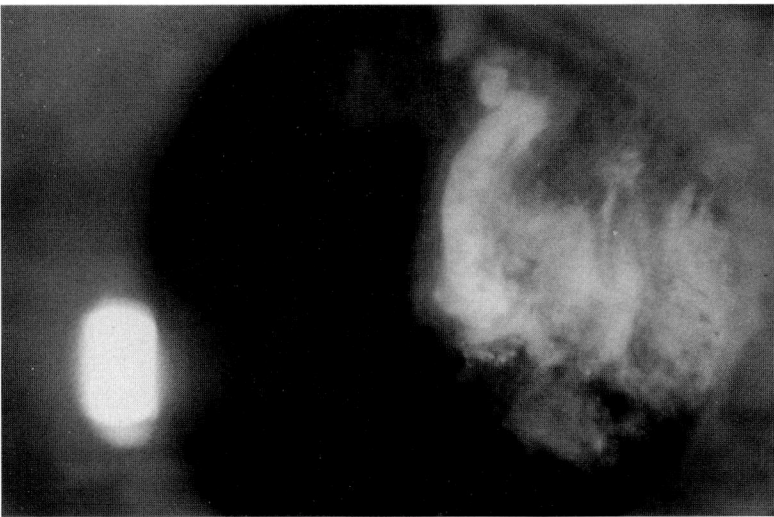

*FIGURE 16–17.* Residual cortex entrapped behind IOL.

is mistaken for a normal PCO and a laser capsulotomy is performed, bacteria can be driven into the vitreous and encourage fulminant endophthalmitis.[76–79]

## Clinical Presentation and Assessment

Patients with PCO often state, "I saw well right after the surgery, but now my vision is as bad as it was with the cataract." They complain of decreased visual acuity, but glare in bright lights may be the major symptom. Clinically, there may be a minor to significant decrease in Snellen visual acuity, but glare acuity is usually very poor.

Further examination of a patient in whom PCO is suspected is very similar to that of a preoperative cataract patient. Specifically, slit lamp and dilated fundus examinations should be used to identify the posterior capsule opacity and/or any other source of the vision loss. Thorough evaluation of the peripheral fundus to ensure that the retina is intact is also critical before considering Nd:YAG capsulotomy. We perform a potential acuity test (Super Pinhole, Microsurgical Technology, Inc, Kirkland, WA) to determine whether it is probable that the patient will have improved visual acuity following a capsulotomy. The patient is carefully counseled and informed consent is obtained before performing a capsulotomy. (See Appendix 8.)

## Treatment, Follow-up, and Prognosis

The severity of a central capsular opacity may be classified (see Chapter 4). When a capsular opacity reaches the point that visual function is impaired, a capsulotomy is indicated. Capsulotomies are performed with a Nd:YAG laser. With this technique, the laser is focused directly behind the posterior capsule and short pulses of laser energy are used to make an opening in the posterior capsular opacity (Figures 16–18 and 16–19). If the laser is focused at or near the IOL surface, pits may form in the IOL. If the laser is focused inside the IOL, lens cracks occur. A few small laser pits are common and do not have a significant visual effect, but IOL cracks may cause significant glare. In general, as the capsule thickens, more laser energy is required to perform the capsulotomy. The energy is transmitted through the vitreous and may encourage complications.

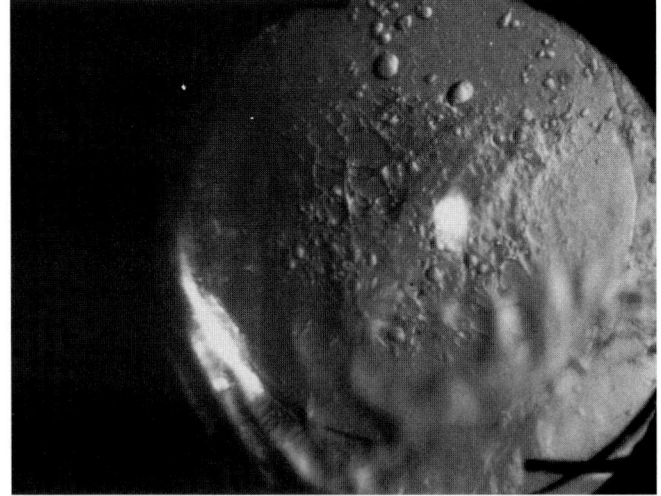

FIGURE 16–18. Posterior capsular opacity, pretreatment with Nd:YAG laser.

The most common complication of laser capsulotomy is transient or late elevation of IOP, which is possibly due to blocking of the trabecular meshwork by debris and/or shock wave–induced damage to the trabecular meshwork.[80,81] Intraocular pressure spikes may occur in up to 39% of patients receiving a laser capsulotomy.[82] Investigators report the average rise in IOP at approximately 5 to 15 mm of mercury. The peak IOP is usually obtained 2–6 hours following treatment.[83,84] There is evidence that eyes with capsular bag-fixated IOLs have minimal Nd:YAG–induced IOP rises.[80] Apraclonidine HCl 1% (Iopidine) is an α-adrenergic agonist that is commonly used to help prevent postlaser IOP spikes.[82,85] It appears to work by reducing aqueous production. One drop of the drug is instilled prior to laser treatment and another drop may be applied immediately after the procedure. The onset of drug action is within 1 hour of instillation and maximum effect (approximately 40% reduction in IOP) occurs in 3–5 hours. Side effects include eyelid retraction, conjunctival blanching, and mydriasis. Topical beta-blockers and oral CAIs may also be used for the same purpose, but they have been used less commonly to control postlaser pressure spikes since the introduction of apraclonidine HCl 1%.

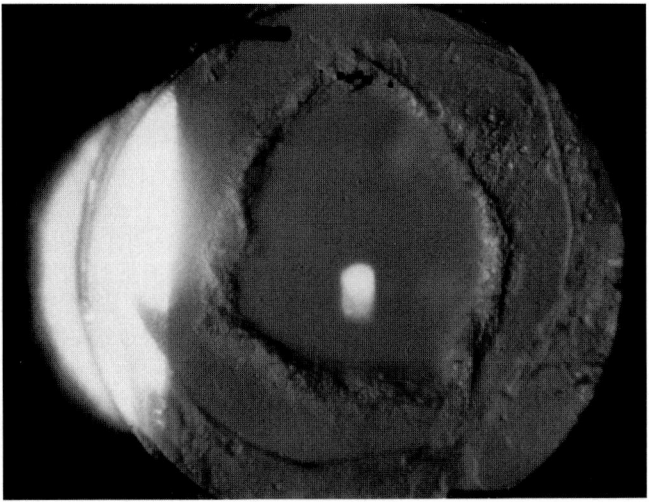

FIGURE 16–19. Same posterior capsular opacity as in Figure 16–18 posttreatment with Nd:YAG laser.

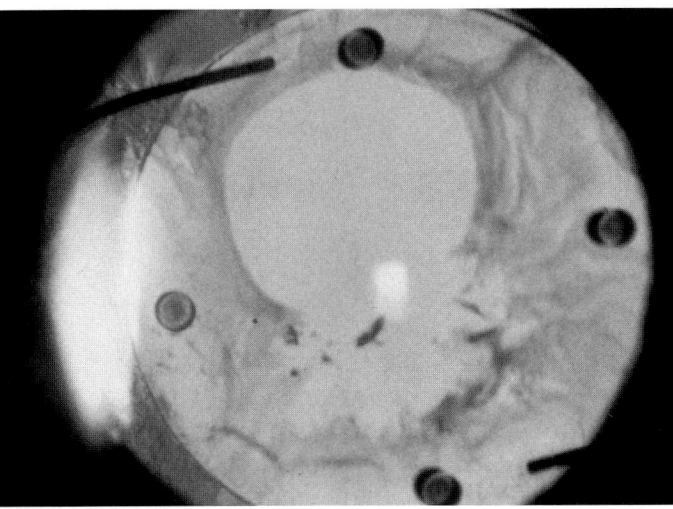

*FIGURE 16–20. A small anterior capsulotomy that was enlarged to eliminate glare symptoms.*

Finally, in addition to the previously mentioned problems, including exacerbation of localized endophthalmitis, other complications of Nd:YAG laser therapy include IOL dislocation/decentration, CME, and retinal detachment.[72,86] In a large random study using selected Medicare beneficiaries who had undergone ECCE in 1986–1987, Javitt et al found that out of over 57,000 patients, the risk of retinal detachment or tear was 3.9 times greater in patients undergoing Nd:YAG capsulotomy versus cataract patients not receiving Nd:YAG.[87] However, Van Westenbrugge et al repudiate these findings on the grounds of flaws in methodology and the fact that previous studies reviewed patients who received cataract extraction with posterior chamber IOLs prior to widespread acceptance of capsulorhexis and reliable placement of IOLs in the capsular bag.[88]

Our protocol for treatment of patients in whom significantly symptomatic posterior capsule opacification is identified is to obtain informed consent, instill one to two drops of apraclonidine HCl 1%, perform the laser with the lowest energy and fewest pulses, and then to advise them of postoperative symptoms such as blur, pain, flashes, and floaters that necessitate immediate return to the clinic. Otherwise, we recommend follow-up in 1–7 days and again in 1–2 months. The patient should be examined for all potential complications and the pupil dilated at both visits or as symptoms warrant. (See Appendix 8.)

The goal of an Nd:YAG capsulotomy is to create an opening in the posterior capsule slightly larger than the patient's natural pupil diameter.[89] When this occurs, the patient should never experience symptoms nor need additional treatment related to the posterior capsule again. Occasionally, however, an off-centered capsulotomy or capsular remnant that thickens continues to cause symptoms following capsulotomy. In addition, rarely, pearl formation may continue after capsulotomy, and create a scaffolding onto the IOL surface. In these cases, repeat Nd:YAG capsulotomy may be performed (Figures 16–20 and 16–21).

## PSEUDOPHAKIC (APHAKIC) CYSTOID MACULAR EDEMA

Cystoid macular edema (CME) has long been identified as a complication of cataract surgery. It was first noted in the literature by Irvine in 1953[90] and Gass and Nordan in 1966.[91] It has led to the recognition of the Irvine-Gass syndrome

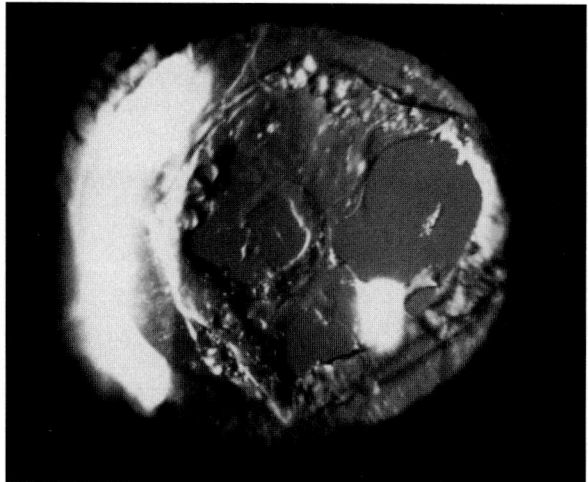

**FIGURE 16–21.** Recurrent posterior capsule opacification secondary to continuing pearl formation directly on the posterior IOL surface creating a "scaffolding."

in which CME with or without vitreous to the wound is associated with cataract surgery. Presently CME is one of the most common reasons for postoperative acuity loss in pseudophakia with or without intraoperative complications.

## Background

### Clinical Versus Angiographic CME

Fluorescein angiography is the definitive clinical test for the diagnosis of CME. Fluorescein angiographic studies in patients with cystoid macular edema have led to two terms describing the presence of dye leakage with or without reduced visual acuity: The term *clinical cystoid macular edema* is used for a patient with reduced visual acuity and positive macular fluorescein leakage, where *angiographic cystoid macular edema* is used when positive angiographic fluorescein leakage occurs without reduced visual acuity. Stark and associates have defined clinical CME as visual acuity loss of one or more chart lines at distance or near and positive fluorescein leakage or observable cystic macular changes.[92]

Angiographic CME occurs more frequently and therefore presents an opportunity to study the prevention of CME. Jaffe et al reported an incidence of 2.9% angiographic CME versus 0% clinical CME in a series of uncomplicated cases of ECCE and intracapsular cataract extraction (ICCE).[93] In the same series, a 29.5% angiographic CME versus 18% clinical CME was reported in cases complicated by capsular rupture and vitreous loss. Other investigators have found a high incidence (16%) of angiographic CME in uncomplicated cataract surgery with posterior chamber IOLs.[94] Studies have used angiographic CME as a suggestive indicator of the macular inflammatory response to IOL characteristics and the effectiveness of prophylactic postoperative anti-inflammatory medications.[95,96] These studies have pointed out that although the incidence of angiographic CME was statistically significant, there was no significant difference in patient Snellen visual acuity. Even though angiographic CME does not correlate well with a patient's visual acuity, it will continue to be studied owing to its much higher incidence compared with clinical CME. Smith and Lindstrom have pointed out, however, that caution must be used when making major therapeutic changes based on angiographic CME studies.[97]

### Epidemiology

Reports show visual loss from CME occurring in approximately 3% to 5% of cases with uncomplicated ECCE and IOL implantation. Most of the uncomplicated cases show spontaneous resolution and improved vision with only a small percentage (1% or less) resulting in persistent edema and visual loss.[92] Some patients have preexisting conditions that make them more prone to CME, such as epiretinal membranes and diabetic macular edema. In addition, the use of topical epinephrine compounds for intraocular pressure control has been shown to induce aphakic cystoid macular edema.[98] The incidence of CME may also be affected by the type of surgery and the ability of the surgeon to avoid complications. Cystoid macular edema is higher in patients with surgical complications such as loss of vitreous, uveitis, rupture of the anterior hyaloid membrane, and vitreous to the wound. The incidence rises as high as approximately 30% when these complications occur. Surgeons have reported a lower incidence of CME in ECCE versus ICCE.[99–101] There also are reports that IOL features, such as ultraviolet-absorbing versus non–ultraviolet-absorbing lenses may affect the development of CME. In a study of 301 patients, Kraff et al[95] found a much higher rate of angiographic CME in non–ultraviolet-absorbing versus ultraviolet-absorbing IOLs (18.8% versus 9.5%).[95] These investigators pointed out, however, that there was no significant difference in final postoperative visual acuity.

Despite the low incidence and frequent spontaneous resolution, CME is still an important cause of persistent vision loss in postoperative cataract patients owing to the large number of cataract surgeries performed annually. This low incidence translates into a significantly large patient morbidity. Therefore, the prevention and treatment of CME are very important.

## *Etiology*

The definite cause of CME is unknown. However, when occurring in a postoperative cataract patient, it is most likely due to intraoperative trauma and/or postoperative inflammatory response. Cystoid macular edema has been shown to be more common in cataract surgery patients with intraocular complications compared with those with uneventful surgery.[93] Direct trauma to the macular region such as macular vitreous traction may also contribute to CME.[102,103] However, indirect inflammatory response mediated by prostaglandins remains the most commonly accepted etiologic pathway for CME.[97,104]

Cystoid macular edema is associated with a change in the permeability of parafoveal capillaries. Fine and Brucker have shown an abnormal parafoveal endothelial change in fluorescein angiographically proven CME, whereas the classic presentation is fluid accumulation in the outer plexiform layer (Henle's layer).[105] Other investigators have found that fluid may accumulate in other intraretinal spaces.[106] Histologic studies of patients with CME from a variety of causes show both intracellular swelling[107] and extracellular accumulation of serous fluid.[108]

Even though the exact mechanism of CME is still in debate, an important aspect of fluid accumulation has been shown to be a breach in the blood-retinal barrier secondary to the inflammatory process.[109] Surgical trauma causes a release of inflammatory mediators such as prostaglandins and leukotrienes. These substances are associated with a variety of physiologic changes seen in patients with CME, such as increased perifoveal capillary permeability and serous leakage.[104] It is thought that with chronic fluid accumulation there is eventually distortion of retinal structures leading to permanent changes that may reduce retinal sensitivity.

## *Prophylaxis*

It is common practice to use topical corticosteroids during the postoperative period to reduce inflammation from surgical trauma. This is the conventional strategy for the prevention of CME. Many surgeons use a periocular subconjunctival injection of steroid at the conclusion of surgery and then administer topical steroids postoperatively.

Nonsteroidal anti-inflammatory drugs (NSAIDs) have been used preoperatively or in conjunction with steroidal therapy postoperatively to reduce the incidence of uncomplicated CME. Klein and associates administered oral indomethacin and found a decreased incidence of clinical CME over a 6-week postoperative period.[110] Kraff and associates reduced the incidence of angiographic CME from 18.5% to 9.6% in a large study of patients undergoing ECCE with IOL implantation by adding topical 1% indomethacin.[111]

Although there are many studies suggesting that NSAIDs are of benefit in reducing angiographic CME in postoperative patients with or without an IOL, there is no large clinical study that shows decreased clinical CME or improved visual acuity outcome by using NSAIDs alone or in conjunction with topical steroids.

## Clinical Presentation and Assessment

A typical patient with CME undergoes an uneventful surgery with good visual acuity for 4–36 weeks followed by a vision loss to the 20/50 to 20/200 range. Seventy-five percent of cases of CME present within the 4-week to 6-month postoperative interval. Vision loss may be the only symptom or it may be accompanied by photophobia, mild injection, and anterior chamber reaction. Therefore, a careful examination to rule out complications that may increase the likelihood of iridocyclitis, such as vitreous to the wound, pupillary capture, lens remnants, or history of chronic iridocyclitis, should be performed in patients suspected of CME.

Retinal examination shows thickening of the macular area and may include small parafoveal hemorrhages, yellowing of the macular area, and disc edema. The classic finding is a cystic honeycomblike formation with retinal thickening. Wrinkling of the internal limiting membrane may also be present. The doctor's view is facilitated by maximum mydriasis and a stereoscopic view of the fundus with a thin slit beam retroilluminating the affected area. Cystoid macular edema is often difficult to visualize. Therefore, fluorescein angiography is useful for a definitive diagnosis. The fluorescein angiography typically shows a normal mid-venous phase. Five to ten minutes later, there is a characteristic hyperfluorescent leakage from the parafoveal capillaries that accumulates in a petalloid pattern. The late phases may show slow accumulation of intraretinal fluid (Figures 16–22 and 16–23). Miyake et al have used a grading system to quantify the severity of late fluorescein leakage[112] (Table 16–13).

**TABLE 16–13. SEVERITY OF FLUORESCEIN STAINING IN CYSTOID MACULAR EDEMA**

| Grade | Appearance |
| --- | --- |
| 0 | No dye leakage |
| 1 | Trace of leakage |
| 2 | Stellate pattern (incomplete–complete) |
| 3 | Atypical stellate pattern |

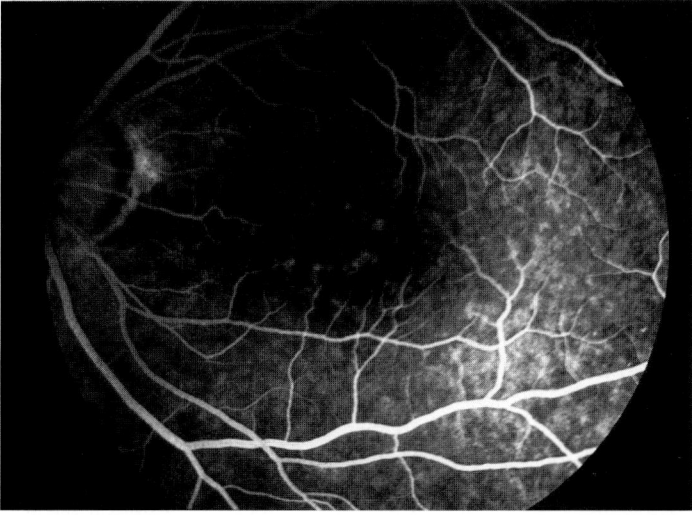

*FIGURE 16–22.* Cystoid macular edema—early phase fluorescein angiography.

## Differential Diagnosis

When presented with a case of presumed CME, the doctor should do a thorough dilated ocular examination ruling out sources of decreased vision from corneal edema, uveitis, capsular clouding, and retinal disease or detachment. A revealing study by Lakhanpal and Schocket reported a series of 17 eyes of patients being followed by ophthalmologists for CME, who after referral, were found to have retinal detachment.[113] In reviewing these cases, these investigators pointed out that the best way to avoid misdiagnosis is to do a thorough eye examination with indirect ophthalmoscopy after maximum mydriasis. They also recommended the use of confrontation or Goldmann visual field testing as well as fluorescein angiographic studies and ultrasound analysis.

It should be remembered that there are other causes of CME such as retinal vascular disease, uveitis, and subretinal neovascularization. As mentioned earlier, CME associated with uveitis necessitates ruling out other causes for the inflammation such as vitreous to the wound, pupillary capture, retained lens

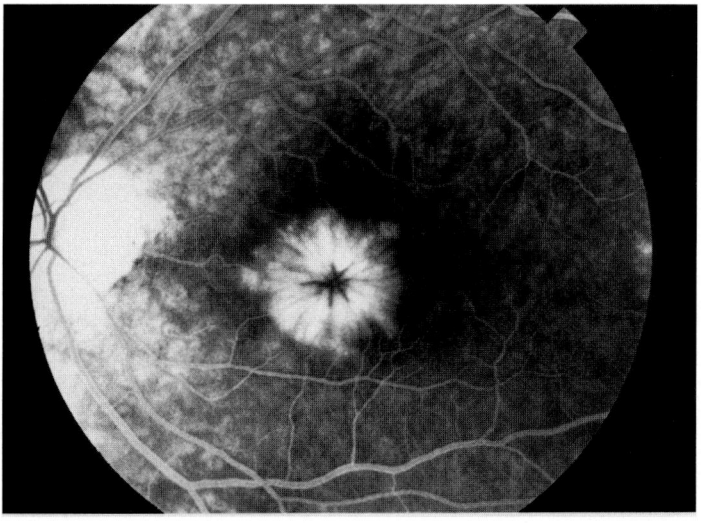

*FIGURE 16–23.* Cystoid macular edema—late phase fluorescein angiography.

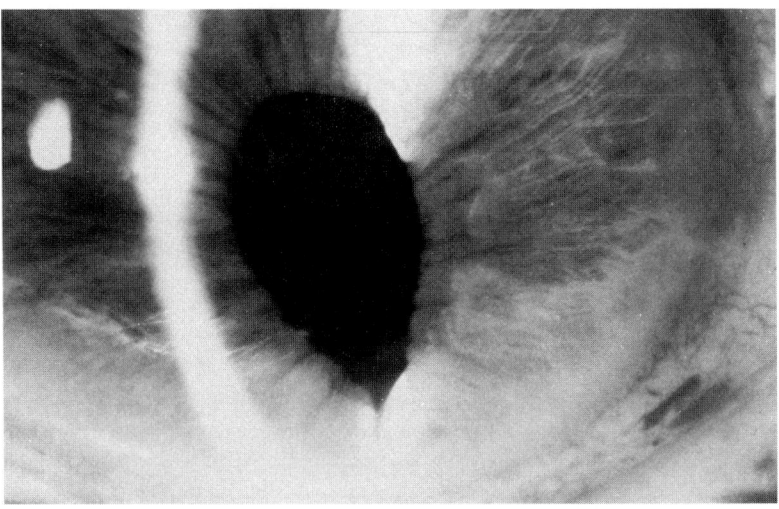

**FIGURE 16–24.** Vitreous to the wound.

material, and/or history of chronic iritis. When the other sources of visual loss such as retinal detachment and retinal vascular disease have been ruled out, the patient should be considered for fluorescein angiography to diagnose CME definitively.

## Treatment, Follow-up, and Prognosis

### Complicated Intraoperative Surgery

Cystoid macular edema is more common in surgery complicated by posterior capsular rupture, especially with vitreous loss and vitreous to the wound. A multicentered prospective study headed by Fung showed visual improvement in patients with chronic CME complicated by vitreous to the wound treated surgically with vitrectomy.[114] There have also been reports of visual improvement in patients with complicated CME following Nd:YAG laser vitreolysis of vitreous to the wound[115,116] (see Chapter 14) (Figures 16–24 to 16–26). Smith and Lindstrom recommend a treatment regimen of a 4- to 6-week trial of topical

**FIGURE 16–25.** Vitreous to the wound.

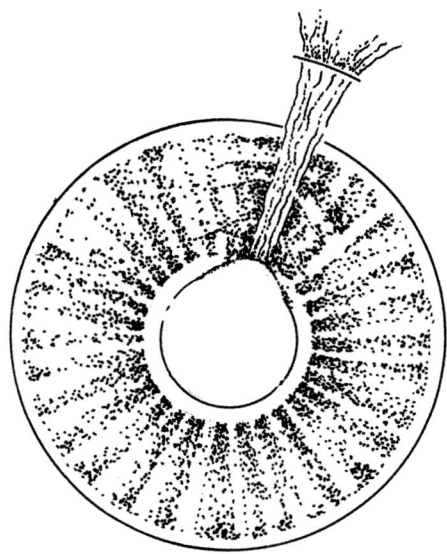

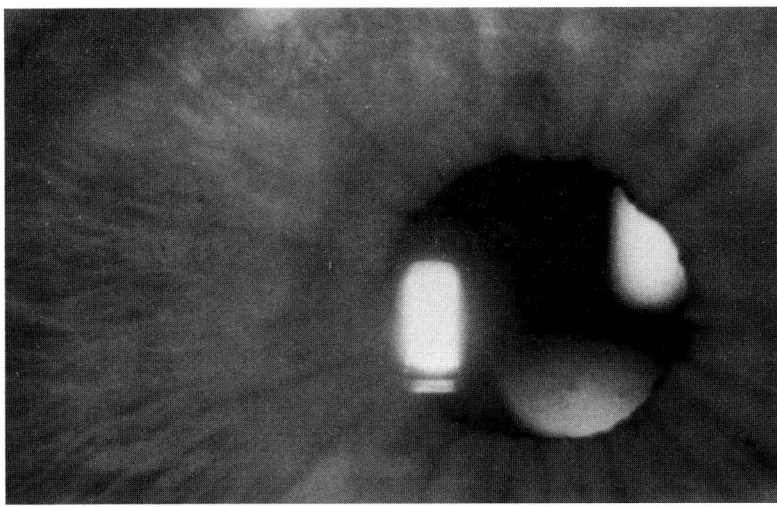

**FIGURE 16–26.** Vitreous to the wound following Nd:YAG lysis.

steroids and/or topical NSAIDs. They add 1 mL of a combination of betamethasone acetate and sodium phosphate (Celestone Soluspan) subconjunctivally in severe cases or if there was no improvement in topical therapy.[97] Oral steroid therapy can be considered in cases without improvement for 4–6 weeks of the above treatment. If topical and oral therapy fails, Nd:YAG laser vitreolysis is attempted in patients with definable vitreous strands and the patient is followed for 4–6 more weeks. Failing this, the patient is considered for anterior vitrectomy and/or lens exchange with vitrectomy (Table 16–14).

### Uncomplicated Intraoperative Surgery

In acute cases of CME, topical steroids alone have been reported to be of benefit.[117–119] These studies suggest that increased IOP with topical steroid use may be a direct or indirect benefit in the resolution of macular edema. There also are reports of success with periocular and oral corticosteroid use.[120,121] Additionally, oral nonsteroidals such as indomethacin have been reported to have no effect on chronic CME resolution, whereas topical ketorolac has been shown to have some promise.[122,123]

**TABLE 16–14. COMPLICATED CYSTOID MACULAR EDEMA: TREATMENT OPTIONS**

Topical corticosteroid: prednisolone acetate 1%, one drop every 2–4 h
Topical nonsteroidal anti-inflammatory drugs: suprofen 1% or diclofenac 0.1%, one drop every 4 h
Cycloplegics: scopolamine 0.25% or homatropine 5%, one drop twice a day (optional)
If there is no improvement with topical agents, subconjunctival corticosteroid may be injected: 0.5 mL, 40 mg triamcinolone acetatonide suspension
Oral steroids: 60–80 mg by mouth for 1 week, then taper
Oral carbonic anhydrase inhibitors (eg, acetazolamide) are controversial
Nd:YAG vitreolysis for well-defined vitreous incarceration to wound
If no improvement, consider the following:
    Surgical vitrectomy if persistent vitreous to the wound
    Iris surgery if iris to the wound

**TABLE 16-15. UNCOMPLICATED CYSTOID MACULAR EDEMA: TREATMENT OPTIONS**

**Without Anterior Chamber Reaction**
Mild
    Option of no treatment; follow for 3 wk
    Topical steroids: prednisolone acetate 1%, one drop four times daily
    Topical NSAIDs: suprofen 1% or diclofenac 0.1%, one drop four times daily
    Both topical steroids and nonsteroidal anti-inflammatory drugs (as above)
Moderate to Severe
    Treat topically, as stated above for mild cystoid macular edema
    If no improvement, consider subconjunctival corticosteroids: 0.5 mL, 40 mg triamcinolone acetonide suspension
    Oral prednisone: 60–80 mg for 3 d, then taper

**With Anterior Chamber Reaction**
Mild
    Topical steroids: prednisolone acetate 1%, one drop four times daily
    Topical NSAIDs: suprofen 1% or diclofenac 0.1%, one drop four times daily
Moderate
    Treat topically, as stated above
    Add subconjunctival corticosteroid: 0.5 mL, 40 mg triamcinolone acetatonide suspension
Severe
    Oral prednisone: 60–80 mg for 3 d, then taper

Patients with biomicroscopic findings of CME may be advised that the condition may resolve without treatment. Nevertheless, the most common treatment involves topical, subconjunctival injections, and/or oral steroids and may also include topical and/or nonsteroidal anti-inflammatories (Table 16–15). In our clinics, we commonly use prednisolone acetate 1%, four times a day, along with a topical NSAID such as suprofen 1% (Profenal) or diclofenac 0.1% (Voltaren), four times a day, for 2–4 weeks. We reevaluate the patient in 1–3 weeks and in nonresponsive cases add a steroidal injection, oral steroids, or oral NSAID. In most cases, the signs and symptoms of clinical CME resolve in 3–12 weeks with this treatment regimen. Follow-up visits are scheduled based on extent of vision decrease, with more frequent follow-up on more severe loss. All patients have a dilated ocular examination on return visits to ensure that no other retinal complications exist.

Occasionally, one encounters a patient with chronic CME following uncomplicated cataract extraction. Jaffe et al have extensively reviewed the treatment of CME and concludes, "despite the inconclusive nature of some of these reports, a trial of systemic, topical, or periocular corticosteroids and systemic nonsteroidal anti-inflammatory drugs (NSAIDs) should be used in cases of established cystoid macular edema."[124]

## — RETINAL DETACHMENT

Retinal detachments associated with cataract surgery usually occur within 6 months of the operation. However, they may occur at any time thereafter, especially in patients with predisposing factors, including axial myopia, lattice degeneration, and a history of retinal detachment in the opposite eye. Such patients must be followed for life with regular dilated fundus examinations and be educated as to the symptoms of retinal detachment.

## Background

Extracapsular cataract extraction is associated with a lower incidence of detachment compared with intracapsular technique where the posterior capsule has been removed and the vitreous potentially disturbed. For similar reasons, it is believed that Nd:YAG capsulotomy also increases the risk of retinal detachment, primarily in eyes with axial myopia, lattice degeneration, or a history of retinal detachment in the fellow eye.[125–128] Retinal detachment, therefore, may be a manifestation during the later postoperative period after Nd:YAG capsulotomy is performed. There has been some controversy regarding the actual incidence of retinal detachment following Nd:YAG capsulotomy. Studies stemming from larger-volume cataract surgery practices that utilize the technique of phacoemulsification with continuous circular capsulorhexis indicate a rate averaging approximately 1%. It is thought that capsulorhexis significantly decreases the likelihood of postoperative complications, including post–Nd:YAG capsulotomy retinal detachments. Thorough preoperative evaluation combined with appropriate patient education regarding the symptoms of detachment is highly recommended for all patients undergoing Nd:YAG capsulotomy (see discussion of posterior capsular opacities and Nd:YAG capsulotomy on page 210). (See Appendix 8.)

## Clinical Presentation and Assessment

The clinical presentation and assessment of retinal detachment manifesting during the intermediate to late postoperative period is similar to that of the early postoperative period (see discussion of retinal break/detachment in Chapter 14). However, the doctor should attempt to determine the duration of the retinal detachment. This is especially indicated in asymptomatic patients who present with a detachment after the first 2 weeks following cataract surgery.

Long-standing detachments, for example, may extend from ora to optic nerve head and have radially oriented alternating bullae and folds. The retina itself will appear opaque and a pigmented demarcation line may be seen at the posterior border of the detachment (Figures 16–27 and 16–28). Such a demarcation line often appears in stationary detachments after approximately 3

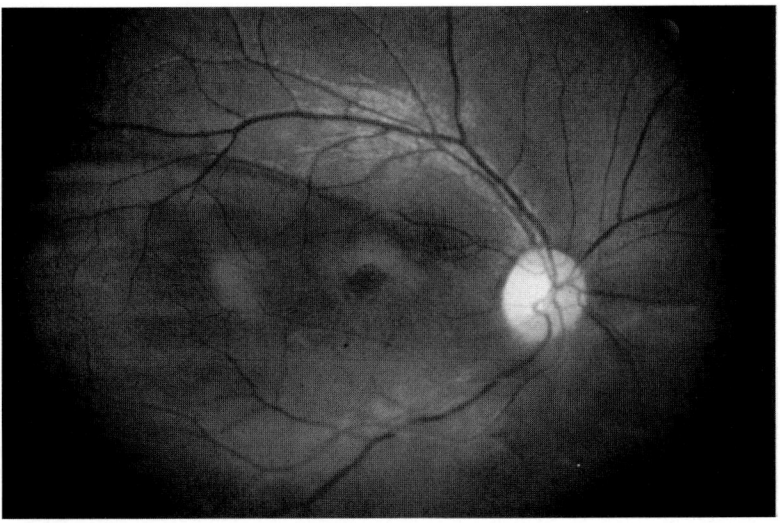

**FIGURE 16–27.** Long-standing retinal detachment involving macula. Note taut surface, loss of choroidal detail, and pigmented demarcation line at posterior edge.

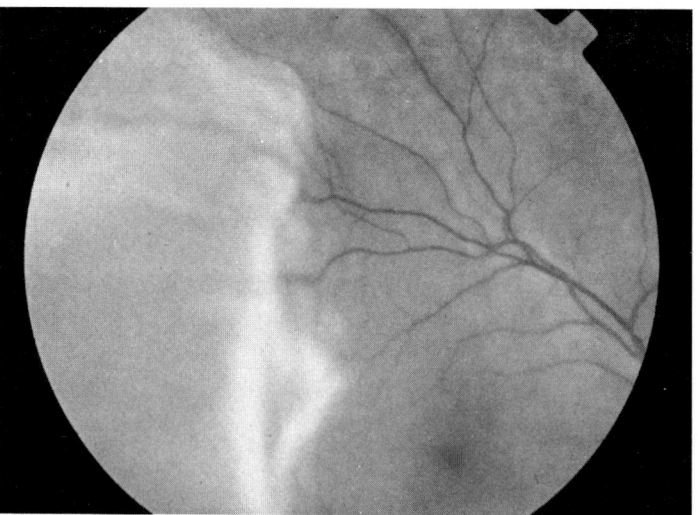

**FIGURE 16–28.** Long-standing retinal detachment with opaque, necrotic detached tissue.

months. Other signs of long-standing detachment include a taut surface with minimal undulation on eye movements, fixed retinal folds, atrophy and necrosis of the detached tissue, and the presence of cream-colored intraretinal or subretinal exudates.

### Differential Diagnosis

The differential diagnosis of rhegmatogenous retinal detachment includes other causes of retinal elevation: exudative and tractional retinal detachment, retinoschisis, and choroidal detachment in which the retina is elevated but not separated from the pigment epithelium.

### Treatment, Follow-up, and Prognosis

All retinal detachments, whether they are recent or long standing, early or late in the postoperative course, require an immediate referral to a retinal specialist for consultation and appropriate treatment. Prognosis for vision will depend on whether the macula has been involved, the duration of detachment, and whether or not macular pucker or CME develops. Surgical intervention and follow-up protocol for intermediate and late retinal detachments are similar to those described for early postoperative retinal detachments (see discussion of retinal break/detachment in Chapter 14).

## — OPTICAL CONSIDERATIONS

Postoperative refractive errors following cataract surgery may be some of the most challenging problems that a clinician will encounter. Since the patient often judges the success of cataract surgery by the vision obtained through postoperative correction, unsuccessful management of these patients often leaves the patient feeling that the surgery itself was a failure. Most postoperative refractive problems are the result of astigmatism, anisometropia, aphakia, diplopia, or dislocated or malpositioned IOLs.

## Astigmatism

Postoperative astigmatism has been a surgical challenge since the advent of cataract extraction. For many years, surgeons, optometrists, and patients accepted the notion that cataract surgery would induce an unpredictable amount of astigmatic error. This astigmatic error was believed to be the result of incision size, incision location, suturing method, and suture tension.[129]

Controlling postoperative astigmatism has been the topic of much ophthalmic surgical research and has resulted in the development of new types of incisions and suturing methods. Historically, when large wounds and interrupted sutures were used, removing sutures to adjust astigmatism at 6 to 8 weeks postoperatively was commonplace. Some surgeons have advocated the induction of small amounts of myopic astigmatism to enhance depth of focus.[130,131] Recently, the use of a scleral tunnel small incision with one-stitch or no-stitch closure has been shown minimally to alter the corneal curvature and induce astigmatism.[132,133] It has also proven to be stable and predictable allowing more successful refractive management of the patient postoperatively.

In addition to new types of incisions and new suturing methods, relaxing corneal incisions and wound revision (astigmatic keratotomy [AK]) have been used by some surgeons to reduce preexisting corneal toricity.[134] At this time, corneal relaxing incisions have had limited success, with radial and arcuate keratotomy showing more promise than trapezoidal[135] (Figures 16–29 and 16–30). With additional study, this technique may evolve into a useful tool in controlling postoperative corneal astigmatism. Nevertheless, in our clinic, we have had good success reducing corneal astigmatism with astigmatic keratotomy (Figure 16–30). On patients with greater than 2 diopters of corneal cylinder, we perform corneal topography and offer astigmatic keratotomy.

New incision techniques and wound closure methods, however, do little for the patient who has already had cataract extraction and has problematic postoperative astigmatism. Correcting astigmatism postoperatively is best approached by first determining whether the astigmatism is regular or irregular. Astigmatism following modern cataract surgery is usually regular and easily correctable with spectacle lenses. Often postoperative astigmatism is "against-the-rule" (minus axis vertical), which may result in vertical anisometropia requiring slab-off prism or asymmetric bifocals (Table 16–16).

Occasionally, uneven suture tension, an irregular wound, preexisting corneal disease, or postoperative corneal problems will result in irregular astigmatism. This astigmatism is often difficult to quantify, but it may be qualitatively assessed by several methods. The easiest method of determining the pres-

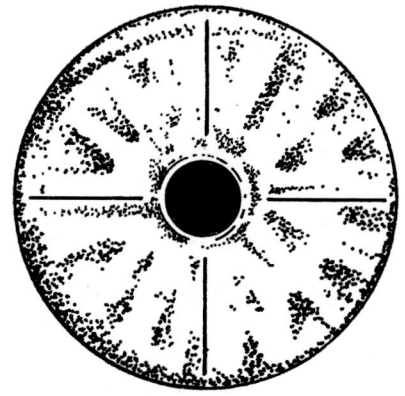

**FIGURE 16–29.** Radial keratotomy.

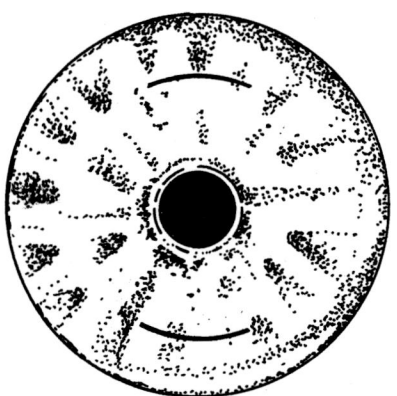

**FIGURE 16–30.** Astigmatic keratotomy. The cuts are made in the steepest meridian of the cornea.

ence of irregular astigmatism is through photokeratoscopy and/or keratoscopy. These instruments, however, are not readily available to many practitioners in a primary care setting; therefore, their use must be foregone for more available and practical instruments. Carefully observing the keratometric mires for irregularity will give the diagnosis of irregular astigmatism. In addition, a scissors-like retinoscopic reflex will aid in determining the presence of corneal irregularity. Improvement in best vision with refraction over a diagnostic rigid contact lens is also of value in qualitatively assessing corneal irregularity that may be missed with either keratometry or retinoscopy.

Irregular corneal astigmatism is usually not adequately corrected with spectacle lenses and most often requires correction with rigid contact lenses. (Rarely, penetrating keratoplasty is required.)

## Anisometropia

Anisometropia may be a source of considerable frustration for both the patient and the practitioner. It occurs when the desired pseudophakic refractive error is not achieved postoperatively. It also occurs in unilateral cataract extraction with a high refractive error in the fellow eye.

Although most patients may be corrected with spectacle lenses if the anisometropia is not greater than 3 diopters, any increase in anisometropia resulting in a total refractive difference of 1 diopter or greater may induce refractive aniseikonia. This can cause symptoms of diplopia, asthenopia, headache, photophobia, near-point problems, and many others.[136] Bartlett gives an excellent current review of the causes, clinical assessment, and spectacle management of the aniseikonic patient.[137] Spectacle management has been reported to relieve symptoms in a high percentage of these patients.[138] Many times in general practice the best conventional lenses are prescribed with attention to optical center alignment and frame adjustment. If the patient then presents with symptoms, changes in spectacle vertex distance, lens thickness, or, more

**TABLE 16–16. OPTIONS FOR POSTOPERATIVE TREATMENT OF INCREASED ASTIGMATISM**

Spectacle correction
Rigid contact lens
Astigmatic keratotomy

**TABLE 16–17. TREATMENT OPTIONS FOR POSTOPERATIVE ANISOMETROPIA**

Spectacle lenses if tolerated
Slab-off prism for reading addition
Separate correction for distance and near
Spectacle monovision to reduce anisometropia
Contact lens correction
Aniseikonic spectacle lenses
IOL replacement
Radial keratotomy
Anterior corneal sculpting
Cataract surgery on fellow eye

commonly, lens base curves are employed to reduce spatial distortion. Contact lenses may also be considered.

In some situations, an anisometropic result is expected or desired such as to create a monovision correction. It may be wise to fit the patient with contact lenses preoperatively in order to determine his or her ability to tolerate this before surgery establishes a monovision correction permanently. In cases of anisometropia with intolerance to the spectacle or contact lens prescription, the practitioner may undercorrect one eye to create better tolerance. If undercorrection of one eye is attempted, it is best either to undercorrect the nondominant eye or undercorrect the more myopic (or least hyperopic) eye if strong dominancy is not demonstrated. In cases where the best potential acuity differs in the two eyes, the eye with the poorest potential acuity should be undercorrected. Finally, the patient may be referred to an ophthalmic surgeon for consideration of IOL replacement if he or she suffers anisometropic intolerance. If the patient shows no contraindications, he or she may also be a candidate for corneal refractive procedures such as radial keratotomy to equilibrate the refraction difference to a tolerable level (Table 16–17; see Figure 16–29).

## Aphakia

Aphakia following cataract surgery was once the norm but today is rarely seen. In modern cataract surgery, adults are rarely left aphakic unless there are surgical complications, preexisting disease, or high myopia that contraindicates IOL implantation. Surgical aphakia is now most commonly seen in infants and young children, since many surgeons consider IOL implantation to be contraindicated in them.

In persons with preexisting high myopia who are left aphakic following cataract surgery there is little difficulty in postoperative refractive correction, since the refractive error is usually minimal. As with all persons with aphakia (and those with pseudophakia without ultraviolet filtering IOLs), ultraviolet filters should be a part of their postoperative correction.

Adult and pediatric aphakia is usually best corrected with contact lenses. Extended-wear soft or silicone lenses are the lens of choice for pediatric patients. For adult aphakia, extended-wear soft lenses, daily-wear soft lenses, and rigid lenses are all alternatives, with extended-wear lenses being the most convenient.

Spectacle lenses have the limitation of restricting the patient's field of view and are poorly tolerated by many patients. However, in those with bilateral aphakia when proper power adjustments are made for vertex distance and optical centers are well-placed, they do very well.

## Malpositioned Intraocular Lenses

Occasionally, the IOL will decenter postoperatively or will be poorly positioned intraoperatively. Both situations may produce refractive problems. The sunset syndrome, where capsular fixation is lost and gravitational forces decenter the IOL inferiorly, may be pronounced enough to produce symptoms of glare and diplopia. In other situations, where one haptic is within and the other haptic outside of the capsular bag, the IOL frequently decenters resulting in complaints of glare and diplopia.[139] Visual complaints in these cases are due to the edge of the IOL optic orapositioning hole being within the pupillary margin.

Rarely, diplopia and glare of this nature may be treated with miotics, which reduce pupillary size enough to eliminate the effect of the lens edge effectively. A custom-made opaque contact lens with a central aperture may also be designed to eliminate the edge effect of the IOL. In severe cases of IOL dislocation or decentration, the IOL may be surgically repositioned[140,141] (see discussion of diplopia on page 192).

Tilting of the IOL may produce astigmatism that is usually correctable with spectacle lenses.[136] Tilting of the IOL may also occasionally produce unusual symptoms of glare and visual distortion. As with dislocated lenses, miotics or surgical repositioning are sometimes helpful in reducing symptoms.

## — REFERENCES

### Ptosis

1. Hamilton RC, Grizzard WS: Complications. In Gills JP, Hustead RF, Grizz WS (eds): *Ophthalmic Anesthesia*. Thorofare, NJ: Slack, 1993:195.
2. Paris GL, Quickert MH: Disinsertion of aponeurosis of the levator palpebrae superioris muscle after cataract extraction. *Am J Ophthalmol*. 1976;**81**:337–340.
3. Alpar JJ: Acquired ptosis following cataract and glaucoma surgery. *Glaucoma*. 1982;**4**:66–68.
4. Feibel RM, Custer PL, Gordon MO: Postcataract ptosis—A randomized, double-masked comparison of peribulbar and retrobulbar anesthesia. *Ophthalmology*. 1993;**100**:660–665.
5. Loeffler M, Solomon LD, Renaud M: Postcataract extraction ptosis: Effect of the bridle suture. *J Cataract Refract Surg*. 1990;**16**:501–504.
6. Girard LJ: Bridle suture in postoperative ptosis. *J Cataract Refract Surg*. 1991;**17**:109 (letter).
7. Kaplan LJ, Jaffe NS, Clayman HM: Ptosis and cataract surgery—A multivariant computer analysis of a prospective study. *Ophthalmology*. 1985;**92**:237–242.
8. Rainin EA, Carlson BM: Postoperative diplopia and ptosis—A clinical hypothesis based on the myotoxicity of local anesthetics. *Arch Ophthalmol*. 1985;**103**: 1337–1339.
9. Yagiela JA, Benoit PW, Buoncristiani RD, et al: Comparison of myotoxic effects of lidocaine with epinephrine in rats and humans. *Anesth Analg*. 1981;**60**:471–480.
10. Foster AH, Carlson BM: Myotoxicity of local anesthetics and regeneration of the damaged muscle fibers. *Anesth Analg*. 1980;**59**:727–736.
11. Linberg JV, McDonald MB, Safir A, et al: Ptosis following radial keratotomy—Performed using a rigid eyelid speculum. *Ophthalmology*. 1986;**93**:1509–1512.
12. Waller RR, McCord CD, Tanenbaum M: Evaluation and management of the ptosis patient. In McCord CD, Tanenbaum M (eds): *Oculoplastic Surg*. New York: Raven Press; 1987:325–375.
13. Arden RL, Moore GK: Complete post-traumatic ptosis: A mechanism for recovery? *Laryngoscope*. 1989;**99**:1175–1179.

## Diplopia

14. Ellingson FT: Explantation of 3M diffractive intraocular lenses. *J Cataract Refract Surg.* 1990;**16**: 697–702.
15. Magramm I, Schlossman A: Strabismus in patients over the age of 60 years. *J Pediatr Ophthalmol Strabismus.* 1991;**28**:28–31.
16. Hamed LM: Strabismus presenting after cataract surgery. *Ophthalmology.* 1991;**98**: 247–252.
17. Metz HS: Complications following surgery for thyroid ophthalmopathy. *J Pediatr Ophthalmol Strabismus.* 1984;**21**:220–222.
18. Hamed LM, Lingua RW: Thyroid eye disease presenting after cataract surgery. *J Pediatr Ophthalmol Strabismus.* 1990;**27**:10–15.
19. Hamed LM, Helveston EM, Ellis FD: Persistent binocular diplopia after cataract surgery. *Am J Ophthalmol.* 1987;**103**:741–744.
20. Kushner BJ: Abnormal sensory findings secondary to monocular cataracts in children and strabismic adults. *Am J Ophthalmol.* 1986;**102**:349–352.
21. Pratt-Johnson JA, Tillson G: Intractable diplopia after vision restoration in unilateral cataract. *Am J Ophthalmol.* 1989;**107**:23–26.
22. Catalano RA, Nelson LB, Calhoun JH, et al: Persistent strabismus presenting after cataract surgery. *Ophthalmology.* 1987;**94**:491–494.
23. Burns CL, Seigel LA: Inferior rectus recession for vertical tropia after cataract surgery. *Ophthalmology.* 1988;**95**:1120–1124.
24. Foster AH, Carlson BM: Myotoxicity of local anesthetics and regeneration of the damaged muscle fibers. *Anesth Analg.* 1980;**59**:727–736.
25. Yagiela JA, Benoit PW, Buoncristiani RD, et al: Comparison of myotoxic effects of lidocaine with epinephrine in rats and humans. *Anesth Analg.* 1981;**60**:471–480.
26. Rainin EA, Carlson BM: Postoperative diplopia and ptosis. A clinical hypothesis based on the myotoxicity of local anesthetics. *Arch Ophthalmol.* 1985;**103**:1337–1339.
27. Erie JC: Acquired Brown's syndrome after peribulbar anesthesia. *Am J Ophthalmol.* 1990;**109**:349–350.

## Ocular Hypertension/Glaucoma

28. Radius RL, Schultz K, Sobocinski K, et al: Pseudophakia and intraocular pressure. *Am J Ophthalmol.* 1984;**97**:738–742.
29. Onali T, Raitta C: Extracapsular cataract extraction and posterior chamber lens implantation in controlled open-angle glaucoma. *Ophthalmic Surg.* 1991;**22**:381–387.
30. Cinotti DJ, Fiore PM, Maltzman BA, et al: Control of intraocular pressure in glaucomatous eyes after extracapsular cataract extraction with intraocular lens implantation. *J Cataract Refract Surg.* 1988;**14**:650–653.
31. Kooner KS, Dulaney DD, Zimmerman TJ: Intraocular pressure following secondary anterior chamber lens implantation. *Ophthalmic Surg.* 1988;**19**:274–276.
32. Bartlett JD, Jaanus SD: *Clinical Ocular Pharmacology,* 2nd ed. Boston: Butterworth; 1989:178–195.
33. Shields MB: Steroid-induced glaucoma. In *Textbook of Glaucoma.* Baltimore, MD: Williams & Wilkins, 1987:312–317.
34. Drews RC: Management of postoperative inflammation: Dexamethosone versus flurbiprofen, a quantitative study using the new flare cell meter. *Ophthalmic Surg.* 1990;**21**:560–562.
35. Nussenblatt RB, Palestine AG: *Uveitis: Fundamentals and Clinical Practice.* Chicago: Year Book Medical, 1989:152.
36. Moses L: Complications of rigid anterior chamber implants. *Ophthalmology.* 1984;**91**:819–825.

37. Gelender H: Corneal endothelial cell loss, cystoid macular edema, and iris supported intraocular lenses. *Ophthalmology.* 1984;**91**:841–846.
38. Woodhams JT, Lester JC: Pigmentary dispersion glaucoma secondary to posterior chamber intraocular lenses. *Ann Ophthalmol.* 1984;**16**:852–855.
39. Tomey KF, Traverso CE: The glaucomas in aphakia and pseudophakia. *Surv Ophthalmol.* 1991;**36**:79–112.
40. Polaski SA, Willis WE: Angle-supported intraocular lenses: A goniophotographic study. *Ophthalmology.* 1984;**91**:838–840.
41. Evans RB: Peripheral anterior synechiae overlying the haptics of posterior chamber lenses—Occurrence and natural history. *Ophthalmology.* 1990;**97**:415–423.
42. Van Buskirk EM: Late onset, progressive, peripheral anterior synechiae with posterior chamber intraocular lenses. *Ophthalmic Surg.* 1987;**18**:115–117.

## Chronic Corneal Edema/Corneal Decompensation

43. Robin JB, Gindi JJ, Kohl K, et al: An update of the indications for penetrating keratoplasty: 1979 through 1983. *Arch Ophthalmol.* 1986;**104**:87–89.
44. Brady SE, Rapuano CJ, Arensten JJ, et al: Clinical indications for and procedures associated with penetrating keratoplasty, 1983–1988. *Am J Ophthalmol.* 1989;**108**:118–122.
45. Rao GN, Stevens RE, Harris JK, Aquavella JV: Long-term changes in corneal endothelium following intraocular lens implantation. *Ophthalmology.* 1981;**88**:386–397.
46. Kraff MC, Sanders DR, Lieberman HL: Endothelial cell loss and trauma during intraocular lens implantation: A specular microscopic study. *Am Intraocular Implant Soc J.* 1978;**4**:107–109.
47. Menchini V, Scialdone A, Fantaguzzi S, et al: Clinical evaluation of the effect of acetylcholine on the corneal endothelium. *J Cataract Refract Surg.* 1989;**15**:421–424.
48. Olson RJ, Kolodner H, Riddle P, Escapini H: Commonly used intraocular medications and the corneal endothelium. *Arch Ophthalmol.* 1980;**98**:2224.
49. Glasser DB, Osborn DC, Nordeen MS, Min YI: Endothelial protection and viscoelastic retention during phacoemulsification and intraocular lens implantation. *Arch Ophthalmol.* 1991;**109**:1438–1440.
50. Bourne WM, Liesegang TJ, Waller RR, Ilstrup DM: The effect of sodium hyaluronate on endothelial cell damage during extracapsular cataract extraction and posterior chamber lens implantation. *Am J Ophthalmol.* 1984;**98**:759–762.
51. Kraff MC, Sanders DR, Lieberman HL: Specular microscopy in cataract and intraocular lens patients: A report of 564 cases. *Arch Ophthalmol.* 1980;**98**:1782–1784.
52. Stark WJ, Worthen DM, Holladay JT, et al: The FDA report on intraocular lenses. *Ophthalmology.* 1983;**90**:311–317.
53. Chambless WS: Incidence of anterior and posterior segment complications in over 3000 cases of extracapsular cataract extractions, intact and open capsules. *Am Intraocular Implant Soc J.* 1985;**11**:146–148.
54. Apple DJ, Brems RN, Park RB, et al: Anterior chamber lenses part I: Complications and pathology, and a review of designs. *J Cataract Refract Surg.* 1987;**13**:157–174.
55. Coli AF, Price FW, Whitson WW: Intraocular lens exchange for anterior chamber intraocular lens-induced corneal endothelial damage. *Ophthalmology.* 1993;**100**:384–393.
56. Kozarsky AM, Stopak S, Waring GO, et al: Results of penetrating keratoplasty for pseudophakic corneal edema with retention of intraocular lens. *Ophthalmology.* 1984;**1**:1141–1146.
57. Arentsen JJ, Laibson PR: Surgical management of pseudophakic corneal edema: Complications and visual results following penetrating keratoplasty. *Ophthalmic Surg.* 1982;**13**:5:371–373.

## Late Hyphema

58. Johnson SH, Kratz RP, Olson PF: Iris transillumination and microhyphema syndrome. *Am Intraocular Implant Soc J.* 1984;**10**:425–428.

## Chronic Iritis

59. Hooper PL, Rao NA, Smith RE: Cataract extraction in uveitis patients. *Surv Ophthalmol.* 1990;**35**:120–144.
60. Gelender H: Corneal endothelial cell loss, cystoid macular edema, and iris-supported intraocular lenses. *Ophthalmology.* 1984;**91**:841–846.
61. Apple DJ, Mamalis N, Loftfield K, et al: Complications of intraocular lenses. A historical and histopathologic review. *Surv Ophthalmol.* 1984;**29**:1–54.
62. Apple DJ: *Intraocular Lenses: Evolution, Designs, Complications, and Pathology.* Baltimore, MD: Williams & Wilkins; 1989:225–254.
63. Poleski SA, Willis WE: Angle-supported intraocular lenses: A goniophotographic study. *Ophthalmology.* 1984;**91**:838–840.
64. Smith SG, Lindstrom RL: *Intraocular Lens Complications and Their Management.* Thorofare, NJ: Slack, 1988:49–81.
65. Lieppman ME: Intermittent visual "white out." A new intraocular lens complication. *Ophthalmology.* 1982;**89**:109–112.
66. Johnson SH, Kratz RP, Olson PF: Iris transillumination and microhyphema syndrome. *Am Intraocular Implant Soc J.* 1984;**10**;425–428.
67. Woodhams JT, Lester JC: Pigmentary dispersion glaucoma secondary to posterior chamber intra-ocular lenses. *Ann Ophthalmol.* 1984;**16**:852–855.
68. Blodi BA, Flynn HW, Blodi CF, et al: Retained nuclei after cataract surgery. *Ophthalmology.* 1992;**99**:41–44.
69. Piest KL, Kincaid MC, Tetz MR, et al: Localized endophthalmitis: A newly described cause of the so called toxic lens syndrome. *J Cataract Refract Surg.* 1987;**13**:498–510.
70. Ormerod LD, Ho DD, Becker LE, et al: Endophthalmitis caused by the coagulase-negative staphylococci. *Ophthalmology.* 1993;**100**:715–723.
71. Lindstrom RL, Smith SG: Malpositioned posterior chamber lenses: Etiology, prevention, and management. *Am Intraocular Implant Soc J.* 1985;**11**:584–591.

## Posterior Capsular Opacities/ Nd:YAG Capsulotomy

72. Apple DJ, Solomon KD, Tetz MR, et al: Posterior capsule opacification. *Surv Ophthalmol.* 1992;**37**:73–116.
73. Sterling S, Wood TO: Effect of intraocular lens convexity on posterior capsule opacification. *J Cataract Refract Surg.* 1986;**12**:655–657.
74. McDonnell PJ, Stark WJ, Green WR: Posterior capsule opacification: A specular microscopic study. *Ophthalmology.* 1984;**91**:853–856.
75. Cobo LM, Eiichi O, Chandler D, et al: Pathogenesis of capsular opacification after extracapsular cataract extraction: An animal model. *Ophthalmology.* 1984;**91**:857–863.
76. Meisler DM, Palestine AG, Vastine DW, et al: Chronic Propionibacterium endophthalmitis after extracapsular cataract extraction and intraocular lens implantation. *Am J Ophthalmol.* 1986;**102**:733–739.
77. Piest K, Kincaid M, Tetz M, et al: Localized endophthalmitis: A newly described cause of the so-called toxic lens syndrome. *J Cataract Refract Surg.* 1987;**13**:498–510.
78. Carlson A, Koch D: Endophthalmitis following Nd:YAG posterior capsulotomy. *Ophthalmic Surg.* 1988;**19**:168–170.

79. Tetz M, Apple D, Price FJ, et al: A newly described complication of Neodymium:YAG laser capsulotomy: Exacerbation of an intraocular infection. *Arch Ophthalmol.* 1987;**105**:1324–1325.
80. Gimbel HV, Van Westenbrugge JA, Sander DR, Raanan MG: Effect of sulcus vs capsular fixation on YAG-induced pressure rises following posterior capsulotomy. *Arch Ophthalmol.* 1990;**108**:1126–1129.
81. Fourman S, Apisson J: Late-onset elevation of intraocular pressure after neodymium-YAG laser post capsulotomy. *Arch Ophthalmol.* 1991;**109**:511–513.
82. Silverstone DE, Brint SF, Olander KW, et al: Prophylactic use of apraclonidine for intraocular pressure increase after Nd:YAG capsulotomies. *Am J Ophthalmol.* 1992;**113**:401–405.
83. Richter CH, Arzeno G, Pappar HR, et al: Intraocular pressure elevation following Nd:YAG laser posterior capsulotomy. *Ophthalmology.* 1985;**92**:636–640.
84. Slomovic AR, Parrish RK: Acute elevations of intraocular pressure following Nd:YAG laser posterior capsulotomy. *Ophthalmology.* 1985;**92**:973–976.
85. Pollack IP, Brown RH, Crandall AS, et al: Prevention of the rise in intraocular pressure following neodymium-YAG posterior capsulotomy using topical 1% apraclonidine. *Arch Ophthalmol.* 1988;**106**:754–757.
86. Milamed S, Barraguer E, Epstein D: Neodymium:YAG laser iridotomy as a possible contribution to lens dislocation. *Ann Ophthalmol.* 1986;**18**:281–282.
87. Javitt JC, Tielsch JM, Canner JK, et al: National outcome of cataract extraction: Increased risk of retinal complications associated with Nd:YAG laser capsulotomy. *Ophthalmology.* 1992;**99**:1487–1498.
88. Van Westenbrugge JA, Gimbel HV, Souchek J, Chow D: Incidence of retinal detachment following Nd:YAG capsulotomy after cataract surgery. *J Cataract Refract Surg.* 1992;**18**:352–355.
89. Long WF, Trich LR: Optimal incision diameter in YAG laser capsulotomy. *Am J Optom Physiol Optics.* 1987;**64**;324–328.

## Pseudophakic (Aphakic) Cystoid Macular Edema

90. Irvine SR: A newly defined vitreous syndrome following cataract surgery: Interpreted according to recent concepts of the structure of the vitreous. *Am J Ophthalmol.* 1953;**36**:599–619.
91. Gass JDM, Norton EWD: Cystoid macular edema and papilledema following cataract extraction: A fluorescein funduscopic and angiographic study. *Arch Ophthalmol.* 1966;**76**:646–661.
92. Stark WJ, Maumenee AE, Fadadau W, et al: Cystoid macular edema in pseudophakia. *Surv Ophthalmol.* 1984;**28**(suppl):452–461.
93. Jaffe NS, Clayman HM, Jaffe MS: Cystoid macular edema after intracapsular and extracapsular cataract extraction with and without an intraocular lens. *Ophthalmology.* 1982;**89**:25–29.
94. Wright PL, Wilkinson CP, Balyert HD, et al: Angiographic cystoid macular edema after posterior chamber lens implantation. *Arch Ophthalmol.* 1988;**106**:740–744.
95. Kraff MC, Sanders DR, Jampol LE, Lieberman HL: Effect of an ultraviolet filtering intraocular lens on cystoid macular edema. *Ophthalmology.* 1985;**92**:366–369.
96. Flach AJ, Stegman RC, Graham J, Kruger LP: Prophylaxis of aphakic cystoid macular edema without corticosteroids. *Ophthalmology.* 1990;**97**:1253–1258.
97. Smith SG, Lindstrom RL: *Intraocular Lens Complications and Their Management.* Thorofare, NJ: Slack; 1988:173–176.
98. Michels RG, Maumenee AE: Cystoid macular edema associated with topically applied epinephrine in aphakic eyes. *Am J Ophthalmol.* 1975;**80**:379–388.
99. Miami Study Group: Cystoid macular edema in aphakic and pseudophakic eyes. *Am J Ophthalmol.* 1979;**88**:45–48.

100. Moses L: Cystoid macular edema and retinal detachment following cataract surgery. *Am Intraocular Implant Soc J.* 1979;**5**:326–329.
101. Percival P: Clinical factors relating to cystoid macular edema after lens implantation. *Am Intraocular Implant Soc J.* 1981;**7**:43–45.
102. Tolentino FL, Schepens CL: Edema of the posterior pole after cataract extraction: A biomicroscopic study. *Arch Ophthalmol.* 1965;**74**:781–786.
103. Schepens CL, Avila MP, Jalkh AE, et al: The role of the vitreous in cystoid macular edema. *Surv Ophthalmol.* 1984;**28**(suppl):499–504.
104. Flach AJ: Cyclo-oxygenase inhibitors in ophthalmology. *Surv Ophthalmol.* 1992;**36**:259–284.
105. Fine BS, Brucker AJ: Macular edema and cystoid macular edema. *Am J Ophthalmol.* 1981;**92**:466–481.
106. Tso MOM: Pathology of cystoid macular edema. *Ophthalmology.* 1982;**89**:902–915.
107. Yanoff M, Fine BS, Brucker AJ, Eagle RC: Pathology of human cystoid macular edema. *Surv Ophthalmol.* 1984;**28**(suppl):505–511.
108. Gass JDM, Andersen DR, Davis EB: A clinical, fluorescein angiographic, and electron microscopic correlation of cystoid macular edema. *Am J Ophthalmol.* 1985;**100**:82–86.
109. Cunha-Vaz JG, Travasso SA: Breakdown of the blood-retinal barriers and cystoid macular edema. *Surv Ophthalmol.* 1984;**28**(suppl):485–492.
110. Klein RM, Katzin HM, Yannuzzi LA: The effect of indomethacin pretreatment on aphakic cystoid macular edema. *Am J Ophthalmol.* 1979;**87**:487–489.
111. Kraff MC, Sanders DR, Jampol LM, et al: Prophylaxis of pseudophakic cystoid macular edema with topical indomethacin. *Ophthalmology.* 1982;**89**:885–890.
112. Miyake K, Sakamura S, Mirura H: Long term follow-up study on prevention of aphakic cystoid macular edema by topical indomethacin. *Br J Ophthalmol.* 1980;**64**:324–328.
113. Lakhanpal V, Schocket SS: Pseudophakic and aphakic retinal detachment mimicking cystoid macular edema. *Ophthalmology.* 1987;**94**:785–791.
114. Fung WE: The national, prospective, randomized vitrectomy study for chronic aphakic cystoid macular edema: Progress report and comparison between control and nonrandomized groups. *Surv Ophthalmol.* 1984;**28**(suppl):569–575.
115. Katzen LE, Fleischman JA, Troxel S: YAG laser treatment of cystoid macular edema. *Am J Ophthalmol.* 1983;**95**:589–592.
116. Steinert RF, Wasson PJ: Neodymium YAG laser anterior vitreolysis for Irvine-Gass cystoid macular edema. *J Cataract Refract Surg.* 1989;**15**:304–312.
117. McEntyre JM: A successful treatment for aphakic cystoid macular edema. *Ann Ophthalmol.* 1978;**10**:1219–1224.
118. Civerchis LL, Balent A: Treatment of pseudophakic cystoid macular edema by elevation of intraocular pressure. *Ann Ophthalmol.* 1984;**16**:890–894.
119. Melberg NS, Olk RJ: Corticosteroid-induced ocular hypertension in the treatment of aphakic of pseudophakic cystoid macular edema. *Ophthalmology.* 1993;**100**;164–167.
120. Gehring JR: Macular edema following cataract extraction. *Arch Ophthalmol.* 1968;**80**:626–631.
121. Stern AL, Taylor DM, Dalburg LA, Cosentino RT: Pseudophakic cystoid maculopathy: A study of 50 cases. *Ophthalmology.* 1981;**88**:942–946.
122. Yannuzzi LA, Klein RM, Wallyn RH, et al: Ineffectiveness of indomethacin in the treatment of chronic cystoid macular edema. *Am J Ophthalmol.* 1977;**84**:517–519.
123. Flach AJ, Jampol LM, Weinberg D, et al: Improvement in visual acuity in chronic aphakic and pseudophakic cystoid macular edema after treatment with topical 0.5% ketorolac tromethamine. *Am J Ophthalmol.* 1991;**112**:514–519.
124. Jaffe NS, Jaffe MS, Jaffe GF: *Cataract Surgery and Its Complications,* 5th ed. St Louis: CV Mosby; 1990:448.

## Retinal Detachment

125. Steinert RF, Puliafito CA, Kumar SR, et al: Cystoid macular edema, retinal detachment, and glaucoma after Nd:YAG laser posterior capsulotomy. *Am J Ophthalmol.* 1991;**112**;373–380.
126. Rickman-Barger L, Florine CW, Larson RS, Lindstrom RL: Retinal detachment after neodymium:YAG laser posterior capsulotomy. *Am J Ophthalmol.* 1989;**107**;531–536.
127. Leff SR, Welch JC, Tasman W: Rhegmatogenous retinal detachment after YAG laser posterior capsulotomy. *Ophthalmology.* 1987;**94**;1221–1225.
128. Ober RR, Wilkinson CP, Fiore JV Jr, Maggiano JM: Rhegmatogenous retinal detachment after neodymium–YAG laser capsulotomy in aphakic and pseudophakic eyes. *Am J Ophthalmol.* 1986;**101**:81–89.

## Optical Considerations

129. Parker WI, Clorfeine GS: Long-term evolution of astigmatism following planned extracapsular cataract extraction. *Arch Ophthalmol.* 1989;**107**:353–357.
130. Datiles MB, Gancayco T: Low myopia with low astigmatic correction gives cataract surgery patients good depth of focus. *Ophthalmology.* 1990;**97**:922–926.
131. Samusch MR, Guyton DL: Optimal astigmatism to enhance depth of focus after cataract surgery. *Ophthalmology.* 1991;**98**:1025–1029.
132. Steinert RF, Brint SF, White SM, Fine IH: Astigmatism after small incision cataract surgery. *Ophthalmology.* 1991;**98**:417–424.
133. Busin M, Schmidt J, Koch J, Spitzans M: Long-term results of sutureless phacoemulsification with implantation of a 7-mm polymethylmethacrylate intraocular lens. *Arch Ophthalmol.* 1993;**111**:333–358.
134. Geary TY: Modification of post-cataract astigmatism by wound revision. *Int Ophthalmol Clin.* 1983;**23**:111–126.
135. Swinyer CA: Postoperative astigmatism. *Surv Ophthalmol.* 1987;**31**:219–248.
136. Holiday JT, Rubin ML: Avoiding refractive problems in cataract surgery. *Surv Ophthalmol.* 1988;**32**:357–360.
137. Bartlett JD: Anisometropia and aniseikonia. In Amos JF (ed): *Diagnosis and Management in Vision Care.* Boston: Butterworths; 1989:173–202.
138. Carleton EH, Madigan LE: Relationships between aniseikonia and ametropia. *Arch Ophthalmol.* 1937;**18**:237–247.
139. Apple DJ, Lichtenstein SB, Heerlein K, et al: Visual aberrations caused by optic components of posterior chamber intraocular lenses. *J Cataract Refract Surg.* 1987;**13**:431–435.
140. Apple DJ, Mamalis N, Leftfield K, et al: Complications of intraocular lenses: A historical and histopathological review. *Surv Ophthalmol.* 1984;**29**;51–54.
141. Jaffe JS, Jaffe MS, Jaffe GS: *Cataract Surgery and Its Complications,* 5th ed. St Louis: CV Mosby; 1990:232–242.

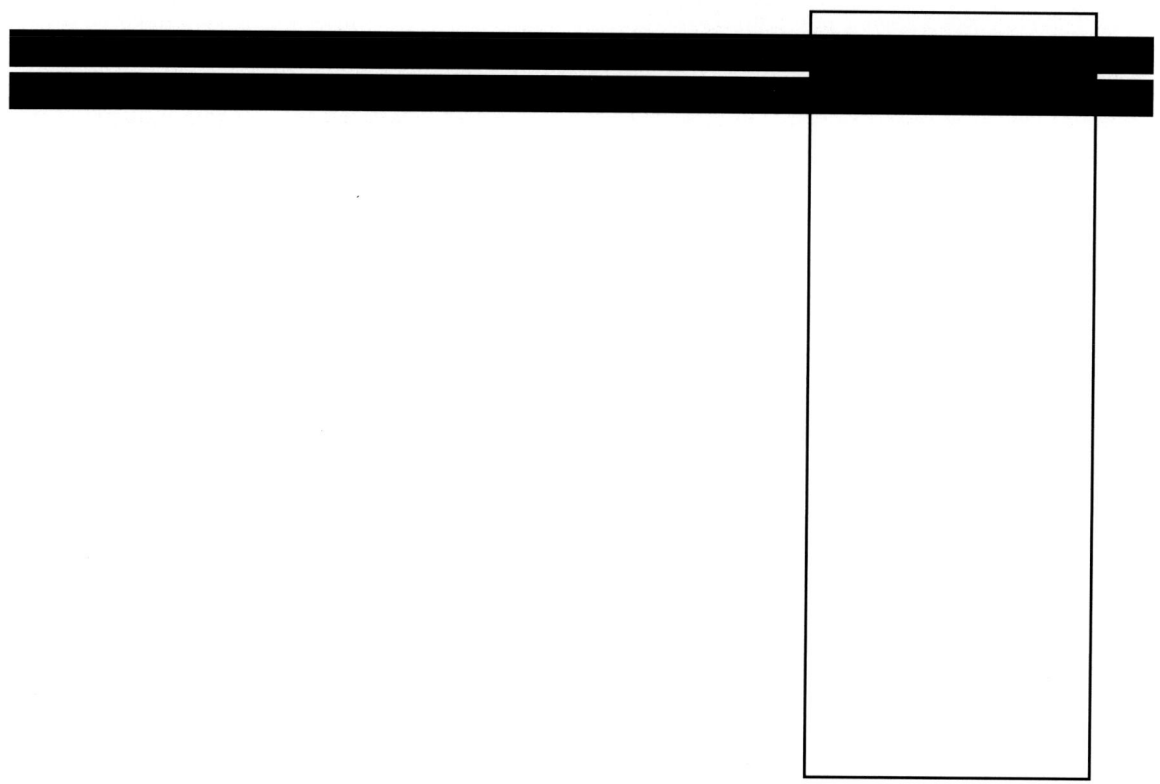

# Appendices

# APPENDIX 1

## Comanagement Patient Communication Aids*

### Cataract Surgery

#### What Is a Cataract?
The lens of your eye, about the size of a baby aspirin and located behind the iris, focuses light on the retina to produce an image. A cataract is a clouding or crystalization of this lens. It distorts the flow of light to the retina causing dim or blurry vision. A cataract can form within a few months or it may take years to develop.

#### What Causes a Cataract?
The most common cause of cataract is aging. Cataract development may also be related to exposure to ultraviolet radiation from the sun. Although you can protect yourself from the sun, there is little you can do to stop the aging process. Just as hair turns gray with time, the lens of the eye turns cloudy with age.

#### What Are the Symptoms of Cataract?
There is no pain, itching, or redness associated with cataracts. However, if you are developing a cataract, you may notice some of these symptoms:

- Blurry or dim vision becoming progressively worse
- Glare or halos around lights at night
- Faded colors
- Filmy or foggy vision
- Difficulty driving at night due to headlight glare and reduced night vision
- Poor vision in bright light
- Glasses seem dirty but cleaning doesn't help
- Difficulty reading, sewing, doing needlework or watching TV
- Stronger glasses fail to improve vision

#### When Should a Cataract Be Removed?
A cataract may be removed when it begins significantly to affect your work or lifestyle. Because of the safety of modern cataract removal, it is not necessary to wait for a cataract to "ripen" until you are nearly blind. Research shows that excessive delay of cataract surgery may result in a greater chance of complications, thereby resulting in poorer vision after surgery. You and your eye doctor are the ones who ultimately determine when you should have your cataract removed.

#### What Surgical Technique Is Used?
PCLI surgeons use the latest method of cataract removal called "phacoemulsification" or ultrasound. With this procedure the cloudy lens is gently washed away. The thin membrane around the lens is left in place and a new plastic lens is implanted. The eye self-heals without stitches—a technique called "no-stitch" surgery. Because this method is quick and uses a very tiny incision without sutures, the eye heals rapidly and allows you to resume your normal activities immediately.

---

*Pacific Cataract and Laser Institute

### Before Surgery Instructions

*The Evening Before or the Morning of Surgery*

- Take a shower and wash your hair.

*The Day of Surgery*
- Dress in clean clothes—You will not have to remove them for surgery.
- You may eat a light meal before your surgery.
- DO NOT TAKE PILOCARPINE EYEDROPS.
- If you are diabetic, take your insulin and eat normally.
- Take all your other usual medications.
- Write down all the medications you are taking on "My Medications" card.
- PLEASE BRING THE CARD WITH YOU.
- HAVE A FRIEND OR FAMILY MEMBER DRIVE YOU TO PCLI.
- Someone should drive you home after surgery and to your examination the next day.
- It is not wise to drive with your eye patched or until your vision is improved.

*On Arrival*
- Please inform the receptionist you are here for your cataract surgery.
- Family and friends are welcome to watch your procedure in the viewing theater.
- If you do not want anyone to view your surgery, please let us know.

### After Surgery Instructions

For the next 24 hours your eye requires little care.

## Activity

- You may do what you normally do.
- You may bend over, sleep on your side, watch TV, dine or whatever you wish.

## Medication

- Cephalexin, 250 mg (if you have allergies to this medication or penicillin, please let the doctor know).
- The day of surgery: Take one capsule at bedtime.
- The day after surgery: Take one capsule at 8:00 AM, noon, 4:00 PM, and 8:00 PM.
- If you have minor discomfort: Take Tylenol, Advil, or whatever you normally take for headaches.

## Pain

- A scratchy feeling or itching is normal.
- If you have severe pain and lose the vision you have, please call us immediately.

## Removing Your Patch

- You may remove your patch before going to bed the night of surgery.
- Your vision may be variable or even poor for a few days as a normal part of the healing process.
- You may shower, shampoo your hair, and wash around your eye.

# APPENDIX 2

## Standard Abbreviations

| | |
|---|---|
| A | Angle of anomaly |
| A | Atropine (eg, A-1%) |
| Abd | Abduction |
| Abn | Abnormal |
| AC | Anterior chamber |
| a.c. | before meals, "ante cibum" |
| ACA | Accommodation–convergence ratio |
| Acc | Accommodation |
| Add | Adduction |
| AION | Anterior ischemic optic neuropathy |
| ALT | Argon laser trabeculoplasty |
| Alt | Altitudinal (as in field Alt defect) |
| AMBL | Amblyopia |
| AODM | Adult onset diabetes mellitus |
| APD | Afferent pupil defect (ie, Marcus Gunn pupillary defect) |
| AR | Against the rule (as in AR astigmatism) |
| ARC | Anomalous retinal (cortical) correspondence |
| ARMD | Age-related macular degeneration |
| AS | Arteriosclerosis |
| A.S. | Anterior synechiae (see PAS) |
| ASC | Anterior subcapsular cataract |
| ASCVD | Atherosclerotic cardiovascular disease |
| ASHD | Atherosclerotic heart disease |
| | |
| BD | Base down |
| BO | Base out |
| BU | Base up |
| bid | Twice a day (also × 2), "bis in die" |
| BAK | Benzalkonium chloride |
| BDR | Background diabetic retinopathy |
| BI | Base in |
| BIO | Binocular indirect ophthalmoscopy |
| BP | Blood pressure |
| BRAO | Branch retinal artery occlusion |
| BUT | Break up time (see TBUT) |
| BRVO | Branch retinal vein occlusion |
| | |
| C | Cells (as in cells in the AC) |
| c̄ | With, "cum" |
| CA | Carcinoma |
| CA | Convergence-accommodation ratio |
| CAD | Coronary artery disease |
| CAG | Closed-angle glaucoma (see NAG) |
| Caps | Capsule |
| CAT(s) | Cataract(s) |
| CBC | Complete blood count |
| CC | Chief complaint |
| c̄c | With correction |
| CCC | Central corneal clouding |
| C/D | Cup to disk ratio |
| CF | Central fixation |

| | |
|---|---|
| CF | Count fingers (see FC) |
| Cj | Conjunctiva |
| CL | Contact lens |
| CME | Cystoid macular edema |
| CNAG | Chronic narrow-angle glaucoma (see CA and NAG) |
| CNVM | Choroidal neovascular membrane |
| c/o | Complaint of, complains of |
| COAG | Chronic open-angle glaucoma |
| CONG | Congenital |
| COPD | Chronic obstructive pulmonary disease |
| CR | Chorioretinal (eg, CR lesion) |
| CRAO | Central retinal artery occlusion |
| CRVO | Central retinal vein occlusion |
| CS | Cortical sclerosis |
| CSME | Clinically significant macular edema |
| CSR | Central serous retinopathy |
| CT | Cover test |
| CT | Computed tomography |
| CV | Color vision |
| CVA | Cerebral vascular accident |
| CVC | Chief visual complaint (see CC) |
| CVF—FTFC | Confrontational visual field—full to finger counting |
| CxR | Chest x-ray |
| | |
| D | Disk |
| D | Distance |
| D | Diopter |
| DC | Discontinue |
| D/C | Deep and clear (as in AC–D/C) or discontinue, eg, to D/C a medication |
| DCR | Dacryocystorhinostomy |
| DDX or d.d. | Different diagnosis |
| DFE | Dilated fundus examination |
| DIPL | Diplopia |
| DM | Diabetes mellitus |
| D/Q | Deep and quiet (as in AC–D/Q) |
| DR | Diabetic retinopathy (see BDR, IRMA, NVD, PDR, PPDR) |
| DV | Distance vision |
| Dx | Diagnosis |
| | |
| E | Esophoria at 6 m (infinity) |
| E′ | Esophoria at 33 cm |
| ECCE | Extracapsular cataract extraction |
| EEG | Electroencephalogram |
| EF | Eccentric fixation |
| EKC | Epidermic keratoconjunctivitis |
| EKG/ECG | Electrocardiogram |
| Elix | elixir |
| EOG | Electro-oculogram |
| EOM | Extraocular muscles |
| EOM | Extraocular motility |
| ERG | Electroretinogram |
| ERM | Epiretinal membrane (see SWR) |
| ET | Esotropia at 6 m (infinity) |
| ET′ | Esotropia at 33 cm |

| | |
|---|---|
| ETOH | Ethanol (eg, on breath/abuse) |
| EWCL | Extended-wear contact lens |
| | |
| F | Field (as in visual field) |
| FA | Fluorescein angiography |
| FB | Foreign body |
| FBS | Fasting blood surgar |
| FC | Finger counting |
| FOcHx | Family ocular history |
| FHx | Family history |
| FROM | Full range of motion (motility) |
| f/u | Follow-up |
| Funct | Functional |
| Fx | Findings |
| Fxn | Function |
| | |
| Glc | Glaucoma |
| GPC | Giant papillary conjunctivitis |
| gt(t) | Drop(s), "guttae" |
| GVF | Goldman visual field |
| | |
| h | hour |
| H/A or Ha | Headache |
| HCL | Hard contact lens |
| HCTZ | Hydrochlorothiazide |
| HEM | Hemorrhage |
| Hgb | Hemoglobin |
| H/H | Hemoglobin/hematocrit |
| HLA | Human leukocytic antigen (ie, B27) |
| HM | hand motion |
| H/O | History of |
| HPPM | Hyperplastic persistent pupillary membrane |
| HR | Hypertensive retinopathy |
| h.s. | Bedtime, "hora somni" |
| HSK | Herpes simplex keratitis |
| HSV | Herpes simplex virus |
| HTN | Hypertension |
| HVF | Humphrey visual field |
| Hx | History |
| Hyst | Hysterical |
| HZV | Herpes zoster virus |
| | |
| ICCE | Intracapsular cataract extraction |
| IDDM | Insulin dependent diabetes mellitus |
| IK | Interstitial keratitis |
| int | Intermittent |
| IOL | Intraocular lens |
| IOP | Intraocular pressure |
| IOT | Intraocular tension |
| IPD | Interpupillary distance |
| IRMA | Intraretinal microvascular abnormalities |
| | |
| J | Jaeger near acuity (eg, J-1, J-5) |
| JODM | Juvenile-onset diabetes mellitus |

| | |
|---|---|
| K | Keratometry |
| KCS | Keratoconjunctivitis sicca |
| KP | Keratic precipitate |
| | |
| L | Lid (eg, LLL—left lower lid, RUL—right upper lid) |
| Lat | Lateral |
| LE | Lupus erythematosus (see SLE) |
| LIA | Laser interference acuity |
| LP | Light perception |
| LP c̄ proj | Light perception with projection |
| LPI | Laser peripheral iridectomy (see PI) |
| LR | Lateral rectus |
| LTP | Laser trabeculoplasty (see ALT) |
| LV (A) | Low vision (aid) |
| | |
| M | Macula |
| M | Manifest refraction |
| ME | Macular edema |
| Merid | Meridional |
| MG | Marcus Gunn (see APD) |
| MFS | Monofixation syndrome |
| MHx | Medical history |
| MIO | Monocular indirect ophthalmoscopy |
| MOT | Motility |
| MR | Medial rectus |
| Mx | Management |
| | |
| N | Near |
| NAG | Narrow-angle glaucoma (see CAG) |
| NI | No improvement |
| NLP | No light perception (amaurosis) |
| NOC | Night |
| NPA | Near point of accommodation |
| NPC | Near point of convergence |
| NRC | Normal retinal (cortical) correspondence |
| NVD | Neovascularization at disk |
| NVE | Neovascularization elsewhere (ie, not at disk) |
| NVM | Neovascular membrane |
| NS | Nuclear sclerosis (grade 0–4+) |
| Nutr | Nutritional |
| NV | Near vision |
| | |
| OA | Optic atrophy |
| OAG | Open-angle glaucoma |
| OD | Optic disk |
| OD | Right eye, "oculus dexter" |
| ODM | Ophthalmodynamometry |
| OGTT | Oral glucose tolerance test |
| Oc HTN | Ocular hypertension |
| Oc Hx | Ocular history |
| OKN | Optokinetic nystagmus |
| ON | Optic nerve |
| ONA | Optic nerve atrophy |
| ORG | Organic |
| OS | Left eye, "oculus sinister" |

| | |
|---|---|
| OU | Both eyes, "oculus uterque" |
| OZ | Optical zone |
| | |
| P | Pulse |
| P | Periphery |
| P | Corneal pachymetry |
| PAM | Potential acuity meter |
| PAS | Peripheral anterior synechiae (see AS) |
| PASK | Peripheral anterior stromal keratopathy |
| PC | Postcycloplegic |
| pc | After meals, "post cibum" |
| PCF | Pharyngeal conjunctival fever |
| PCO | Posterior capsular opacity |
| PD | Interpupillary distance (see IPD) |
| PDR | Proliferative diabetic retinopathy |
| PEE | Punctate epithelial erosion |
| PEK | Punctate epithelial keratitis (keratopathy) |
| PERRLA | Pupils equal, round, react to light and accommodation |
| PH | Pinhole |
| Phaco | Phacoemulsification |
| PHPV | Persistent hyperplastic primary vitreous |
| PI | Peripheral iridectomy (see LPI) |
| PLT | Preferential looking technique |
| PMMA | Polymethylmethacrylate (CL) |
| PO | By mouth |
| POHS | Presumed ocular histoplasmosis syndrome |
| PPDR | Preproliferative diabetic retinopathy |
| PPLOV | Painless progressive loss of vision |
| PPM | Persistent pupillary membrane |
| PRN | As needed (necessary), "pro re nata" |
| PRP | Panretinal photocoagulation |
| PS | Posterior synechiae |
| PSC | Posterior subcapsular cataract (grade 0–4+) |
| PSI | Punctate subepithelial infiltrate |
| PSRT | Photostress recovery test |
| Px | Prognosis |
| | |
| q | Every (eg, q2h) |
| qd | Daily (or ×1), "quaque die" |
| qh | Hourly |
| qid | Four times daily (or ×4), "quater in die" |
| qod | Every other day, "quaque altera die" |
| qs | Sufficient quantity, "quantum satis" |
| | |
| R | Retinoscopy |
| RA | Rheumatoid arthritis |
| RD | Retinal detachment |
| RF | Rheumatoid factor |
| R/O | Rule out |
| R+R | Recess and resect |
| Rx | Prescription |
| | |
| s | Without, "sine" |
| sC | Without correction |
| SCL | Soft contact lens |

| | |
|---|---|
| SEI | Subepithelial infiltrate |
| SI | Sector iridectomy (keyhole pupil) |
| Sig | Label or let it be imprinted, "signa" |
| SLE | Slit lamp examination (biomicroscopy) |
| SLE | Systemic lupus erythematosus |
| SLK | Superior limbic keratoconjunctivitis |
| SMD | Senile macular (choroidal) degeneration |
| SO | Superior oblique |
| SOAP | Subjective, objective, assessment, and plan |
| SOS | One time only |
| S/P | Status post |
| SPK | Superficial punctate keratitis |
| SR | Superior rectus |
| SRNVM | Subretinal neovascular membrane |
| SS | One half |
| Stat | Immediately, "statim" |
| Stereo | Stereopsis |
| Strab | Strabismus |
| STT 1 | Schirmer tear test 1 |
| STT 2 | Schirmer tear test 2 |
| SWR | Surface wrinkling retinopathy (see ERM) |
| Sx(s) | Symptom(s) |
| | |
| TA | Temporal arteritis |
| TAIR | Tonometry by air |
| TAP | Tonometry by applanation |
| TBUT | Tear break-up time (see BUT) |
| TIA | Transient ischemic attack |
| tid | Three times daily (or ×3), "ter in die" |
| Tox | Toxic |
| Tx | Treatment or therapy |
| | |
| ung | Ointment |
| | |
| V | Vasculature |
| VA | Visual acuity |
| VA c̄C | Visual acuity with correction |
| VA s̄C | Visual acuity without correction |
| VDRL | Venereal Disease Research Laboratory |
| VEP | Visual evoked potential |
| VER | Visual evoked response |
| VF | Visual field |
| VKH | Vogt-Koyanagi-Harada syndrome |
| | |
| w/ | With |
| w-4-D | Worth four dot |
| WC/LS | Warm compresses/lid scrubs |
| WD | Working distance |
| WNL | Within normal limits |
| w/o | Without |
| | |
| XT | Exotropia |

# APPENDIX 3

## Doctor-to-Doctor Communication Aids

### *Preoperative Evaluation**

Patient _____ Date _____
    ( )Baseline evaluation    ( )Pre-surgical evaluation

Chief visual complaint:
    ( )Reading    ( )Hobbies    ( )_____
    ( )Driving    ( )Glare    ( )_____

Medical problems:
    ( )Hypertension  ( )Diabetes    ( )_____

Eye history:
    ( )Injury _____    ( )Surgery _____
    ( )Glaucoma _____    ( ) _____

Previous visual acuities
19____ OD 20/____    19____ OD 20/____
     OS 20/____          OS 20/____

Refraction:  Date _____
OD _____ – _____ × _____ 20/_____
OS _____ – _____ × _____ 20/_____

Pinhole acuity:
OD  20/____
PS  20/____

Tonometry:    ( )air ( )applanation
OD _____mm Hg    OS _____mm Hg

Visual field enclosed: ( )yes  ( )no
Comments: _____
_____
_____

( ) PCLI to make patient appointment  phone # ( ) ___ - _____
( ) Patient scheduled at PCLI on _____ at _____
                           Date          Time
                          _____, O.D.

---

* Pacific Cataract and Laser Institute

**Follow-up\*: Cataract** ☐   **YAG** ☐   **Other** ☐

NAME: _____ Exam Date: _____

Symptoms:   OD: _____   OS: _____

|  OD  |  OS  |
|---|---|

Date of Surgery: _____   Date of Surgery: _____
Visual Acuity _____      Visual Acuity _____
    with/without RX:  20/_____       with/without RX:  20/_____
    Pinhole:          20/_____       Pinhole:          20/_____
IOP: (Air/AP) _____             IOP: (Air/AP) _____
Keratometry:_____/_____@_____         Keratometry:_____/_____@_____
Refraction: ____−____×____ 20/____    Refraction: ____−____×____ 20/____

**Examination:** (check if normal)    **Post-Op Visit:**

|                    | OD | OS |          | OD | OS |
|---|---|---|---|---|---|
| Patient comfort    | ☐ | ☐ | 1 day    | ☐ | ☐ |
| Wound              | ☐ | ☐ | 1 week\* | ☐ | ☐ |
| Conjunctiva        | ☐ | ☐ | 3 weeks  | ☐ | ☐ |
| Cornea             | ☐ | ☐ | 5 weeks\*| ☐ | ☐ |
| Anterior chamber   | ☐ | ☐ | 3 months\*| ☐ | ☐ |
| Pupil              | ☐ | ☐ | 6 months\*| ☐ | ☐ |
| IOL                | ☐ | ☐ | Yearly\* | ☐ | ☐ |
| Capsule            | ☐ | ☐ | _____  | ☐ | ☐ |
| Fundus             | ☐ | ☐ | _____  | ☐ | ☐ |
| Visual fields      | ☐ | ☐ |          |   |   |
| Motility           | ☐ | ☐ | \* Dilation for YAG—1 wk, 3 mo |
| Lid position       | ☐ | ☐ | \* Dilation for Cataract—5 wk, 6 mo, 1 yr |

REMARKABLE FINDINGS: _____

PLAN/ADVISE TO PATIENT: _____

MEDICATION: _____

QUESTIONS TO SURGEON: _____

_____

_____, O.D./M.D.
Please print or write legibly

---

\* Pacific Cataract and Laser Institute

# APPENDIX 4

## Professional Correspondence

### Example of Letter from Doctor of Optometry to Surgery Center, Requesting Evaluation of Patient with Cataracts

**To:** Dr. M.D.

**Date:** July 9, 1994

**Patient Name:** A.F.

**Exam Date:** May 6, 1994

**Chief Complaint:** Blurred vision OU

**Patient Profile:** 77-year-old white female, retired

**Fields:** Each eye is full on the Synemed automated perimeter.

**EOM:** Versions and vergences were full.

**Pupils:** Each eye reacts normally to light both direct and consensually. There is no Marcus-Gunn pupil.

**Biomicroscopy:** Lids, lashes, conjunctiva and cornea were clear. Anterior chambers were normal depth with no cells or flare. Angles appear open, irides are blue, flat, and form round pupils. Lenses exhibit cataracts OU. Vitreous is clear.

**Tensions:** Appl 18/18

**Ophthalmoscopy:** Posterior poles are unremarkable with sharp foveal reflexes and apparently normal cup/disk ratio. Peripheral retinas were unremarkable.

**Consultation:** Cataract consultation July 20, 1994, with Dr. M.D.

### Example of Letter from Surgery Center to Referring Doctor of Optometry, Concerning Patient with Cataracts

July 22, 1994

Re: A.F.
Date of Exam: 7-20-94

Dear O.D.:

Thank you for referring A.F. to our clinic for an evaluation of cataracts. The following is a summary of our exam:

**Subjective:** Patient complains of difficulty with a gradual increase of fuzzy vision and trouble with night driving, glare, and halos. Ocular and medical histories are unremarkable.

**Objective**

| Visual Acuity: | Contrast testing: | Potential acuity: |
|---|---|---|
| OD   20/30-1 | OD   20/200 | OD   20/20-3 |
| OS   20/40-1 | OS   20/200 | OS   20/25-3 |

IOP by NCT: 18 OD, 20 OS
Pupils: Without afferent pupillary defect OU
Slit lamp evaluation: Clear and quiet OU
Lens:   **OD** 2-3+ NS, 2+ CS and trace PSC   **OS** 3+ NS, 2+ CS and trace PSC

Vitreous: PVD OD

Dilated fundus examination: Cup/disk ratio of 0.4 OD and 0.5 OS with normal retinal vessels, macula and periphery OU

**Assessment**
1. Cataracts OU, OS>OD
2. PVD OD

**Plan**
1. Following a discussion of pros/cons of cataract surgery including potential risks, benefits and complications, A.F. elected to proceed with cataract extraction for her left eye. Surgery was scheduled.

Again, thank you for referring this patient to our office. If you have any questions do not hesitate to call.

Sincerely,

## Cataract Work-up

Name: _____ Date: _____

Chart # _____ Age _____ City, State _____

**Ref. Dr:** _____ **Family Dr:** _____

**Complaints:** READING/DRIVING/DISTANCE/GLARE/HALOS

_____

_____

Hx of cataracts: _____

**Ocular Hx:** GLC/ARMD/CAT/AMB/CXE/INJ

_____

**Ocular Surgeries** _____

_____

**Medical Hx:** DIA/HBP/KID/ASTHMA/LUNG/HRT

**Meds:** Ocular _____
**Meds:** Systemic _____

_____

**Allergies** _____

                              OD                      OS

**Present Glasses:** _____   _____

**Visual Acuity** w/c wo/c      20/_____ J _____  20/_____ J _____

**Glare**/contrast acuity:        20/_____  20/_____

**Refraction:**                   20/_____  20/_____

**Potential acuity** w/c wo/c w/tf 20/_____  20/_____

**Intraocular Pressure** (AIR/APP) _____ _____

**Pupils:** _____ NMG _____ Size _____ / _____ M & N: O _____ @ _____

**Motility:** WNL _____ OU  OD _____ OS _____

**CVF:** _____

**ECC** Readings:     OD _____ OS _____

**K-Readings:**                                  OD        OS

                                            AL _____ _____

                                           SRK _____ _____

                                             _____ _____

                                         PLAN _____ _____

## Cataract Work-up (Continued)

Date _____  Name _____

|  OD  |  OS  |
|---|---|

L/L _____  _____
&AD: _____  _____
C: _____  _____
AC: _____  _____
Iris: _____  _____
Lens: NS _____ CS ____ PSC _____   NS _____ CS _____ PSC _____
_____  _____

V: _____  _____
C/D: _____  _____
_____  _____
Vessels: _____  _____
M: _____  _____
_____  _____

P: _____ W/BIO _____   _____ W/BIO _____

No additional finding affecting VA ☐   No additional finding affecting VA ☐
Impression: _____
_____
Cataract surgery indicated OD ☐ OS ☐ _____
Pros/cons of cataract surgery discussed by doctor including potential risks, benefits and complications ☐
Potential limitations of vision due to _____ discussed ☐
Follow-up with doctor and schedule discussed ☐ Refraction by: _____
Discussion: _____
_____
_____
_____

Plan: _____

Ins. Counselor _____
_____ O.D. _____ M.D.   First Eye _____
Second Eye _____

☐ Second eye scheduled _____

## APPENDIX 5

## Example of Verbal Preoperative Instructions to the Patient

An example of patient counseling might go like this: "You've been found to have a cataract that is significantly affecting your ability to do the things you wish to do. A cataract is a clouding of the natural lens that sits behind the pupil. It is a normal change that happens to everyone. When this cloudy lens affects your ability to do the things you wish to do, it may be removed by surgery. Another alternative would be to not remove the cataract if you feel that you can function with your vision as it is. Removing the cataract is not an emergency; it is not like heart or any surgery that must be performed to save your life. The cataract, actually, is not damaging the eye by being there, it is merely obstructing your vision. In making this decision as to whether or not to have surgery, we have to remind you that all surgeries have their risks. In cataract surgery, there is a risk of 1 in 5000 of having a serious complication such as bleeding or infection that might leave your vision worse.[1] There is a 1% to 2% chance of having some minor problem following surgery that may need to be treated with some type of medication, extra visits, laser, or additional surgery.[2]

"As in any surgery, your best results will be obtained from the surgeon with the most experience. Therefore, I am recommending doctors: _____, _____, and _____. They are located at _____. If you decide to have the surgery, this is what you can expect:

- You should eat normally and dress comfortably.
- You will be at the surgery center for about 3 hours total. The surgery itself will take 10–15 minutes.
- When you walk in, your clothes, head, and feet will be covered and the side of your face will be numbed for the surgery.
- An opening will be made that is about an eighth to one quarter inch in size. Through that opening, an instrument will be inserted that will vibrate with sound waves (ultrasound). It will liquefy, then vacuum away the cataract. A small lens implant will be placed in the eye to give the eye its focus back. Following that, because of the technique used, the opening made for the surgery will self-seal. This is called no-stitch surgery.
- Your eye will be patched and you'll remove this patch before bedtime and you'll be checked the following day.
- Your follow-up will include several check-ups—usually, 1 week later, 3 weeks later, and 5 weeks later following surgery. Sometime after 5 or 6 weeks, you'll be able to get a new lens for your glasses. You will still need to wear glasses afterwards, and they'll probably be similar to what you are wearing (eg, bifocals, trifocals).

You've also been found to have _____ problem and this will place some limitation on your vision. The treatment for this problem is _____, and we will do this before/after the cataract removal."

## REFERENCES

1. Pacific Cataract and Laser Institute.
2. Revicki DA, Brown RE, Adler MA: Patient outcomes with comanaged postoperative care after cataract surgery. *J Clin Epidemiol.* 1993;**46**:5–15.

## APPENDIX 6

## Informed Consent for Cataract Extraction with Posterior Chamber Intraocular Lens*

### Patient Statement

The basic procedure for cataract surgery and its advantages, disadvantages, risks, possible complications, alternative treatments and the follow-up care options have been explained to me. Although it is impossible to inform me of every possible complication which may occur, all my questions have been answered to my satisfaction.

I give permission for medical data concerning my operation and subsequent treatment to be submitted to the lens manufacturer and to the FDA for clinical study.

I have read the four pages of this informed consent or it has been read to me. I fully understand the possible risks, complications and benefits that may result from the surgery.

Patient's Name (printed) _____

1. I wish to have a cataract extraction with an intraocular lens implanation on my RIGHT / LEFT eye.
2. Since my cataract was previously removed and I have been informed by my doctor that my eye is medically acceptable for lens implantation, I wish to receive an intraocular lens implant on my RIGHT / LEFT eye.
3. ☐ I elect to be seen for follow-up care by the doctors at PCLI for approximately 4 weeks after surgery. I understand that I will then be referred to the Doctor of Optometry whom I choose for my continued follow-up care and prescription of new glasses.
4. ☐ I elect to return to a Doctor of Optometry for follow-up care immediately after my 1-day postoperative examination at PCLI. I understand that my doctor will remain in close contact with the doctors at PCLI regarding my recovery, and that I may contact PCLI doctors at any time with questions or concerns. Please schedule my additional post-operative visits with Dr. _____.

Patient's Signature _____
Legally Responsible Person _____
relationship
Date _____ Time _____ Place _____

Witness' Signature _____
Doctor's Signature _____

### Informed Consent for Cataract Operation, and/or Implantation of Intraocular Lens

#### Introduction

This information is given to you so that you can make an informed decision about having eye surgery. Take as much time as you wish to make your decision about signing this informed consent. You have the right to ask questions about any procedure before agreeing to have the operation.

After your doctor has told you that you have a cataract, you and your doctor are the only ones who can determine if or when you should have a cataract operation . . . based on your own visual needs and medical consideration.

---

* Pacific Cataract and Laser Institute

Except for unusual problems, a cataract operation is indicated only when you cannot function adequately due to poor sight produced by the cataract. You must remember that the natural lens within your own eye even with a slight cataract, although not perfect, has some distinct advantages over any man-made lens.

## *Alternative Treatments*

I understand that I may decline to have a cataract operation at all. However, should I decide to have an operation, I understand that these are the three methods of restoring useful vision after the operation:

1. **Intraocular Lens.** This is a small plastic artificial lens surgically placed inside the eye. It is intended to be permanent. With the intraocular lens, there is no apparent change in the size of the object seen. Conventional eyeglasses with bifocals (not cataract spectacles) are usually required in addition to an intraocular lens. Intraocular lenses are presently the most common method of correcting vision after cataract surgery.
2. **Spectacles (Glasses).** Cataract spectacles required to correct your vision are usually thicker and heavier than conventional eyeglasses. Cataract spectacles increase the size of objects by about 25%, and clear vision is obtained only through the central part of cataract spectacles, which means you must learn to turn your head to see clearly on either side. Cataract spectacles usually cannot be used if a cataract is removed from only one eye (and the other is normal) because they may cause double vision.
3. **Contact Lens.** A hard or soft contact lens increases the apparent size of objects only about 8%. Handling of a contact lens is difficult for some individuals, and not everyone can tolerate them. For near tasks, reading glasses (not cataract spectacles) will be required in addition to contact lenses.

## *Consent for Operation*

In giving my permission for cataract extraction and/or possible implantation in my eye of an intraocular lens, I declare that I understand the following information:

1. Cataract surgery, by itself, means removal of the natural lens of the eye by a surgical technique. In order for an intraocular lens to be implanted in my eye, I understand that cataract surgery must first be done.
2. If an intraocular lens is implanted, it is done by surgical method. It is intended that the small plastic lens will remain permanently in my eye.
3. My doctor may include, as part of the procedure, surgical treatment of astigmatism (an imperfection in the shape of my eye) by modifying the incision or by making additional incisions.
4. The results of surgery in my case cannot be guaranteed.
5. At the time of surgery, my doctor may decide **not** to implant an intraocular lens in my eye even though I may have given prior permission to do so.
6. Complications of Surgery to Remove the Cataract: As a result of the surgery, it is possible that my vision could be made worse. In some cases, complications may occur weeks, months, or even years later. Complications may include hemorrhage (bleeding), loss of corneal clarity, infection, detachment of the retina, glaucoma, and/or double vision. These and other complications may occur whether or not a lens is implanted and may result in poor vision, total loss of vision, or loss of the eye.

7. Specific Complications of Lens Implantation: Insertion of an intraocular lens may induce complications which otherwise would not occur. In some cases, complications may develop weeks, months or even years later. Complications may include, but are not limited to, loss of corneal clarity, infection, uveitis, iris atrophy, glaucoma, bleeding in the eye, inability to dilate the pupil, dislocation of the lens and retinal detachment.
8. At some future time, the lens implanted in my eye may have to be repositioned or removed surgically.
9. Complications of Surgery in General: As with **all** types of surgery, there is the possibility of other complications due to anesthesia, drug reactions or other factors which may involve other parts of my body, including a possibility of brain damage or even death. Since it is impossible to state every complication that may occur as a result of surgery, the list of complications in this form is incomplete.

## *Follow-up Care*

On the day after surgery, my eye will be examined by one of the doctors at PCLI. The remainder of my follow-up care will be arranged for me by PCLI. I may choose one of the following options:

1. I may be seen for some of my additional follow-up care at the PCLI facility which is most convenient for me. After approximately 4 weeks, I will be referred to the Doctor of Optometry I choose. I will then be seen by this doctor for the remainder of my 90-day postoperative period and for the fitting of my new glasses. The doctors at PCLI and my doctor will maintain close communication regarding my recovery and progress. If any complications should develop, I will be cared for in the most appropriate manner determined by all doctors involved.

or

2. After I am examined at PCLI on the day after surgery, I will return to the Doctor of Optometry I choose for my additional follow-up care. I will be seen by this doctor for the remainder of my 90-day postoperative period and for the fitting of my new glasses. The doctors at PCLI and my doctor will maintain close communication regarding my recovery and progress. If any complications should develop, I will be cared for in the most appropriate manner determined by all doctors involved.

I understand that a Doctor of Optometry is not a medical doctor, but is trained and licensed to perform specific postsurgical care procedures including those which would be required for my follow-up care after cataract surgery. Any conditions requiring further specialty care will be referred back to Pacific Cataract and Laser Institute.

I understand that doctors at Pacific Cataract and Laser Institute are available 24 hours a day, 7 days a week for consultation and that they will see me should any questions arise that need their expertise. I may call anytime with questions or concerns.

# APPENDIX 7

## Postoperative Instructions to the Patient*

For the next 24 hours your eyes require little care.

### *Activity*
You may bend over, sleep on either side, read, watch TV, go out to dinner, or whatever you feel like doing.

### *Medication*
Cephalexin, 250 mg (antibiotic)

- Take one capsule at bedtime
- Take one capsule tomorrow at 8:00 AM, 12:00 noon, 4:00 PM and 8:00 PM

If you have minor discomfort, you may take Tylenol, aspirin, Advil, or whatever you normally take for headache. Take your regular medication as ordered.

### *Pain*
Scratchy feeling or itching is of little concern, but should you experience severe pain and loss of the vision you have, please call immediately: 1-800-888-9903 toll free (number is answered 24 hours)

### *Remove Your Patch Tonight Before Bed*
You may experience blurry or double vision after removing the patch. Do not be alarmed. Vision will often be variable or even poor for a few days as a normal part of the healing process.

You may shower and shampoo and wash around your eye.

## If You Have a Problem

Please call the PCLI Center nearest you. Telephones are answered 24 hours a day.

| | |
|---|---|
| Bellevue, WA | Lewiston, ID |
| (206) 462-7664 | (208) 746-2025 |
| 1 800 926-3007 | 1 800 926-3008 |
| La Grande, OR | Kennewick, WA |
| (503) 963-9093 | (509) 736-0826 |
| 1 800 926-3009 | 1 800 888-9904 |
| Chehalis, WA | Tacoma, WA |
| (206) 748-8632 | (206) 756-9440 |
| 1 800 888-9903 | 1 800 888-9905 |

---

* Pacific Cataract and Laser Institute

## APPENDIX 8

## Nd: YAG Informed Consent and Postoperative Instructions*

### Explanation of the Procedure

Prior to cataract surgery a thin transparent membrane, called the capsule, surrounds the cataract. During cataract removal the surgeon leaves most of this membrane in place and inserts the intraocular lens inside the membrane. Many of these membranes will become cloudy with time and blur the vision. The YAG laser is used to create an opening in the cloudy membrane to clear the image. This opening is called a capsulotomy.

### Alternatives (to a YAG capsulotomy)

1. Conventional eye surgery can also create an opening in the cloudy membrane, but this requires local anesthesia and is riskier than laser treatment.
2. No treatment is an alternative for an early cloudy membrane, however, the cloudier the membrane becomes, the more laser energy is required, increasing risk.

### Risks and Complications

The following may occur after a YAG capsulotomy:

1. Retinal detachment
2. Retinal swelling
3. Elevated eye pressure
4. Floaters
5. Pitting of the implant

### Benefits

The YAG capsulotomy procedure in most cases restores the vision which has been lost due to the formation of the cloudy membrane, however, in some instances refinement of spectacle correction may be needed.

### Warning Signs

If you should notice any of the following, please contact your doctor for an examination:

1. Flashing lights
2. Black shadow or curtain in vision you can't see through
3. Increase in floaters
4. Blurry vision
5. Pain

### Consent

I understand that there is no guarantee of improvement in vision. Also, I have read the above and understand the procedure and its potential complications and consent to have Dr. _____ perform this procedure on my right / left eye.

SIGNATURE: _____
DATE: _____
WITNESS: _____

*Pacific Cataract and Laser Institute

Discharge instructions given to.  ( ) PATIENT   ( ) FAMILY
Discharged to: _____
Tech/Writer: _____

## YAG Capsulotomy Postoperative Instructions

*Patient Name:*_____
*Date:* _____

If you notice any of the following, please contact your doctor for an examination:

1. Flashing lights
2. Black shadow or curtain in vision you can't see through
3. Increase in floaters
4. Blurry vision
5. Pain

| PACIFIC CATARACT & LASER INSTITUTE: 1-800-926-3007 or 462-7664 (24 HOURS A DAY) |
|---|

REFERRING DOCTOR OF OPTOMETRY:_____
            PHONE NUMBER:_____

# Index

## A

Abbreviations, standard, 240–245
Acetazolamide, 71
    for choroidal detachment, 180–181
    for ocular hypertension, 126, 129, 132, 138, 170
Activity, postoperative, 238, 254
Adrenaline. *See* Epinephrine
AION. *See* Anterior ischemic optic neuropathy
AK. *See* Astigmatic keratotomy
Akinesia, prolonged, postoperative, 160
Alphachymotrypsin, injection, for intracapsular cataract extraction, 88
Altitudinal field loss, due to ischemic optic neuropathy, 183, 184f
Ambulatory surgery center, 3, 71
American Optometric Association, co-managed care study, 6–7
Amsler grid, 48
ANA test. *See* Antinuclear antibody test
Anesthesia, 71f, 71–72. *See also specific block*
    myotoxicity from, strabismus caused by, 194
Angiography, fluorescein
    of cystoid macular edema, 216, 218, 218t, 219f
    for preoperative evaluation, 48
Aniseikonia, refractive, 226

Anisometropia, postoperative, 226
    treatment of, 226–227, 227t
Anterior capsular contraction, 211, 211f
Anterior chamber
    examination of, postoperative, 116–117, 119, 121–122
    shallow or flat
        reformation of, 137–138
        wound leaks with, 134t, 134–138
            clinical presentation and assessment of, 135f–136f, 135–137
            differential diagnosis of, 137
            treatment of, 137–138, 138t
    well-formed, wound leak with, 160–162
        clinical presentation and assessment of, 160–161, 161f
        differential diagnosis of, 161
        treatment, follow-up, and prognosis, 162, 162t
Anterior chamber cells, grading system for, 24, 24t, 25f
Anterior chamber flare
    grading system for, 24, 26t, 26f–27f
    postoperative, 116, 119, 121
Anterior chamber intraocular lens(es)
    early, 62f, 62–63
    examination of, postoperative, 127–128
    explanation of, 99, 100f
    modern, 64–66, 65f
        characteristics of, 65, 66t
    secondary, implantation of, 95–98, 97f

        advantages and disadvantages of, 98
        complications of, 98
        preoperative examination for, 53f, 53–54, 95–96
        vitrectomy prior to, 96f, 96–97
Anterior chamber reaction, 24
Anterior ischemic optic neuropathy, 181–186
    arteritic form of, 183, 184f
        treatment of, 185, 185t
    clinical presentation and assessment of, 182–183, 182t–183t, 183f–184f
    differential diagnosis of, 185
    etiology of, 181
    incidence of, 181–182
    nonarteritic form of, 183, 183f
        treatment of, 185t
    risk factors for, 182
    treatment, follow-up, and prognosis, 185t, 185–186
Anterior segment examination, preoperative, 45–46
Antibiotics, 91, 118. *See also specific drug*
    for hyphema, 169
    for infectious endophthalmitis, 142
    for wound leak, 162
Anticoagulants, risk of postoperative hyphema with, 166–167
Antiglaucoma therapy
    for chronic corneal edema, 204
    for ocular hypertension, with hyphema, 170

---

Page numbers followed by *t* and *f* indicate tables and figures, respectively.

Antiglaucoma therapy (cont.)
  for open angle glaucoma, 197
  for uveitis, 176
Anti-inflammatory agents. See also specific drug
  postoperative use of, 118
Antinuclear antibody test, with anterior ischemic optic neuropathy, 183
Aphakia, postoperative, 227
Aphakic eye, secondary lens implantation in, 97f, 97–98
  vitrectomy prior to, 96f, 96–97
Aphakic spectacles, versus secondary intraocular lens implantation, 98
Applanation tonometer, for postoperative screening, 128, 136
Apraclonidine
  for acute corneal edema, 165
  for ocular hypertension, 129
    with hyphema, 170
    with laser capsulotomy, 214–215
ASC. See Ambulatory surgery center
A-scan ultrasonography, 39, 39f, 48
Aspirin, risk of postoperative hyphema with, 166–167
Astigmatic keratotomy, 91, 225, 226f, 226t
Astigmatism
  induced, and incision closure, 89–90, 123
  postoperative, 225–226
    due to malpositioned intraocular lens, 228
    irregular, diagnosis of, 225–226
    management of, 225, 225f–226f, 226t
Atrophy, iris, 46, 47f
Atropine, for choroidal detachment, 180

## B

Balanced salt solution
  capsulorhexis with, 77
  hydrodissection with, 87
  intraocular lens implantation with, 80, 97
Bar grids, for contrast sensitivity, 36
Baron, André, 62
Basement membrane, embryology of, 13
BAT. See Brightness Acuity Tester
Batelle Human Affairs Research Centers, comanaged care study, 6–7
Beta-blockers
  for acute corneal edema, 164–165
  dosage and administration, 91
  for ocular hypertension, 128–129, 132–133
    with hyphema, 170
    with laser capsulotomy, 214
  for open angle glaucoma, 197
  for UGH syndrome, 199, 209
Betamethasone, for cystoid macular edema, 221
Betaxolol (Betagan), 91

Binkhorst, C. D., 64
Binkhorst formulas, 39
Binkhorst intraocular lenses
  iridocapsular, 63, 64f
  iris-fixated, 63
Binocular diplopia, 192
Binocularity, preoperative evaluation of, 45
Biomicroscopy, postoperative
  at first visit, 115t, 115–118, 116f–117f
  at second visit, 119–120, 120f
  at third and fourth visits, 122
Blue field entoptic phenomena, 38–39
Bridle sutures, 193, 193f
  complications of, 193
Brightness Acuity Tester, 35, 36f
B-scan ultrasonography, 39–40, 48
BSS. See Balanced salt solution

## C

CAIs. See Carbonic anhydrase inhibitors
Canthotomy, lateral, for retrobulbar hemorrhage, 106, 106f
Capsular bag
  intraocular lens placement in, 66, 80, 84f–85f, 87, 101
  posterior chamber intraocular lens in, 148, 148f
  rupture of, during phacoemulsification, 107, 108f, 128
    cystoid macular edema with, 220–221, 220f–221f
Capsular debris, in anterior chamber, postoperative, 116
Capsulorhexis, 5
  nuclear expression with, 86
  phacoemulsification with, 79
    with trabeculectomy and intraocular lens implantation, 100–101
  technique for, 77–78, 78f–79f
Capsulotomy
  can-opener, 5, 78–79, 86, 87f
    intraocular lens dislocation with, 148
  continuous-tear, 5
    instrumentation, 73–74
    phacoemulsification with, 79
      with trabeculectomy and intraocular lens implantation, 101
    technique for, 77, 78f
  posterior, by Nd:YAG laser
    complications of, 214–215
    for endocapsular hematoma, 171, 172f
    informed consent and postoperative instructions for, 256–257
    for opacification, 213–215, 214f–216f
    retinal detachment with, 223
Carbonic anhydrase inhibitors, 91, 133
  for acute corneal edema, 165
  for choroidal detachment, 180–181
  for ocular hypertension, 214

  for UGH syndrome, 199, 209
  for uveitis, 177
Case conclusion, 91–93
Cataract(s). See also specific type
  age-related, 14
  definition of, 14
    for patient, 237
  grading of, 18–24, 21f
  hereditary factors influencing, 14
  prevalence of, 3
  symptoms of, description of, to patient, 237
Cataract care, 3, 4t
  history of, 3–5
  outcome
    definition of, 6
    factors influencing, 6t, 6–7
  trends in, 3–8
Cataract extraction. See also Extracapsular cataract extraction; Intracapsular cataract extraction
  combined procedures for, 99–102
  description of, to patient, 237
  without intraocular lens, 98–99
Cataractogenesis, 14–16, 14f–16f
  description of, to patient, 237
Cataract work-up, 249–250
CBC. See Complete blood count
Celestone Soluspan. See Betamethasone
Cephalexin
  dosage and administration, 71, 91–93, 118, 238, 254
  for wound leak, 162
Choroidal detachment, 179–181, 180f
  classification of, 179
  clinical presentation and assessment of, 180
  differential diagnosis of, 180
  treatment, follow-up, and prognosis, 180–181, 181t
Choroidal hemorrhage, intraoperative, 107
Choyce, Peter, 63
Ciliary sulcus, intraocular lens fixation at, 66
Ciprofloxacin (Ciloxan), prophylactic use of, for wound leak, 162
CME. See Cystoid macular edema
Comanagement, 9–12
  definition of, 9
  medicolegal responsibilities in, 10
  studies of, 5–7
Communication
  in comanaged care, 10–12
  doctor-to-doctor, 10–12
    aids for, 246–247
  patient, 10–11
    aids for, 237–239
Complete blood count, with anterior ischemic optic neuropathy, 183
Complications. See also specific complication
  intraoperative, 105–109

*Page numbers followed by t and f indicate tables and figures, respectively.*

postoperative
　　early (1–14 days)
　　　　emergent, 125–158
　　　　less emergent, 159–188
　　　　intermediate to late, 189–234
Congenital lens dislocations, 103, 103f
Conjunctival edema, postoperative, 115, 120
Conjunctival injection, postoperative, 115, 117, 120, 122, 126
Conjunctival replacement, over self-sealing incision, 81, 85f
Consultation, definition of, 9
Contact lenses
　　for anisometropia, 227
　　for aphakia, 227
　　hard, central corneal clouding with, 18
　　soft, postoperative use of, 118
Continuous suturing, 90, 91f
Contrast, definition of, 36
Contrast sensitivity testing, 36
　　for preoperative evaluation, 45
Copeland intraocular lenses, 63
Cornea, examination of
　　postoperative, 115, 116f, 119, 120f, 121, 121f
　　preoperative, 45–46, 46f
Cornea guttata, 18, 20f, 46f
　　endothelial cell counts in, 40
　　phacoemulsification for, duration of, 79, 81–82
　　preoperative evaluation of, 57, 57t
Corneal abrasion, postoperative, 115, 117f
　　treatment of, 118
Corneal bullae, 19f
Corneal clouding, central, 18
Corneal decompensation, 202–205
　　clinical presentation and assessment of, 203
　　differential diagnosis of, 203–204
　　etiologies of, 200, 200t
　　pathogenesis of, 202, 202t
　　treatment, follow-up, and prognosis, 204t, 204–205
Corneal disease, and preoperative cataract examination, 48, 49t
Corneal edema, 18, 20f
　　acute, 162–163
　　　　clinical presentation and assessment of, 163, 163f–164f
　　　　differential diagnosis of, 164
　　　　etiology of, 162–163
　　　　treatment, follow-up, and prognosis, 164–165, 165t
　　chronic, 202–205
　　　　clinical presentation and assessment of, 203
　　　　differential diagnosis of, 203–204
　　　　etiologies of, 200, 200t
　　　　pathogenesis of, 202, 202t
　　　　treatment, follow-up, and prognosis, 204t, 204–205
　　microcystic, 19f
　　postoperative, 115, 126, 127f
Corneal endothelium, damage to, with phacoemulsification, 79, 81

Corneal findings, clinical, grading system for, 18, 18t
Corneal flap, sutureless wound with, 91, 92f
Corneal striae, 19f
Cortex, 14, 14f
　　retained, 206–207, 207f
　　　　trapped behind intraocular lens, 212, 213f
Cortical cataract
　　formation of, 14–15, 14f–16f
　　grading of, 18–24, 21f–23f
Cortical clefts, 15, 15f
Cortical fragments
　　in anterior chamber, postoperative, 116
　　residual, after phacoemulsification, removal of, 80, 81f
Cortical lamellar separations, 15, 16f
Cortical spokes, 15, 15f
Cortical vacuoles, 15, 15f
Cortical wedges, 14f, 15
Corticosteroids. See also specific drug
　　for chronic iritis, 209
　　for ocular hypertension, 129
　　prophylactic use of, for cystoid macular edema, 217
　　for uveitis, 176
Coumadin. See Warfarin
Counseling
　　postoperative, 118, 120, 122–124
　　preoperative, 49–50, 69, 70f, 251
　　for iritis patients, 173
Cyclopentolate, 70
Cycloplegic agents, 118, 133
　　for choroidal detachment, 180
　　for chronic iritis, 209
　　for uveitis, 176
Cystoid macular edema, 215–222
　　clinical, versus angiographic, 216
　　clinical presentation and assessment of, 218, 218t, 219f
　　differential diagnosis of, 219–220
　　epidemiology of, 216–217
　　etiology of, 217
　　with posterior capsular rupture, treatment of, 220–221, 220f–221f, 221t
　　and preoperative cataract evaluation, 48
　　prophylaxis, 217–218
　　with pseudophakic bullous keratopathy, 204–205
　　risk of, with vitreous to wound, 145
　　treatment, follow-up, and prognosis, 220–222, 221t–222t
Cystotome, for capsulotomy, 74

# D

Dacron sutures, 90
Dapiprazole, 132
Descemet's membrane, detachment of, intraoperative, 108, 108f
Descemet's membrane, folds in, postoperative, 115, 163, 164f

Dexamethasone
　　dosage and administration, 91, 118
　　open angle glaucoma induced by, 196t, 196–198
Diabetic retinopathy, patient with, postoperative hyphema in, 171
Diabetic sixth nerve palsy, 193
Diamond blade, 73
Diamox. See Acetazolamide
Diazepam, 71
Diclofenac
　　for cystoid macular edema, 222
　　dosage and administration, 118, 129–130
　　for ocular hypertension, 129–130
Dilated fundus examination, postoperative, 120–122, 128, 153
Diplopia, 114, 160, 192–195, 228
　　binocular, 192
　　classification of, 160, 192
　　clinical presentation and assessment of, 160, 194–195
　　differential diagnosis of, 160, 195
　　monocular, 192
　　preexisting conditions manifesting as, 192–193
　　treatment, follow-up, and prognosis, 160, 195, 195t, 228
Doctor-to-doctor communication, 10–12
　　aids for, 246–247

# E

ECCE. See Extracapsular cataract extraction
Ecchymosis, postoperative, 115
Edema. See also Corneal edema; Cystoid macular edema
　　conjunctival, 115
　　stromal, 18
Elschnig pearls, 211, 212f
Endocapsular hematoma, with hyphema, 171, 171f–172f
Endophthalmitis, 138–142
　　clinical presentation and assessment of, 139–141, 140f–141f, 207–208
　　delayed-onset, 139–140
　　differential diagnosis of, 142
　　etiology of, 139, 140t, 208
　　incidence of, 138–139
　　phacoanaphylactic, 173
　　treatment, follow-up, and prognosis, 142, 142t, 143f
Endothelial cell counts, 40, 40f
Endothelial damage
　　intraoperative, 79, 81, 202
　　postoperative, 203
Entoptic phenomena testing, 38–39
　　for preoperative evaluation, 48
Epinephrine, administration of, with local anesthesia, 71
Epithelial downgrowth, 201–202
Erythrocyte sedimentation rate (ESR), 183
Explantation, of intraocular lenses, 99, 100f
　　in UGH syndrome, 200

Extracapsular cataract extraction, 4–5, 75
  by nuclear expression, 86–87, 86f–88f
    advantages and disadvantages of, 83t, 87
    opening incision for, 77
  with penetrating keratoplasty and intraocular lens implantation, 101–102, 102f
  phacoanaphylactic endophthalmitis after, 173
  by phacoemulsification, 77–85, 80f
    advantages and disadvantages of, 81–82, 83t
  posterior capsular opacification after, 210
  retinal break/detachment after, incidence of, 151, 153t
  with trabeculectomy and intraocular lens implantation, 100f, 100–101
Eye, softening of, preoperative, 72f, 72–73
Eye disease, coexisting. See also specific disease
  preoperative examination with, 48, 49t, 55–58

## F

Facial block, 72
FDA. See Food and Drug Administration
Fibrinoid membranes
  in iritis, 173, 174f
  in uveitis, 175, 175f
Fluorescein, wound examination with, 117, 136–137, 137f, 160
Fluorescein angiography
  of cystoid macular edema, 216, 218, 218t, 219f
  for preoperative evaluation, 48
Fluorometholone
  for chronic iritis, 209
  open angle glaucoma induced by, 196t, 196–198
Fluoroquinolones, prophylactic use of, for wound leak, 162
Flurbiprofen, 197
Flying corpuscle test, 38–39
Food and Drug Administration, CORE study, 7
Fresnel prism spectacles, for diplopia, 195
Frown incision, 76f
Fuchs' dystrophy. See Cornea guttata
Fundus, examination of
  postoperative, 120–122, 128
  for retinal break/detachment, 153
  in uveitis, 175

## G

Ghost cell glaucoma, 171
Glare, with malpositioned intraocular lens, 228

Glare testing, 35–36
  for preoperative evaluation, 45
Glaucoma, 195–202
  closed angle, 200–202
    etiologies of, 200, 200t
  ghost cell, 171
  malignant, 132–133, 133f
    clinical presentation and assessment of, 132–133
    differential diagnosis of, 133
    treatment and prognosis, 133
  open angle, 196–198
    chronic, preoperative evaluation of, 57, 57t
    steroid-induced, 196t, 196–198
      clinical presentation and assessment of, 197
      treatment, follow-up, and prognosis, 197t, 197–198
  patient with
    postoperative ocular hypertension in, 125
    treatment of, 129
    preoperative examination of, 48, 49t
Glaukomflecken, 46
Globe, pressure on, after local anesthesia, 72f, 72–73
Goldmann applanation tonometer, for postoperative screening, 128, 136
Grading system, 17–31
  for anterior chamber cells, 24, 24t, 25f
  for anterior chamber flare, 24, 26t, 26f–27f
  for cataracts, 18–24, 21f
  conventional, 17t, 17–18
  for corneal findings, 18, 18t
  for hyphema, 28, 28f
  for hypopyon, 24–28, 27f
  for posterior capsule opacification, 29, 29t, 29f–30f
Gram-negative species, endophthalmitis caused by, 139–140, 140t

## H

Healon, 138
Hematoma, endocapsular, with hyphema, 171, 171f–172f
Hemorrhage
  choroidal, intraoperative, 107
  retrobulbar, intraoperative, 105–107, 106f
  subconjunctival, postoperative, 115
  vitreous, postoperative, 170–171
Holladay formula, 39
Homatropine, for uveitis, 176
Honan balloon, 72
Horror fusionis, 193
Hyaluronidase, administration of, with local anesthesia, 71
Hydrodissection, 87
Hypermature cataract, 23f

Hyperosmotic agents
  for chronic corneal edema, 204
  for ocular hypertension, 129, 132–133
Hyphema, 116
  clot, 167–168, 168f
  diffuse, 167, 168f
  early, 126, 128f, 165–172
    clinical presentation and assessment of, 167–169, 169f
    complications of, 170t, 170–172
    differential diagnosis of, 169
    incidence of, 165
    prophylactic measures against, 166–167
    risk factors for, 165–166
    treatment, follow-up, and prognosis, 169t, 169–172
  eightball, 28, 28f, 167–168, 168f
    complications of, 170
  and glaucoma, postoperative, 126
  grading system for, 28, 28f
  late, 205
  layered, 167, 168f
Hypopyon
  definition of, 24
  grading of, 24, 27f
  postoperative, 116
  in uveitis, 174

## I

ICCE. See Intracapsular cataract extraction
Incision
  auxiliary, depression of, for ocular hypertension, 129
  closure of, 81, 89–91, 90f–92f
  for intracapsular cataract extraction, 88, 89f
  lateral, 76
  limbal, 76
    closure of, 89–90, 90f
    glaucoma with, postoperative, 126
  opening, 75–77, 76f
    for nuclear expression, 86, 86f
  posterior, 76
  scleral, 76–77
    closure of, 90–91, 91f–92f
  for secondary implantation, 96
  self-sealing, 73, 76f, 77
    closure of, 81, 85f, 91, 92f
  description of, to patient, 237
  superior, 76
Indirect ophthalmoscopy, diagnosis of retinal break/detachment with, 153
Indomethacin, prophylactic use of, for cystoid macular edema, 218
Inflammatory reactions, associated with mechanical effects of intraocular lens, 173
Informed consent, 252–254
  for Nd:YAG laser capsulotomy, 256–257

Instrumentation *See also specific instrument*
  special, 35–41
  surgical, 73–74, 74f
Interferometry, 37
  for preoperative evaluation, 48
Interrupted sutures, 89, 90f
Intracapsular cataract extraction, 4, 75
  disadvantages of, 89
  for dislocated lens, 103
  retinal break/detachment after, incidence of, 151, 153t
  technique of, 88–89, 89f
  for traumatic cataract, 102f, 102–103
Intraocular lens(es), 5. *See also* Anterior chamber intraocular lens(es); Posterior chamber intraocular lens(es)
  cataract extraction without, 98–99
  decentration of, 54, 146, 147f, 148–149, 177f, 177–179
    clinical presentation and assessment of, 178
    differential diagnosis of, 178
    with opacification, 211–212
    refractive errors caused by, 228
    risk factors for, 177f, 177–179
    treatment, follow-up, and prognosis, 178–179, 179t
  dislocation of, 54, 146–151
    clinical presentation and assessment of, 148–149
    definition of, 146
    differential diagnosis of, 149
    etiology of, 148
    treatment of, 150f, 150t, 150–151
  examination of, postoperative, 117, 119, 121–122
  explantation of, 99, 100f
    in UGH syndrome, 200
  history of, 61–68, 62f
  iridocapsular, 64, 64f
  iris-fixated, 63, 64(s)
    pupillary block with, 130f, 130–131
  irritation, ocular hypertension secondary to. *See* UGH syndrome
  malpositioned, refractive errors caused by, 228
  mechanical effects of, inflammatory reactions associated with, 173
  polymethylmethacrylate, 77
  power calculation, 39, 39f
  precipitates, 209–210, 210f
  pupillary capture of. *See* Pupillary capture
  repositioning/exchange of, 228
    with chronic corneal edema, 204
    with chronic iritis, 208
    preoperative examination for, 54–55
Intraocular lens implantation
  history of, 3, 5
  with penetrating keratoplasty and cataract extraction, 101–102, 102f
  posterior chamber, technique for, 80, 83f–85f, 87
  secondary, 95–98, 97f
    advantages and disadvantages of, 98

complications of, 98
preoperative examination for, 53f, 53–54, 95–96
vitrectomy prior to, 96f, 96–97
with trabeculectomy and cataract extraction, 100f, 100–101
Intraocular pressure
  control of, preoperative, 46–48, 72–73
  elevated. *See* Glaucoma; Ocular hypertension
  evaluation of
    in infectious endophthalmitis, 141
    postoperative, 114–115, 119, 122, 127–128
    preoperative, 46–48
    in uveitis, 174
Intraoperative complications, 105–109. *See also specific complication*
IOL. *See* Intraocular lens(es)
IOP. *See* Intraocular pressure
Iopidine. *See* Apraclonidine
Iridectomy, obstruction of, pseudophakic pupillary block due to, 130f, 130–131
Iridocapsular intraocular lenses, 64, 64f
Iridotomy, laser, for pseudophakic pupillary block, 131f, 131–132
Iris
  atrophy of, 46, 47f
  convex, 46f
  damage to, with phacoemulsification, 82
  examination of
    postoperative, 128
    preoperative, 46
  prolapse of, 143–145
    clinical presentation and assessment of, 143–144, 144f, 146f
    etiology of, 143
    treatment, follow-up, and prognosis, 144–145, 145t, 146f
Iris-fixated intraocular lenses, 63, 64f
  pupillary block with, 130f, 130–131
Iris pigment, in anterior chamber, postoperative, 116
Iris synechia, 46, 47f
Iritis. *See also* Uveitis
  chronic, 206–210
    clinical presentation and assessment of, 208
    differential diagnosis of, 208
    etiologies of, 206, 206t
    patient with
      cataract extraction in, 98
      preoperative evaluation of, 56, 56t
    treatment, follow-up, and prognosis, 208–210, 209t
  fibrinoid inflammatory pupillary membranes with, 173, 174f
  postoperative complications associated with, 173
Irvine-Gass syndrome, 215–216
Ischemic optic neuropathy. *See* Anterior ischemic optic neuropathy
Ischemic Optic Neuropathy Decompression Trial, 186

## K

Keflex. *See* Cephalexin
Kelman, Charles, 4, 75
Keratic precipitates, 46, 47f, 208–209
Keratitis, secondary to postoperative medication, 203–204
Keratoconus, 101
Keratometric data, lens implant power calculation with, 39
Keratoplasty, penetrating
  with cataract extraction and intraocular lens implantation, 101–102, 102f
  indications for, 101
  open sky method of, 101, 102f
Keratoscopy, 226
Keratotomy
  astigmatic, 91, 225
  radial, for astigmatism, 225, 225f–226f
Ketorolac, for cystoid macular edema, 221

## L

Laboratory tests, with anterior ischemic optic neuropathy, 183
Laser. *See* Nd:YAG laser
Lens(es). *See also* Contact lenses; Intraocular lens(es)
  anatomy of, 13–14, 14f
  clear, 21
  embryology of, 13
  examination of, preoperative, 46
  subluxated
    congenital, 103, 103f
    preoperative examination of, 52–53, 53f
Lens material, retained, 206–207, 207f
Lids
  evaluation of, postoperative, 115
  upper, anatomy of, 190f
Lid speculum, ptosis caused by, 190
Light projection, for preoperative evaluation, 45, 48
Limbal incision, 76
  closure of, 89–90, 90f
  glaucoma with, postoperative, 126
Local anesthesia, 71f, 71–72, 105
Low-stress atmosphere, for patient preparation, 69
Loyd Superpinkie, 72

## M

Macular disease, and preoperative cataract examination, 48, 49t
Macular edema. *See* Cystoid macular edema
Macular function, evaluation of, preoperative, 48
Maddox rod, for preoperative evaluation, 48
Marcaine, dosage and administration, 71

Mature cataract, 23f
 management of, 46
Maxitrol, dosage and administration, 91, 118
Maxwellian view, 38, 38f
Mechanical compression, of globe, 72
Medical history, consideration of, in preoperative evaluation, 44
Medicamentosa, 203–204
Medications. *See also specific drug*
 postoperative, 118, 120, 123, 238, 254
  keratitis secondary to, 203–204
 preoperative, 70–71, 71f
Medicolegal responsibilities, of eye care providers, 10
Mersilene sutures, 90
Microhyphema, 167, 168f, 205, 205f
Miotic agents
 for acute corneal edema, 165
 contraindications to, 177, 207
 for diplopia, 195, 228
Monocular diplopia, 192
Monocular patients, preoperative evaluation of, 55
Morgagnian cataract, 23f
Mydriatic agents, 118
 for ocular hypertension, 132–133
 for uveitis, 176
Myopia, high, patient with, cataract extraction in, 98–99
Myotoxicity, from anesthetic, strabismus caused by, 194

# N

Nd:YAG laser
 capsulotomy with
  complications of, 214–215
  for endocapsular hematoma, 171, 172f
  informed consent and postoperative instructions for, 256–257
  for opacification, 213–215, 214f–216f
  retinal detachment with, 223
 iridotomy with, for pseudophakic pupillary block, 132
 precipitotomy with, 209–210, 210f
 removal of dislocated lens with, 103
 vitreolysis with, of vitreous to wound and cystoid macular edema, 220–221, 220f–221f
 round pupil after, 144, 145f
Neomycin sulfate, dosage and administration, 91, 118
Neuralgia, postoperative, 115
Nonsteroidal anti-inflammatory drugs, 118
 for cystoid macular edema, 218, 221–222
 for ocular hypertension, 129
 for uveitis, 176
Nuclear cataract
 diagnosis of, 45
 formation of, 15, 16f
 grading of, 18–24, 21f, 23f
Nuclear expression, extracapsular cataract extraction by, 86–87, 86f–88f
 advantages and disadvantages of, 83t, 87
Nuclear sclerotic button, 15, 16f, 45
Nucleus, 14, 14f
 damage to, diplopia caused by, 193
 retained, 207, 207f, 209
Nylon sutures, 90

# O

Objective data, consideration of, in preoperative examination, 44–48
Ocular history, consideration of, in preoperative evaluation, 44
Ocular hypertension, 125–133, 195–202. *See also* Glaucoma
 closed angle, with pupillary block, 130f–131f, 130–132
  clinical presentation and assessment of, 132
  differential diagnosis of, 132
  risk factors for, 130–132
  treatment of, 132, 133t
 factors affecting, 125–126
 with hyphema, 169–170
 incidence of, 125
 with laser capsulotomy, 214
 open angle, 125–130
  clinical presentation and assessment of, 126–128, 127f–128f
  differential diagnosis of, 128
  risk factors for, 125–126, 127f
  treatment of, 128–130, 129t
 secondary to intraocular lens irritation, 198f, 198–200
  clinical presentation and assessment of, 198–199, 199f
  treatment, follow-up, and prognosis, 199–200, 200t
 with uveitis, 176–177
Ocular hypotony, 160
 with shallow or flat anterior chamber, 135–136, 136f
Ocular motility
 in infectious endophthalmitis, 141
 preoperative testing of, 45
Office of Technology Assessment (OTA), comanaged care report, 5–7
Opacification. *See* Posterior capsular opacification
Operative techniques, 75–93. *See also specific technique*
Ophthalmologists
 postoperative care provided by, studies of, 6–7
 role in cataract care, 5, 9–10
Ophthalmoscopy, indirect, diagnosis of retinal break/detachment with, 153
Optical considerations, postoperative, 224–228
Optic nerve decompression, for anterior ischemic optic neuropathy, 185–186
Optic nerve disease, and preoperative cataract examination, 48, 49t
Optic neuropathy. *See* Anterior ischemic optic neuropathy
Optometrists
 postoperative care provided by, studies of, 6–7
 role in cataract care, 5, 9

# P

Pacific Cataract & Laser Institute, hyphema study, 170, 170t–171t
Pain, postoperative, 114–115, 238, 254
PAM. *See* Potential acuity meter
Patch
 postoperative, 91, 92f
  removal of, 113, 239, 254
 pressure, 118, 138, 162
Patient characteristics, affecting treatment outcome, 6, 6t
Patient communication, 10–11
 aids for, 237–239
Patient draping, 73, 73f
Patient education, 9–10
 postoperative, 118, 120, 122–124
 preoperative, 49–50
Patient history
 consideration of, in preoperative evaluation, 44
 preoperative review of, 70
Patient instructions
 postoperative, 238–239, 255
  with Nd:YAG procedures, 256–257
 preoperative, 238
 verbal, 251
Patient preparation, 69–74
 low-stress atmosphere for, 69
PBK. *See* Pseudophakic bullous keratopathy
PCO. *See* Posterior capsular opacification
Pearls, 211, 212f
Pediatric cataracts, preoperative examination of, 51
Penetrating keratoplasty
 with cataract extraction and intraocular lens implantation, 101–102, 102f
 indications for, 101
 open sky method of, 101, 102f
Peribulbar block, 71f, 71–72
 muscle trauma caused by, 193–194, 194f
 ptosis caused by, 72, 159, 189
 versus retrobulbar, 105–106
Peripheral arc of light, postoperative, 115
Phacoemulsification, 4–5, 75
 complications of, 82, 107–108, 202
 description of, to patient, 237

Page numbers followed by *t* and *f* indicate tables and figures, respectively.

duration of, 78–79, 81
endocapsular, 202
extracapsular cataract extraction by, 77–85, 80f
  advantages and disadvantages of, 81–82, 83t
  with trabeculectomy and intraocular lens implantation, 100–101
opening incision, 77
posterior capsule polishing after, 80, 82f
residual cortical material after, removal of, 80, 81f
Phacoemulsification unit, 73–74, 74f
Phenylephrine, topical, 70–71
Photokeratoscopy, 226
Photostress test, for preoperative evaluation, 48
Physical assessment, preoperative, 48
Pilocarpine, 132
  for diplopia, 195
PK. See Penetrating keratoplasty
Plan, preoperative, 49–50
Polymethylmethacrylate (PMMA)
  hard contact lenses, central corneal clouding with, 18
  intraocular lenses, 77
Polymyxin B sulfate, dosage and administration, 91, 118
Posterior capsular opacification, 210–215, 211f–212f
  clinical presentation and assessment of, 213
  etiology of, 211–212, 213f
  grading system for, 29, 29t, 29f–30f
  risk factors for, 210–211
  treatment, follow-up, and prognosis, 213–215, 214f
Posterior capsule, 13–14, 14f
  damage to, during phacoemulsification, 82, 107, 108f, 128
  examination of
    postoperative, 117, 119–120
    preoperative, 46
  polishing of, after phacoemulsification, 80, 82f
  wrinkling of, 119–120, 121f, 123f
Posterior chamber intraocular lens(es)
  in capsular bag, 148, 148f
  decentration of. See Intraocular lens(es), decentration of
  dislocation of. See Intraocular lens(es), dislocation of
  early, 61–62
  examination of, postoperative, 127
  implantation, technique for, 80, 83f–85f, 87
  mechanical effects of, inflammatory reactions associated with, 173
  modern, 65f, 66–67, 66f–67f
    characteristics of, 66t
  placement of
    in capsular bag, 80, 84f–85f, 87, 101
    correct, 148, 148f
  pupillary capture of. See Pupillary capture
  secondary, implantation of, 95

Posterior segment examination, preoperative, 48
Posterior subcapsular cataract
  formation of, 15
  grading of, 18–24, 21f, 23f
Postoperative care
  doctor-to-doctor communication for, 246–247
  uncomplicated, 113–124
    first visit (day 1), 113–118, 114t
    second visit (3–14 days), 118–120, 119t
    third visit (2–4 weeks), 119t, 121–122
    fourth visit (5–8 weeks), 122t, 122–124
Postoperative complications
  early (1–14 days)
    emergent, 125–158
    less emergent, 159–188
  intermediate to late, 189–234
Postoperative instructions, for patient, 238–239, 255
  with Nd:YAG procedures, 256–257
Postoperative medications, 118, 120, 123, 238, 254. See also specific drug
  keratitis secondary to, 203–204
Potential acuity meter, 38, 38f
  for opacification testing, 213
  for preoperative evaluation, 48
Precipitotomy, Nd:YAG laser, 209–210, 210f
Prednisolone acetate
  for chronic iritis, 209
  for cystoid macular edema, 222
  open angle glaucoma induced by, 196t, 196–198
  for UGH syndrome, 199
  for uveitis, 176
Prednisolone phosphate, open angle glaucoma induced by, 196t, 196–198
Preoperative assessment, 48–49
Preoperative evaluation, 43–50, 44t
  of chronic iritis, 56, 56t
  of coexisting eye disease, 48, 49t, 55–58
  of cornea guttata, 57, 57t
  doctor-to-doctor communication for, 246
  of high refractive error, 55–56, 56t
  for intraocular lens repositioning/exchange, 54–55
  of monocular patients, 55
  objective data for, 44–48
  of pediatric cataracts, 51
  of retinal detachment, 58
  for secondary intraocular lens implantation, 53t, 53–54
  subjective data for, 43–44
  of subluxated lenses, 52–53, 53f
  of traumatic cataracts, 51–52, 52f
Preoperative instructions, for patient, 238
  verbal, 251
Preoperative medications, 70–71, 71f. See also specific drug
Preoperative plan, 49–50
Preoperative-postoperative area, arrangement of, 69, 70f
Pressure patch, 118, 138, 162

Prism spectacles, for diplopia, 195
Profenal. See Suprofen
Professional correspondence, 248–250
Prolene sutures, 90
*Propionibacterium acnes*
  colony, that mimics opacification, 212–213
  endophthalmitis caused by, 139–141, 140t
PSC. See Posterior subcapsular cataract
Pseudocapsule, with eightball hyphema, 170
Pseudoexfoliation, 46, 48f
Pseudophakic bullous keratopathy, 101. See also Corneal edema, chronic
Pseudophakic pupillary block, 130f–131f, 130–132
Psychologic stress, with postoperative hyphema, 170
Ptosis, 115
  definition of, 189
  early, 159–160
    clinical presentation and assessment of, 159
    differential diagnosis of, 159–160
    treatment, follow-up, and prognosis, 160
  etiology of, 189
  incidence of, 189
  intermediate to late, 189–192
    clinical presentation and assessment of, 190, 191f
    differential diagnosis of, 190, 191t
    treatment, follow-up, and prognosis, 191–192, 192t
Pupil
  changes in, in infectious endophthalmitis, 141
  examination of
    postoperative, 118–119, 121
    preoperative, 45
  in uveitis, 174–175
  peaked
    with iris prolapse, 145, 146f
    with vitreous to wound, 144, 144f
  round, after Nd:YAG laser vitreolysis, 144, 145f
Pupillary block
  diagnosis of, 45–46
  pseudophakic, 130f–131f, 130–132
Pupillary capture, of intraocular lens, 146, 147f, 149, 177–179
  clinical presentation and assessment of, 178
  differential diagnosis of, 178
  risk factors for, 177–178
  treatment, follow-up, and prognosis, 150–151, 178–179, 179t
Purkinje tree phenomenon, 38

# R

Radial keratotomy
  for astigmatism, 225, 225f–226f
  for anisometropia, 225f, 227, 227t

Referral, definition of, 9
Refractive errors. *See also specific error*
   high, patient with
      and cataract extraction, 98–99
      preoperative evaluation of, 55–56, 56t
   postoperative, 121–123, 224–228
   preoperative, 45
Regression formulas, for lens implant power calculation, 39
Retina, examination of
   in cystoid macular edema, 218
   in infectious endophthalmitis, 142
   postoperative, 118
   preoperative, 48
Retinal break/detachment
   early, 151–155, 152f
      clinical presentation and assessment of, 151–153, 154t
      etiology of, 151, 153f
      incidence of, 151, 153t
      treatment, follow-up, and prognosis, 154t, 154–155
   intermediate to late, 222–224
      clinical presentation and assessment of, 223–224, 223f–224f
      differential diagnosis of, 224
      risk factors for, 222–223
      treatment, follow-up, and prognosis, 224
   preoperative evaluation of, 58
Retinal vascular disease, patient with, postoperative hyphema in, 171
Retinopexy, pneumatic, for retinal break/detachment, 154
Retinoscopic reflex, in infectious endophthalmitis, 141
Retinoscopy, for preoperative evaluation, 45
Retrobulbar block, 72, 105–106
   muscle trauma caused by, 193–194, 194f
   versus peribulbar, 105–106
   ptosis caused by, 159, 189
Retrobulbar hemorrhage, intraoperative, 105–107, 106f
Ridley, Harold, 3, 5, 61, 66, 75
Running bootlace sutures, 91f

## S

Scheerer's phenomena, 38–39
Scleral depression
   contraindications to, 153
   diagnosis of retinal break/detachment with, 153
   indications for, 48
Scleral incision, 76–77
   closure of, 90–91, 91f–92f
Scopolamine, for choroidal detachment, 180
Sedation, preoperative, 71

Seidel test, 117, 136, 137f
Self-sealing incision, 73, 76f, 77
   closure of, 81, 85f, 91, 92f
   description of, to patient, 237
Single-stitch suturing, 90–91, 91f
Sixth nerve palsy, diabetic, 193
Slit lamp examination
   of glaucoma, 126–128, 127f–128f
   of infectious endophthalmitis, 141
   of pupillary capture and lens decentration, 178
   of retinal break/detachment, 153
   of uveitis, 174
   for wound leak
      with shallow or flat anterior chamber, 135, 135f
      with well-formed anterior chamber, 160–161
SOAP format, 11, 43
Sodium hyaluronate, anterior chamber reformation with, 138
Spectacles
   for anisometropia, 226–227
   aphakic, 227
      versus secondary intraocular lens implantation, 98
   for astigmatism, 123, 228
   prism, for diplopia, 195
SRK formula, 39
*Staphylococcus*, endophthalmitis caused by, 139–140, 140t, 141f, 142
Sterile technique, 73, 73f
Steroids, 91, 118, 120. *See also specific drug*
   for anterior ischemic optic neuropathy, 185
   for choroidal detachment, 180
   for chronic corneal edema, 204
   for chronic iritis, 208–209
   for cystoid macular edema, 218, 221–222
   for fibrinoid membranes, in uveitis, 175
   for hyphema, 169
   open angle glaucoma induced by, 196t, 196–198
   for UGH syndrome, 199, 209
   for uveitis, 176–177
Strabismus, postoperative, 192–194
Strampelli, B., 63
*Streptococcus*, endophthalmitis caused by, 139–140, 140t
Stress, psychologic, with postoperative hyphema, 170
Stroma
   examination of, preoperative, 45
   thickening/folds, with corneal edema, 20f
Stromal edema, 18
Subconjunctival hemorrhage, postoperative, 115, 120
Subjective data, consideration of, in preoperative evaluation, 43–44

Subluxated lenses, preoperative examination of, 52–53, 53f
Sunset syndrome, 148, 149f, 228
   treatment of, 150
Super Pinhole, 37f, 37–38
   diagnostic use of
      postoperative, 114
      preoperative, 48
Suprofen
   for cystoid macular edema, 222
   dosage and administration, 71, 118
Surgical considerations, special, 95–104
Surgical instrumentation, 73–74, 74f
Surgical misadventure, 99
Surgical wound construction, 73
Sutural cataract, 22f
Suture(s)
   bridle, 193, 193f
      complications of, 193
   continuous, 90, 91f
   interrupted, 89, 90f
   material for, 90
   running bootlace, 91f
   single-stitch, 90–91, 91f
   testing of, postoperative, 117
Suture cutting, for induced astigmatism, 90, 123
Synechiae
   iris, 46, 47f
   lenticular, 46
Synechial angle closure, 200–201

## T

Telephone conversation, in comanaged care, 11
Telephone follow-up, postoperative, 93
Thermal cautery, 166
Thyroid orbitopathy, 192–193
Tonometers, for postoperative screening, 126, 128
Tonopen, 128
Toxic lens syndrome, 173
Trabeculectomy, with cataract extraction and intraocular lens implantation, 100f, 100–101
Trabeculitis, postoperative, 126
Traumatic cataract, 23f
   preoperative examination of, 51–52, 52f
   removal of, 102f, 102–103
Treatment plan, 49–50
Tropicamide, 71
   for ocular hypertension, 132
Two-point discrimination, preoperative evaluation of, 48

## U

UGH syndrome, 63, 98, 198–200, 206
   clinical presentation and assessment of, 198–199, 199f

Page numbers followed by *t* and *f* indicate tables and figures, respectively.

etiology of, 206
treatment, follow-up, and prognosis, 199–200, 200t, 209
Ultrasonography
A-scan, 39, 39f, 48
B-scan, 39–40, 48
Uveitis, 172–177, 174f. *See also* Iritis
clinical presentation and assessment of, 174–175, 175f
differential diagnosis of, 176
risk factors for, 172–173
treatment, follow-up, and prognosis, 176t, 176–177
Uveitis glaucoma hyphema syndrome. *See* UGH syndrome

# V

Valium. *See* Diazepam
Viscoelastics
capsulorhexis with, 77–78, 79f
intraocular lens implantation with, 80, 87
secondary, 97–98
phacoemulsification with, 79
and postoperative glaucoma, 126
retained, complications of, 173
Visual acuity
with anterior ischemic optic neuropathy, 185
with infectious endophthalmitis, 141
with uveitis, 174
Visual acuity charts, for contrast sensitivity, 36
Visual acuity testing
postoperative, 115, 119, 121
preoperative, 45
Visual field loss
with anterior ischemic optic neuropathy, 185
with ischemic optic neuropathy, 183, 184f

Visual field testing, postoperative, 118, 121–122
Visual function tests, 35–36
Visual potential devices, 37–39
Vitrectomy, prior to second implantation, 96f, 96–97
indications for, 96
Vitreolysis, Nd:YAG laser, of vitreous to wound
and cystoid macular edema, 220–221, 220f–221f
round pupil after, 144, 145f
Vitreous
examination of
in infectious endophthalmitis, 142
postoperative, 117–118
preoperative, 48
in uveitis, 175
to wound, 143–145
clinical presentation and assessment of, 144, 144f–145f
cystoid macular edema with, treatment of, 220–221, 220f–221f
etiology of, 143
treatment, follow-up, and prognosis, 144–145, 145t
Vitreous hemorrhage, postoperative, 170–171
Vitreous loss
with broken posterior capsule, 107, 108f, 117, 128
risk of retinal detachment with, 151, 153f
Vitreous wick syndrome, 82, 117, 144
Voltaren. *See* Diclofenac

# W

Warfarin, risk of postoperative hyphema with, 166–167
White-out syndrome. *See* Microhyphema

Windshield wiper syndrome, 98
treatment of, 150
Worst Medallion intraocular lenses, 63
Wound examination
at first visit, 115, 116f, 117
at second visit, 120, 120f
at third visit, 121, 122f
at fourth visit, 122, 123f
for leaks, 117, 136–137, 137f, 160–161
Wound leak
with shallow anterior chamber, 134t, 134–138
clinical presentation and assessment of, 135f–136f, 135–137
differential diagnosis of, 137
treatment of, 137–138, 138t
with well-formed anterior chamber, 160–162
clinical presentation and assessment of, 160–161, 161f
differential diagnosis of, 161
treatment, follow-up, and prognosis, 162, 162t
Written correspondence, professional, 11, 248–250

# X

Xylocaine, dosage and administration, 70–71

# Y

Y sutures, 13–14

# Z

Zonular rupture, intraoperative, 107–108